ISBN 9789390371365 (Int. Edition)

Published by : **Associated Publishing Company**®
A Division of
Astral International Pvt. Ltd.
– ISO 9001:2015 Certified Company –
4736/23, Ansari Road, Darya Ganj
New Delhi-110 002
Ph. 011-43549197, 23278134
E-mail: info@astralint.com
Website: www.astralint.com

Digitally Printed at : Replika Press Pvt. Ltd.

Animal Oncology

S. Sivaseelan

2020
Associated Publishing Company®
A Division of
Astral International Pvt. Ltd.
New Delhi – 110 002

Animal Oncology

The Author

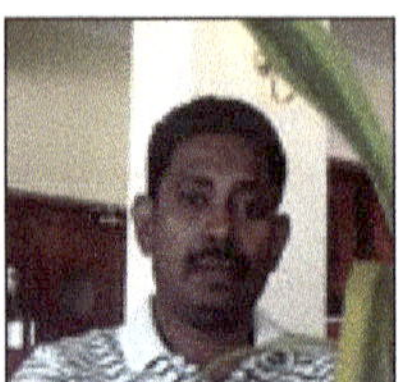

Dr S. Sivaseelan, M.V.Sc., Ph.D., is a Veterinary Pathologi involving in the teaching, research and extension services Veterinary Pathology and Oncology for the past 22 years a currently serving as a Professor and Head inTamil Nadu Veterina and Animal Sciences University. He has prepared a "Colour At of Animal Tumours" under the guideline of Indian Council Agricultural Research. He has guided several M.V.Sc., studen and published 103 Research Articles in reputed Indian and international Journals. has also prepared four manuals and several booklets on various aspects of Veterina Pathology for the benefit of undergraduate and postgraduate Veterinary Students. is responsible for establishing cytological diagnosis not only in neoplasms, but also various infectious diseases at Veterinary College and Research Institute, Namakk Tamil Nadu.

Institute of Molecular and Cell Biology
A*STAR

IMCB
(Institute of Molecular and Cell Biology)
61 Biopolis Drive
Proteos
Singapore 138673
www.imcb.a-star.edu.sg

Foreword

In modern world, cancer causes a greatest challenge in biomedical field. After three centuries of light microscopy, the specialty of veterinary pathology is blooming in science and supports the hidden truth of disease progression in veterinary cancer therapy.

Most of the pathology books have explanatory information with few photographs of tumours from domestic animals, making the readers to imagine the lesions and resulting in lack of interest in reading. Limited availability of books, mostly of foreign origin, is not sufficient to cover the need of veterinary students who want to lead their career as the veterinary pathologist. Non-availability of such informative materials clobbers the veterinarians who practice the veterinary profession in remote areas elsewhere in India. These are the issues that have yet to be resolved.

Great people who have done spectacular things in their career centred around one brilliant concept. Prof. Sivaseelan is one such rare personality who delivered his works in veterinary pathology profession into a book, Animal Oncology. He has done a great favour to the next generation of veterinary pathologist and researchers by collating the important veterinary oncology materials from his efforts into a most informative textbook. He also brings this new volume in broad perspective, honed by many years engaged in the veterinary profession.

Most of the tumours evaluated in animal practice setting are discussed in a concise manner in Animal Oncology. Details of specific neoplasms of different animal species are illustrated with colourful photographs in this book. This supports the diagnosis approach as a ready reckoner. It also allows practitioners and pet owners to easily refer for possible treatment options for a particular tumour. This book also stands as a bulwark behind the endeavours discussed and leaves an enormous value to veterinary students.

In recent decades, progressively, more veterinary pathologists have found employment and made their careers in pharmaceutical industries. This book fulfils the need for scientific information on comprehensive and diverse knowledge related to veterinary neoplasms. Using this book as a reference, anatomic pathologist is then able to make their diagnosis proficiently.

I feel, "Animal Oncology", should be on the desk of every pathology students, veterinary clinical practitioner and researchers and this book could stand as one of the foundation cornerstones for animal oncology in the 21st century in India.

Dr.R.Ravisankar, BVSc, MVSc, PhD. Diplomate. ABT.

Project Leader, (Pathology & Toxicology)
Advanced Molecular Pathology Unit,
Institute of Molecular and cell Biology,
Agency for Science, Technology and Research,
Singapore -138673.

Preface

Veterinary Oncology is considered as a mystery by the veterinary students as well as practitioners owing to the fact that a completely comprehensive book written in simple language covering the pertinent information is highly lacking.

I have self-experienced that veterinary students are not in the position to understand this aspect of pathology just by imaginations alone. Hence, clear illustrations on each and every aspect of veterinary oncology would inculcate better knowledge on this subject.

This book has two portions namely General Oncology and Special Oncology. General Oncology deals with the general concepts of neoplasms in 14 Chapters. Special Oncology illustrates specific neoplasms pertaining to different body systems in 35 Chapters. Special Oncology has been fortified with 155 colour photographs that have been taken from various tumour cases diagnosed by me over a period of more than 10 years. These photographs with their legends will make students and practitioners to understand about almost all neoplasms that occur in Livestock and Poultry easily. Research articles published by us pertaining to certain tumours have also been included for the interest of oncology researches.

Confirmation of tumour has been remaining as a Herculean task even today, because to finalize a tumour, an experienced Pathologist should observe and analyze so many parameters like cell type, size, shape, its relation with adjacent cells, status of inter-cellular space, presence of inflammatory cells and their type, RBCs, parasites, bacteria, any other pathogen, status of cytoplasm, nucleus, nucleolus, presence of mitotic figures and inclusions *etc.*

The World Health Organization and World Health Animal Organization-approved, Gold standard technique to finalize a growth/swelling/mass/tumour is Histopathological reading that must be done by a pathologist, not even by a highly sophisticated machine right now in the world. This fact would be well understood by any veterinary student or practitioner who is reading this book.

I am grateful to Dr. G.A. Balasubramaniam, Dr. P Srinivasan, Dr. P. Balachandran, Dr. R. Thangathurai, Dr. A. Arulmozhi and Dr. R. Madheswaran of Department of Veterinary Pathology, Veterinary College and Research Institute, Namakkal for their help rendered to convert my experience into this book.

I am highly indebted to Dr. M. Murugan, Professor of Poultry Science, TANUVAS: Tamil Nadu Veterinary and Animal Sciences University who continuously motivated me to write this book. My sincere thanks are expressed to Dr. R. Ravisankar, Project Leader, Institute of Molecular and Cell Biology, Singapore, who has been kind enough to write the Foreword of this book.

I am thankful to Dr. S. Dharmaceelan, Dr. P. Vasan, Dr. M. Palanisamy, Dr. N. Mohana and other technical staff members of Veterinary College and Research Institute, Namakkal for their help extended during certain case documentation.

I owe special thanks to my wife Santhanalakshmi and my sons Ramkarthik and Sivaram for their support and encouragement rendered throughout to complete this book.

I am dedicating this book to my parents S. Soundarapandian and S. Rajamani who always wished me to contribute my scientific knowledge to India to my level best.

Dr. S. Sivaseelan

Contents

Part I
General Oncology

1

Certain Terminologies Used in Relation with Neoplasm

Neoplasm

Neoplasm means new growth of cells. It is popularly known as tumour (swelling), but not all swellings are neoplasms. The study of neoplasm is called as oncology, oncos - tumours, logy- study. Malignant neoplasm are commonly called as **"cancers"**, the Latin meaning is crab, because cancer firmly grasps tissues and does not leave it until death and it can spread in any direction by infiltration.

Definition (Mallory, 1914)

- ★ Neoplasm is a new growth of cells, which proliferate continuously without control
- ★ Bears a considerable resemblance to the healthy cells from which they arise
- ★ Have no orderly structural arrangement
- ★ Serves no useful function
- ★ Have no clearly understood cause

Differences between Hyperplasia and Neoplasia

Hyperplasia	Neoplasia
★ Arises due to the need	★ Arises without any need
★ Etiological agents can be identified	★ Etiological agents can not be identified for all the tumours
★ The growth stops after the removal of stimuli	★ Grow even after the cessation of the stimuli
★ Proliferating cells are typical of the parent cells with regular size and shape	★ The proliferating cells may be atypical, anaplastic and pleomorphic in malignant tumours
★ Cells are organised and co-ordinate with the parent cells	★ Cells are disorganised and not co-ordinate with the parent cells
★ Metastasis is not a feature	★ Metastasis is often seen in malignant tumours

Teratoma

- ★ **"Cohnheim's cell rest theory"** explains about the origin of teratoma. During embryonic life some immature pluripotent undifferentiated cells (totipotential cells) may be trapped in some of the organs
- ★ This theory says that all neoplasms arise from such "cell rests". Though this theory may explain teratoma, it cannot explain the occurrence of all the tumours
- ★ Teratoma contains multiple tissues from **different germinal layers** such as epithelium, bone and cartilage. Benign and malignant types are called as, mature and immature teratomas respectively. Ovarian teratomas are cystic (cystic teratoma), whereas testis teratomas are solid (solid teratoma) in consistency. The most common teratomas are the human ovarian **dermoids** or **dermoid cysts**
- ★ These cysts are lined by squamous epithelium and contain skin components of hair, keratin, and sweat and sebaceous glands. **True teratomas should consist of tissues from two or three germinal layers**
- ★ Canine mixed mammary tumour cannot be considered as a teratoma, since the epithelium and connective tissue are normal components of the mammary gland arising from the same germinal layer, and the bone and cartilage originate from metaplasia of myo-epithelial cells
- ★ Embryonic nephroma (Wilm's tumour) also contains multiple tissues, but it is not a teratoma. It is an aberrant differentiation of embryonic tissues of the kidney, so arising from a single germinal layer

Hamartoma

It is a tissue defect that occurs during development in which abnormal combination of tissues is formed (**Hamartia**), but all the tissues in that combination are normally found in that area. The tumour arising from such tissue defect or hamartia is called as **Hamartoma.**

Choristoma

Tissue defect in which mass of histologically normal tissues found in abnormal location is called as **Chorista**. Tumour arising from such tissue defect or chorista is called as **choristoma**.

Polarity

In epithelial tissues, the cells are arranged in a particular order bearing a distinct relation to the adjacent cells. This is called as polarity.

e.g. In the intestinal epithelium, the long axis of the cells is arranged perpendicular to the lamina propria. If these cells are arranged parallel or at different angles of the lamina propria it is called as **loss of polarity**. Loss of polarity is one of the important features in malignant neoplasm in which the cells are dividing haphazardly and so are arranged without a definite order.

Anaplasia

"Ana" means backward in Latin. Reversion to embryonic type due to lack of differentiation through inadequate maturation is known as anaplasia.

Salient features of Anaplasia are:

- Large sized hyperchromatic nuclei
- Increased nuclear, cytoplasmic ratio (indicative of rapid growth)
- Increased size of nucleolus with increase in nucleolar, nuclear ratio (Also an indicative of rapid growth)

Anisocytosis / pleomorphism - Variation in the size of the cells

Anisokaryosis - Variation in the size of the nuclei

Poikilocytosis - Variation in the shape of the cells

Poikilokaryosis - Variation in the shape of the nuclei

Multinucleated cells

Rapid nuclear division that is not followed by cytoplasmic division makes the neoplastic cell as a multinucleated cell, which is a feature of malignant neoplasms. It is also called as "Tumour Giant cell".

Carcinoma *in situ*

An actively dividing tumour in which though all the features of carcinoma are seen, breakage of lamina propria is not found, indicating locally invasive nature without metastasizing to distant areas. *e.g.* Basal cell tumour (previously designated as basal cell carcinoma).

Dysplasia

Alteration in size, shape and orientation of adult cells is called as dysplasia. *e.g.* In normal epidermis, stratum corneum st.lucidum st. granulosum st. spinosum and basal cell layer are arranged from below upwards of basal cell layer. Each layer is also composed of definite number of rows of cells and the cells are uniform in size and shape, but in dysplasia, the number of rows of cells in each layer is increased and the size and shape of cells are altered. In glandular epithelium and columnar epithelium loss of polarity can also be seen.

Differences between Benign and Malignant Tumours

Criteria	Benign	Malignant
Growth rate	Slow over a period of time	Rapid
Mitotic figures	Less than ten	More than ten (multinucleated tumour cells can also be seen)
Mode of growth	Grow by expansion, spherical in shape, causes pressure to the surrounding and so capsulated. Fibrous capsule is formed due to slow growth. Some may lack the capsule also.	It grows by expansion and also by invasion and infiltration. No time is permitted for the fibrous tissue formation and so the capsule is not formed.

Criteria	Benign	Malignant
	e.g. Haemangioma. The capsule cannot stop the growth, but it restricts the growth.	In a tissue section extension of growth below the basement membrane is the adequate evidence of malignancy.
Continuance of growth	Grow slowly and indefinitely, stop growing after some time. Some even show regression spontaneously.	Grow continuously and finally causes death of the host.
Metastasis	Does not occur (it is the phenomenon of formation of secondary tumour due to the transport of malignant cells through blood, lymph or cavities)	Occur
Clinical course	Harmless, except by their 1. Location Benign tumours of brain are always serious and fatal. 2.Complication Severe haemorrhage of papilloma of urinary or alimentary tract or uterus may occur. 3. Eexcessive hormone production ★ Adenoma of pituitary gland causes gigantism ★ Adenoma of Islets of Langerghans causes hypoglycemia	It can cause clinical defects similar to benign variety. In addition to this, infiltration and metastasis to other organs may cause very dangerous defects to bring about death invariably.
Recurrence	Will not recur	Recur after removal and death is an invariable outcome
Structure	Proliferating cells resemble closely the parent cells	Anaplasia is the feature
Histology	★ Anisocytosis and Anisokaryosis are noticed, but the cells will resemble the parent cells (normal N / C ratio of 1:4 to 1:6 is changed as 1:2 or even 1:1) ★ Nuclear membrane will be regular and uniform. Hyperchromatic nuclei indicate high prolificacy ★ Nucleolus size is increased ★ Very few blood vessels are seen ★ Most of the tumours maintain polarity	★ In addition to the size, Poikilocytosis and Poikilokaryosis are also noticed (Anaplastic). ★ Folding of nuclear membrane and indentation of nucleus can be observed. ★ In addition, multiple unequal nucleoli can be noticed ★ Malignant tumours grow fast that require abundant blood supply, so very thin walled numerous blood vessels are seen. In some tumours, the blood supply is not adequate, so the cancer cells undergo necrosis. ★ Loss of polarity

2

Nomenclature and Classification of Tumours

Cytological or histological classification

In this, the suffix "oma" is added to the tissue of tumour origin

e.g. Fibroma

Behaviouristic classification

This is based on the clinical behaviour of tumour. It classifies tumours as whether harmless (benign) or dangerous (malignant). Benign and malignant denote innocent and dangerous in Latin respectively.

TNM classification

- ★ The **WHO** has adopted an international system of grouping and staging of cancers for both human as well as animals
- ★ The system allows from the fact that the survival rates is higher for cases in which the disease is localised, than for those in which the cancer has extended beyond the organ of origin. These groups were referred as "early cases" and "late cases".
- ★ The principle purpose of this classification is to provide the method of conveying one person's clinical observation to others without ambiguity.

Objectives

- ★ To aid the clinician in planning treatment
- ★ To give prognosis of cancers
- ★ To assess the treatment effects

- ★ To facilitate the exchange of information between treatment centres
- ★ To contribute information for the comparison of human and animal cancers
- ★ To contribute information to the cancer research

General rules of TNM classification

- ★ In all cases, confirmation of malignancy by histological or cytological examination is obligatory
- ★ Any cases not proved as a cancer by this method is recorded separately
- ★ TNM groups must be identified prior to treatment for all the cases.
- ★ The histopathological observation is considered as obligatory investigation and the other diagnostic procedures including surgery and radiological examination are considered as refinements that can be added even after planning the treatment
- ★ After assessing the TNM category they are grouped into clinical stages

TNM categories

- ★ **"T"** - Extent of primary tumour (size of the tumour)
- ★ **"N"** condition of regional lymphnode
- ★ **"M"** presence or absence of distant metastasis
- ★ Addition of numbers to these **TNM** components indicated the extent of the malignant disease

"T" category

Size of tumour (T) and possible involvement of contiguous structures

Size	T1	T2	T3	T4
	<3cm	3-5cm	>5cm	
Skin	Minor involvement			Major Involvement
Fascia, muscle thoracic abdominal wall involvement	With or without fascia or muscle fixation			Thoracic or abdominal wall fixation

T1, T2, T3 and T4 indicate the increasing degrees or extent of the primary tumours (T1-less than 3 cm; T2-3-5 cm; T3 and T4-more than 5 cm)

- ★ The number of these T categories may vary according to the size of the tumour, but in general, the maximum size should not exceed four
- ★ Circumscribed and pedunculated visible tumours are easily measured and the T category is assigned

- ★ The second situation arises where the tumour is not so circumscribed, in this circumstance, the approximate size may be indicated
- ★ Tumours of visceral organs are measured by means of radiography. Size can also be assigned when the tumour is seen by surgical procedures
- ★ In multiple tumours, the number of tumours should be counted and the size of the largest tumour should be recorded. The maximum size should be indicated and the numbers of tumours can be shown within the parenthesis
- ★ Those tumours, which are occurring in the hollow viscera or cavities in which the exact numbers cannot be assessed or categorised, the suffix "m" is used just after "T" to indicate more than one. In this case also, the largest tumour size should be indicated
- ★ T-0 (T-zero) indicates no evidence of primary tumour. This category is necessary to cover cases where metastasis occurs, but the primary neoplasm remains occult
- ★ Tx indicates impossible to assess the full extent of primary tumour
- ★ Tis indicates carcinoma *in situ*

"N" category

- ★ N1, N2 and N3 indicate the characteristic of lymphnode, which may be assessed by palpation, lymphangiography or other procedures
- ★ Number of these "N" categories varies according to the site
- ★ N-0 (N zero) indicates no palpable regional lymphnode is observed. This denotes no involvement of regional lymphnode or lymph node appears to be normal
- ★ N1 indicates involvement of movable one lymphnode
- ★ N2 denotes involvement of movable two ipsilateral or contralateral
- ★ lymphnodes
- ★ N3 indicates immovable fixed lymph nodes
- ★ Histological information can be added by biopsy or surgery
- ★ N+ (N plus) and N– (N minus) denotes involvement and noninvolvement of distant regional lymphnode respectively
- ★ Nx denotes, impossible to assess the metastasis to distant lymphnode

Other symbols of N are

- ★ Absence of visible growth in / on the involved lymphnode - N1a
- ★ Presence of visible growth in / on the involved lymphnode - N1b
- ★ The same is applicable to N_2 and N_3 also

"M" category

- ★ M-0 indicates no metastasis is detectable clinically
- ★ M1 denotes metastasis to other than regional lymphnode
- ★ Mx conveys the meaning of impossible to assess the presence/absence of metastasis

Histopathological Extent of tumour (P)

- ★ "P" category is applicable to only hallow organs like intestine
- ★ P1 indicates that tumour is confined to mucosa only
- ★ P2 specify the involvement of mucosa, submucosa and serosal, but the tumour has not penetrated out through the serosa
- ★ P3 denotes the tumour has penetrated the serosa with or without invasion of contiguous structures
- ★ P4 indicates that the tumour involves diffusely the entire thickness of wall without obvious boundaries

Pathological grading of malignancy (G)

- ★ G1 - low grade malignancy
- ★ G2 - medium grade malignancy
- ★ G3 - high grade malignancy

TNM staging

- ★ With four possible degrees of T, three degrees of N and two degrees of M, the number of groups extends from T1 N0 M0 at one end of the scale to T4 N3M1 at the other end is 32
- ★ Recording of individual case in these groups is simple, but the demerit is unrelated groups are grouped in the same clinical stage, example - in stage III, 12 TNM groups are grouped ranging from T1 N2 M0 to T4N3M0. In these groups, the one year survival of the first group may be sixty per cent, whereas the last group is 15 per cent. This shows the limitation of staging dissimilar groups, but the overall merit is incredible.

Writing TNM categories

TNM Groups		Clinical stages	Number of groups per stage
T1N0M0	T2N0M0	I	2
T1N1M0	T2N1M0	II	2
T1N2,3M0 T3N0,1,2,3M0	T2N2,3M0 T4N0,1,2,3M0	III	12
Any TNM symbol +M1		IV	16
Total			32

- ★ Animal details, anatomical location of the tumours and region involved should be indicated first
- ★ Method of observation like palpation, radiological procedures and surgical methods should be supplemented
- ★ Shorthand notation of the tumour should follow these informations

Anatomical locations

- ★ Skin excluding lymphosarcoma and mastocytoma
- ★ Skin mastocytoma
- ★ Mammary gland tumour
- ★ Head and neck
- ★ Alimentary system including pancreas and liver
- ★ Neurological system excluding CNS
- ★ Genital and urogenital system
- ★ Bones and joints
- ★ Lymphoid and haemopoietic tissue including lymphosarcoma of skin
- ★ Respiratory system
- ★ Endocrine glands

Tumours of eye, CNS, heart and endocrine glands (Adrenal and thyroid) are not included, because it is difficult to classify them clinically at present and many of these tumours are locally invasive.

3

Etiology of Neoplasms – Intrinsic and Extrinsic Factors

Intrinsic / Predisposing factors

Hereditary factor

Inheritance plays a vital role in causing several neoplasms. In some strains of animals and human families higher incidences of certain cancers have been recorded. In human, neuroblastoma, adenocarcinoma of colon, retinoblastoma and zeroderma pigmentosum have been recorded. Elimination of avian leucosis complex in certain strains of layers can be quoted as examples. By selection, a highly resistant strain of chicken has been developed in which incidence of ALC is very low, which indicates the inheritance of certain traits could predispose the animals to tumours.

Experimentally it is possible to breed a strain of mice, which are highly susceptible to neoplasms. It has been found that simple Mendelian recessive factor is acting a key role in causing neoplasms.

Zeroderma pigmentosum

This denotes highly pigmented dried skin, which occurs in children due to the defect that involves in the synthesis of enzymes needed for nucleotide excision repair, so that the deficient children are extremely sensitive to sunlight and susceptible to various kinds of skin neoplasms in childhood, which can be said as an example for the inherited defect. As on date, no responsible gene is identified, but it can be reasonably inferred that there is distinct genetic control in tumour production based on the above example

Age

Cancer age is the average period of life at which cancers are commonly appearing in human as well as in animals. It varies among different species of animals.

e.g.

- ★ Human after 50 years
- ★ Cattle 8 -10 years
- ★ Dogs after 5 years

Congenital tumours like nephroblastoma and sarcoma appear in young animals, whereas, carcinomas are common in older ones. In general cancer is the disease of older ages.

The governing factors are as detailed below

- ★ Decrease in the cell metabolism
- ★ More opportunity for exposure to carcinogens
- ★ High latent periods for the action of carcinogen
- ★ Sometimes all these three factors may act together

Pigmentation

Melanin protects the skin from actinic rays of sun. Thus, cutaneous cancers are seldom seen in pigmented animals. Malignant melanoma is very frequently observed in gray and white horses. If these animals are allowed to survive till older ages, they would invariably develop malignant melanoma. Incidence of squamous cell carcinoma of eye is more in Hereford cattle when compared to the Aberdeen angus cattle reared in the same location of southern USA.

Hormones

Certain organs in the body are under the influence of hormones. Hyper production of these hormones may lead to the hyperplasia and in turn to cancers.

The basic structure of estrogen, progesterone, testosterone and adrenocorticoids is similar to that of benzanthracene and benzypyrene, which are powerful chemical carcinogens. The phenanthrene group is the basic structure found in all these hormones and chemical carcinogens. It is suspected that these hormones may be changed into the active chemical carcinogens within the body. Similarly cholic acid and cholesterol may be converted into methyl cholanthrene, which also contain the phenanthrene group.

Hormonal carcinogenesis appears to be independent of chemical or ionizing radiation induced initiation. Involvement of inherited genetic predisposition to hormone induced tumours is the important feature. Estrogen induced tumours in dogs has been proved beyond doubts. Pan-hysterectomy in dogs before the first oestrus caused mammary neoplasm in 1/100 of dogs and the incidence after first estrus was 1/12 and after second estrus it was 1/4. Administration of estrogen induces ovarian carcinomas in female dogs.

Progesterone can produce mammary hyperplasia in female cats. Treatment of bitches with progesterone can induce over production of growth hormone in the mammary gland and this may play a role in mammary carcinogenesis in dogs by autocrine activity.

Extrinsic Factors

Physical Trauma

Neoplasms can develop from the sites of injury in dogs and man. Burn scar may act as a seat of proliferation of tumour cells. Squamous cell carcinoma, basal cell carcinoma and sarcomas have also been reported that occurred due to trauma. Large breeds of dogs developed osteosarcoma at the healed fractured lines of long bone. Fractures associated sarcomas differ from other osteosarcoma in being diaphysial rather than metaphysial in location. The mean interval between the time of injury and tumour diagnosis was about 8 years.

Chronic irritation

Repeated chronic irritations can cause neoplasm

Clay pipe

Lip cancer is commonly seen among clay pipe smokers. The irritation caused by constant heat of the clay pipe and its pressure on the lip causes cancer of the lips.

Kangri baskets

In order to keep the body warm, a bamboo basket containing a small earthen pot with burning charcoal (Kangri basket) is kept under the cloth touching the abdomen. This practice among the Kashmeres is causing abdomen cancers due to the continuous irritation by the heat.

Reversed chutta

Smoking cigars with the burning end inside the mouth (reversed chutta) has caused palate neoplasm among the Andrapradesh people of India due to constant heat and irritation.

Sharp teeth

Chronic irritation by irregularly pointed teeth can cause neoplasm of gums, inner cheek and tongue.

Gall stones and kidney stones

Cancers can be produced in gall bladder wall and kidney pelvis due to the stones in the respective organs by means of chronic irritation for a prolonged period.

Yoke induced tumours

Constant friction of the yoke in working bullocks may be responsible for horn cancer and skin cancers. Chronic irritation causes degeneration and necrosis of cells, which will be replaced by the actively proliferating new cells. Eventually, these proliferating cells exceed the restraint exerted by the neighboring cells and may lead to the uncontrolled proliferation, but all forms of chronic irritation do not result in neoplasia.

4

Radiation Induced Carcinogenesis

- ★ Radiation includes both ionizing radiations and solar radiation
- ★ Ionizing radiations are produced by various isotopes that emit either electromagnetic radiation including X-rays, gamma rays or particulate radiation of alpha, beta rays, protons and neutrons
- ★ Solar radiation or actinic rays is the UV radiation

Ionizing radiation

- ★ Ionizing radiations caused very many skin cancers and leukemia in a number of earlier radiation workers including Marie Curie.
- ★ Danger of radiation exposure was learnt in the Second World War in which atom bombs were exploded in Japan. Acute myeloid leukemia in survivors was noticed even after ten years of latency. Other neoplasms like thyroid, lung, breast and colon tumours were also observed in that attack
- ★ Similar reports have also come from Marshall Island where hydrogen bomb was exploded. In that incident more thyroid tumours among children due to radioactive iodine was observed out of which five percent were carcinomas
- ★ Focal X-ray irradiation on the hands and arms can cause carcinomas among the X-ray lab workers

Possibilities of ionizing radiation induced tumours

Radiation	Tumour
Strontium 90 Inhalation	Osteosarcoma
Radium painting in watch industry	Osteosarcoma, Leukemia
Uranium inhalation in mines	Pulmonary cancers
Therapeutic radiation for the enlargement of thymus in children	Thyroid adenocarcinoma
Radiation therapy for ankylosing spondylitis of adults	Osteosarcoma, Leukemia

- ★ Ionizing radiation can cause variety of neoplasms in dogs. Gamma irradiation in young dogs has been proved to increase the risk of mesenchymal and epithelial neoplasms in the later ages of life
- ★ Inhalation of plutonium, a source of alpha particles can induce pulmonary neoplasms in dogs
- ★ Radiation therapy can cause very many neoplasms in dogs. Osteosarcoma are more frequent outcome

Mechanism of Ionizing radiation induced neoplasms

Target Theory

Ionising rays target the intracellular organelles like mitochondria as well as nucleus. Defect in organelles can be rectified to certain extent, but if the target is the gene, the defect becomes permanent when the enzymes involved in nucleotide excision repair are also inactivated by the rays. The defective genes with mutation are passed to the subsequent generations of cells. Added mutation may transform the normal cell into neoplastic cells.

Poison Theory

Radiant energy can ionise the water into free hydroxyl and hydrogen radicals, which combine with free oxygen to form HO_2 and H_2O_2, which are highly potent oxidizing agents. These toxic products cause changes in organelles, enzymes including the NER as well as nucleus for the conversion of normal cell into neoplastic cells. Non-lethal hit to the cell is considered as an important event for the conversion. DNA damage is the main event, which can be caused either by direct effect of ionizing radiation or indirectly by producing free radicals. Derangement of NER system should accompany the DNA damage for the neoplastic change.

Solar Radiation induced Carcinogenesis

UV radiation

UV portion of solar spectrum has three wavelength ranges

1. UV - A (320 - 400nm)
2. UV - B (280 - 320nm)
3. UV - C (200 - 280nm)

UV – C is filtered by the earth ozone layer before it reaches the surface. UV – B is a well known cause of cutaneous neoplasia that it can cause

1. Squamous cell carcinoma
2. Basal cell carcinoma
3. Malignant melanoma

UV – A can also cause cutaneous neoplasms to certain extent.

Mechanism of UV Rays induced Carcinogenesis

UV – B produces mutation at sites in DNA where two pyrimidine bases (cytocine and thymine) are occurring tandem. Linking the adjacent cytocine and thymine bases pyrimidine dymers are produced. The acquired mutation is passed to the subsequent generation of cells in which the degree of mutation is added for neoplastic conversion. When the protooncogenes and tumour suppressor gene (^{53}P) regions are affected by forming pyrimidine dymers, the chance of cancer transformation is more.

UV – B also decreases the cell mediated immunity by acting on dividing immunogenic cells, which may be the cause for the active proliferation of bovine papilloma virus to cause bovine ocular squamous cell carcinoma in eyes of white skinned Hereford cattle in southern USA. UV – A may cause DNA damage indirectly through the formation of free radicals and reactive oxygen species. Neoplasm arises in white or less pigmented skin and area of skin that have a thin hair coat.

5

Chemical Carcinogenesis

History

Sir Percivall Pott in the year 1775 reported the relation of coal and cancers in England. He observed scrotal cancers among the chimney sweepers. Cancer was observed on the thighs, scrotum and abdomen of mule spinners also. The lubricants used in spinning industry contained petroleum products that spilled on these places to produce cancers. Lip cancers were observed among the Scottish fisherman who used to hold the tar smeared bone needle thread in between their lips. In 1915, Yamagiwa and Itchikawa in Japan applied tar on the ear of rabbits daily for six months to produce a skin tumour. In1932, Kenneway and Cook observed benzypyrene as a chemical carcinogen fraction in tar. Later on several chemicals like dibenzanthrazene naphthalene, zinc chloride and aflatoxin were proved as important carcinogens.

Definitions

Direct carcinogen

Chemical substance, which do not require the bio-transformation by cytochrome P-450 and glutathione transferase enzymes of smooth endoplasmic reticulum of hepatic cells for its carcinogenicity is called as direct carcinogen. Indirect carcinogen needs the bio-transformation *in vivo.*

Indirect carcinogen or Procarcinogen

Require metabolic conversion *in vivo* by SER enzymes to induce cancer transformation. This is also called as **ultimate carcinogen.**

Complete carcinogen

Chemicals, which possess the capacity of both initiation and promotion are called as complete carcinogen, whereas incomplete carcinogen can cause initiation alone.

Initiation

A permanent irreversible genotoxic event caused by direct or indirect carcinogen is called as initiation. **Initiators** are the substances, which can cause permanent irreversible genotoxic changes of host cell genome by forming covalent bonds with the host cell DNA. Initiation occurs even in a single brief exposure to an initiator.

Promotion

The process of conversion of initiated cells into neoplastic cells is called as promotion. The agents are called as **promoters**. Most promoters are non genotoxic chemicals that do not require metabolic activation and whose effects are reversible. Promoters alter signal transduction within the cells and stimulate clonal replication of initiated cells.

Co-carcinogen

It is a chemical substance, which increases the degree of genotoxic effects when administered simultaneously with initiators. Co carcinogen cannot act as an initiator.

Classification of chemical carcinogens

Type	Example	Mode of action
Initiators Direct acting	**Dibenzanthrazene** (polycyclic aromatic hydrocarbon), a purely synthesized chemical **Benzanthrazene** (polycyclic aromatic hydrocarbon) which is encountered in tobacco smoke **Nitrosamines** (Formed in the stomach from dietary sources) **Naphthalene** (Cyclic hydrocarbon from aniline industry) **Ethylene imine** **Aromatic amines** and **Azo dyes** (ethydium bromide) some of these dyes were used in food industry earlier	Electrophilic organic compounds (direct acting initiators) that covalently bind with nucleophils of host cell) to form covalent adducts to cause genetic damage as a irreversible permanent change (initiation)
Initiators Indirect acting (needs biotransformation to form active compounds)	Aflatoxin B1 (a common contaminant of corn and peanuts) bio-transformed into **epoxide**, a potent carcinogen	Initiate tumour change similar to direct acting initiators
Promoters	**Phenol:** Bile acids (methyl cholanthrene, a potent hydrocarbon carcinogen may form from cholic acid, a normal constitute of the bile) **Saccharin** **Croton oil** **Phenobarbitol** **Methyl sterculate**	Non genotoxic, cannot initiate cancer transformation, but transform the initiated cells by initiators
Co carcinogens	**Ethanol** **Phorbol esters**	Enhance the genotoxic effects of initiators when given simultaneously. It may serve as a promoter also

Type	Example	Mode of action
Immuno suppressor	**Anti lymphocytic sera**	Immunosuppression and virus induced cancers
Inorganic chemicals	**Cadmium** **Nickel** **Chromium** **Arsenic** **Zinc chloride**	Alter DNA replication, but not directly genotoxic, so can predispose the cells for the easy action of initiators.
Hormones	**Estradiol** **Progesterone** **Growth hormone** **Thyroxine**	Alter cell differentiation through endocrine imbalance. They can easily transform initiated cells into cancer (may act as promoters)

Environmental Chemical Carcinogens

Environmental exposure to carcinogenic chemicals can induce cancer in domestic animals. An increased risk of bladder cancer may occur due to frequent contact of the skin with insecticides. Direct inhalation of cigarette smoke can cause pulmonary adenocarcinoma dogs. Ingestion of bracken fern act as a cofactor with papilloma virus, which can lead to neoplasms of the digestive and urinary tract.

Experimental chemical carcinogenesis

Several chemicals have been used to induce experimental carcinogenesis in dogs and laboratory animals. Nitrosamines are potent carcinogens in the canine stomach, lung and liver.

Pulmonary neoplasms can be produced experimentally by exposure to polycyclic aromatic hydrocarbons. Carcinomas in the canine urinary bladder have been induced by dichlorobenzidine. Naphthalene can be used to induce bladder carcinoma.

Cells differ in their susceptibility to cancer development by chemicals. Whatever may be the route of administration the carcinogen may cause cancer always in a particular organ. For example, cancer of mammary gland may be produced in mice by applying the carcinogen to the nasal mucosa.

Models of initiation and promotion in experimental carcinogenesis

Initiator	Promoter	Tissue
Benzypyrene	Croton oil	Mouse skin
2-acetamidofluorene	Phenobarbital	Rat liver
Methyl nitrose urea	Saccharin	Rat bladder
Aflatoxin - B1	Methyl sterculate	Trout fish liver

Mechanism of Chemical Carcinogenesis

The process of carcinogenesis can be divided into **initiation** and **promotion**, initiation occurs when cells are exposed to a chemical that can permanently and irreversibly alter the cellular DNA. Usually a single brief exposure to an initiator is sufficient to produce a mutation by formation of covalent bonds between the chemical and nucleotide of DNA in the host cell.

Initiation is a two-step process. Following the initial genetic damage, replication by mitosis should occur within 72 –96 hrs to fix the mutation as a permanent change. Chemicals that act as initiators are highly reactive electrophils (electron deficient) that form covalent bonds with electron rich target (nucleophils) such as DNA, RNA and protein to form covalent adducts.

Adducts formed with proteins and RNA can lead to cell death. DNA adducts can lead to cell death if the damage is severe or nucleotide excision repair occur if the damage is mild. If the repair mechanism fails is some mild to moderate damage, the DNA mutation becomes permanent that lead to permanent irreversible genetic damage.

A few chemicals are capable of forming adducts directly with DNA without metabolic activation and most of the initiators need metabolic biotransformation before action.

Promoters

Promoters are non-genotoxic chemicals that do not require biotransformation and the effects are reversible. They are not capable of transforming cells by their action alone, but sufficient exposure to promoters after initiation will lead to tumour formation.

Promoters alter signal transduction within cells and stimulate clonal replication of initiated cells. Cell replication occurs quickly due to the deranged signal transduction, which paves way for the accumulation of mutation without nucleotide excision repair. Since mutation accumulates more rapidly, there is an increased risk of tumour formation.

Initiation followed by promotion can only lead to cancer formation. Application of promoter with sufficient frequency for sufficient duration with constant interval is necessary for cancer production owing to the fact that effects of promotion are reversible.

It has been proved in an experiment on mouse skin by using benzypyrene as an initiator and croton oil as a promoter

Initiation and promotion in chemical carcinogenesis

Treatment 1	↓	no tumour
Treatment 2	∇ ∇ ∇ ∇ ↓	no tumour
Treatment 3	∇ ∇ ∇ ∇ ∇	no tumour
Treatment 4	↓ ∇ ∇	no tumour
Treatment 5	↓ ∇ ∇ ∇ ∇	tumour
Treatment 6	↓ ∇ ∇ ∇ ∇	tumour

↓ - initiator

∇ - promoter

6

Parasitic Carcinogenesis

Parasites

Chronic irritation by parasites may lead to tumour transformation.

Schistosoma hematobium

In man, it is considered to cause cancer of urinary bladder. The parasite lives in small veins of urinary bladder, the ova with their spines and lytic enzymes pears through the tissue producing inflammatory reaction resulting in ulceration of mucosa of bladder. The edges of ulcer become hyperplastic and act as a seat of neoplastic transformation.

Cysticercus fasciolaris

Infection of rat liver by *Cysticercus fasciolaris,* the bladder worm of cat tapeworm *Taenia taeniaformis* produces cyst with fibrous tissue may progress to fibrosarcoma with metastasis to lungs.

Spirocerca lupi

Inhabit wall of esophagus and aorta of dogs. The fibrous nodule with worm sometime develops into fibrosarcoma or even into osteosarcoma with metastasis to lung and other viscera.

Eimeria steidae

These coccidian protozoa may cause papillary cystadenoma of bile duct epithelium in rabbits due to mechanical and toxic irritations.

7

Bacterial Carcinogenesis

The bacteria *Helicobacter pylori* has been linked to peptic ulcers, gastric lymphoma and adenocarcinoma in human and dogs. Chronic infection with this bacterium is thought to induce reactive T-cells that cause proliferation of polyclonal B cell population via cytokine reaction.

These T-cell dependant B cells eventually become monoclonal and T-cell independent. The resultant tumour is called as marginal zone lymphoma (maltoma). Before becoming T cell independent such B cells proliferation responds to anti bacterial treatment.

Pathogenic *H. pylori* contain "cag-A" (cytotoxin associated gene A). This "cag-A" gene and a secreting system, which inject the cag- A protein into the host cell can cause the chromosome translocation of 11 and 18 (t: 11-18) and thus causing genetic damage, which can be passed to the daughter cells. Proliferation of these modified cells produce adenocarcinoma.

Another gene associated with the virulence is "vac – A" (Vacuolating gene), which encodes a vacuolating toxin which causes hepatic necrosis.

Mechanism of *H. pylori* induced Lymphoma

↓

Helicobacter pylori

↓

Chronic infection in intestine of human and dog

↓

Stimulate T-lymphocytes of intestinal submucosa

↓

Release of cytokines by activated T-lymphocytes

↓

Stimulate B-lymphocytes

↓

Polyclonal expansion of B-lymphocytes (T-cell dependent)

↓

B-cells acquire T-cell independency

↓

Monoclonal expansion of B-cells

↓

Lymphoma

Mechanism of *H. pylori* induced Adenocarcinoma

↓

H. pylori in the intestine of human and dog

↓

Bacterial "cag A" gene expression

↓

"cag A" protein production

↓

Injection of "cag A" protein into the host intestinal epithelial cells with the help of *H.pylori* secreted enzyme, which act on the cell membrane

↓

Translocation of chromosome 11 and 18 (Genetic damage)

↓

Inheritance of genetic damage to the daughter cells

↓

Proliferation of modified body cells

↓

Adenocarcinoma

8

Viral Carcinogenesis

Oncogenic Viruses

Oncogenic viruses represent a diverse group, including RNA and DNA viruses. All of the RNA viruses that cause neoplasia are retroviruses (oncorna viruses), but only some of the Retroviridae are oncogenic.

Retroviruses have a common life cycle. All retroviruses have an RNA genome that is reverse transcribed via an endogenous enzyme, reverse transcriptase, into a double stranded DNA provirus. As an obligatory part of the normal life cycle of retroviruses, the DNA provirus is integrated, usually at random, into the genome of the infected cell. The three major retroviral genes are ***gag, pol*** and ***env***.

Oncogenes and Tumour Suppressor Genes

Carcinogens induce mutations only in a few hundred of the ten thousand genes thought to comprise the mammalian genome. This few hundred genes can be divided further into two sub classes, **oncogenes** and **tumour suppressor genes**, based on their functional attributes.

Oncogenes

Animals infected with certain viruses (retroviruses) rapidly develop tumours. Such viruses carry genes, termed *oncogenes*, which transform normal cells into tumour cells.

The origin of the oncogenic genes is cellular, not viral. The oncogenic retroviruses have acquired (or transduced) certain cellular genes and incorporated them into their genomes.

The normal cellular counterparts of the retroviral oncogenes are termed *protooncogenes.* They encode proteins that participate in one or more signal transduction pathways. Such signaling pathways regulate cell proliferation and maturation.

Because of their central role in the life cycle of the cell, protooncogenes have been conserved throughout evolution and vary little from yeast to humans.

Once this protooncogene enter into a virus, its original activities are deregulated via mutation or inappropriate expression which leads to activation of cellular DNA to code for the production of transforming protein ends with cancer. These viruses are replication defective.

The protooncogene becoming viral oncogene become mutated during transduction and viral oncogenes are structurally different from protooncogenes. **Thus acquire ability to transform at the expense of ability to replicate**.

Oncogenes are referred using a three-letter nomenclature that is related to the virus from which they were originally identified. For example, the protooncogene *myc* was originally isolated from avian ***mye***locytomatosis virus, and ***erb***A and ***erb***B were isolated from avian *ery*throblastosis virus.

The viral oncogene is usually preceded by a v, as in v-***myc*** to distinguish it from the related protooncogene (often preceded by a c for cellular, as in c-***myc***). It is not the gene, but the encoded protein that leads to cell transformation. The protein encoded by oncogenes is referred to as ***oncoprotein.***

Activation of Protooncogenes

Protooncogenes are activated by one of two means: alteration of gene expression or alteration of gene structure.

I. Alteration of Gene Expression

Gene expression can be altered via

1. Gene amplification
2. Promoter insertion
3. Gene translocation

All these contribute production of altered protein leads to cancer transformation.

1. Gene amplification

Tumour cells often sustain excessive rounds of localized DNA replication that can result in the formation of multiple copies (Gene amplification) of the same gene or genes. The duplicated genes (Amplicon) over produce the protein by abnormal expression.

2. Promoter insertion

Certain retroviruses insert their genome into cellular DNA and deregulate the expression of cellular DNA. When a retrovirus integrates within a region of genomic DNA that flanks a protooncogene, transcription of the protooncogene can be deregulated, leading to cell transformation. In most circumstances, viral insertion events affect the regulation of gene expression, not the function of the gene.

3. Gene translocation

Chromosome translocations may occur spontaneously or induced by carcinogens. Translocation results from movement of portions of one chromosome to another chromosome, or portions may be exchanged between chromosomes in reciprocal translocation events. Translocated genes are oncogenes code for abnormal transcription and cancer transformation.

II. Alteration of Gene structure

Protooncogenes can be transformed into oncogenes following damage to their structure. Structural alterations can occur by mutation of individual nucleotide or alterations that may occur during more global genetic events such as translocation of chromosomes.

Damage to individual nucleotides (point mutation) is the most common structural change sustained by protooncogenes. Chemical carcinogens and some forms of radiation exert their influence this way.

In a normal cell, signal transduction is controlled by ***ras*** gene. Normally, the ***ras*** protein is inactive and is bound to guanine diphosphate (GDP). When the ***ras*** protein is stimulated by signals it exchanges GDP for guanine triphosphate (GTP) and becomes activated by GAP (GTPase activating protein), a protein that enhances the hydrolysis of ***ras*** bound GTP to GDP (returning to normal state).

Point mutation of ***ras*** gene leads to alteration in ***ras*** protein so that it is unable to interact with GAP and remain constitutively activated as a consequence, the proliferative signals that emanate from ***ras*** proceed unchecked leading to cancer formation.

Classification of Oncogenes

1. Growth factors

An example of this category is ***sis*** protooncogene, which encodes the beta chain of platelet-derived growth factor. Simian sarcoma virus (retrovirus) that contains v-***sis*** trigger the fibroblast DNA to encode for the production of platelet derived growth factor which act on platelet derived growth factor receptors on their own cell surface in an autocrine fashion.

2. Growth factor receptors

Oncogenes may encode growth factor receptors. A typical growth factor receptor has three components; an extracellular growth factor binding domain, a transmembranous segment and a cytoplasmic domain with kinase activity. Growth factor receptors encoded by oncogene such as ***erb*** B, are often truncated without extracellular domain.

3. Inracellular signal transducers

They are located in the cytosol (eg. ***abl, raf***) or are membrane associated (***e.g.ras, src***). Point mutations or gross structural alterations can constitutively activate these proteins leading to uncontrolled cell proliferation.

4. Nuclear regulatory proteins

Transcription factors are nuclear proteins that regulate gene expression. They bind to selected sites on DNA, alone or in a complex with other proteins to facilitate gene expression. The oncoproteins encoded by ***myc, jun,*** and ***fos*** are transcription factors that stimulate expression of genes that are necessary for cell division. Abnormal levels of expression or mutations that alter the function of these proteins can compromise growth control.

Oncogene categories

S.No.	Mode of action	Category	Protooncogene
1	Growth factors	Platelet derived growth factor	sis
		Fibroblast growth factor	int2
2	Growthfactor receptors	EGF receptor	erbB
		EGF-like receptor	erbB2
		CSF-1 receptor	fms
		Angiotensin receptor	mas
3	Intracellular signal transducers	GTP-binding protein	ras
		Membrane-associated	src
		Cytosolic	abl
		Cytosolic	raf
		Cytosolic	mos
4	Nuclear regulatory proteins	Transcription factor	myc
		Transcription factor	myb
		Transcription factor	fos
		Transcription factor	jun
5	Cell cycle regulators	Cyclins	cyclin D
		Cyclin-dependent kinase	CDK4

These abnormal receptors do not require growth factor binding for stimulation and are constitutively activated.

5. Cell cycle regulators

Cyclins are a series of proteins that regulate cell cycle. Individual cyclins are expressed for brief intervals at appropriate points in the cell cycle. The cyclins interact with and activate enzymes termed *cyclin dependent kinases* (cdk). The cdks, in turn, activate proteins that are essential for progression through the cell cycle. Disruption in the function of cyclins leads to dysregulated control of cell replication. Several types of tumours in humans have been described with mutations in the genes that encode cyclins or cdks.

Tumour Suppressor Genes

Tumour suppressor genes (TSG) play a critical role in the control of cell growth. They serve as the "brakes" to cell replication. When tumour suppressor genes are inactivated, cells lose regulatory control of cell proliferation. A single intact copy of a tumour suppressor gene is sufficient to maintain control of cell proliferation. When both alleles are lost or damaged the affected cell has a high risk of neoplastic transformation.

For the better understanding of action of TSG, Mitotic cell division events that happen one after another continuously are illustrated. Mitotic cell division, which occurs in all eukaryotic body cells, is the process by which single cells reproduce themselves and multi cellular organisms grow.

Mitotic cell division consists of two interrelated processes:

1. **Mitosis**, the division of nucleus.
2. **Cytokinesis**, the change in the cytoplasm that includes division of the cell proper.

Mitosis is divided into five sequential phases:

1. Interphase (consisting of G_0, G_1, S, G_2 stages) in which the cell prepares itself for mitotic phase.
2. Prophase
3. Metaphase ⟶ Mitotic phase
4. Anaphase
5. Telophase

Mitosis: Cellular events

S.No.	Cell cycle phases	Events	Period
1	G_0 phase	Quiescent stage after mitotic division	Vary
2	G_1 Phase	RNA and proteins are synthesized, but not DNA	6-12 hours
3	S phase	Synthesis of DNA (diploid to tetraploid chromosome)	3-8 hours
4	G_2 Phase	Chromosomes divide as two diploid sets	3-4 hours
5	M Phase	Nucleus divides into two daughter nuclei	Vary

G-Growth, M-Mitotic phase

G_1 / S Check Point (Pause)

When cell sustain injury by radiation or chemical carcinogens, cell cycle is halted between G1 and S phase. During this pause, DNA that has been damaged can be repaired before mutations are passed on to the genomes of daughter cells. A similar checkpoint is present at the transition between G2 and the M phase of the cell cycle.

In cells in which tumour suppressor genes (***p53*** and retinoblastoma, ***Rb*** gene) are absent or not functioning properly, genetic damage is left unrepaired and often leads to genetic instability and additional oncogenic events.

Rb genes and ***p53*** encode nuclear phosphoproteins that regulate cell cycle progression. **p53** can detect cell that sustains genetic damage and arrest the entry of the cell into the S phase from the G1 phase to allow time for the repair of cellular DNA damage. It also induces DNA repair enzymes to aid in elimination of mutations.

Nucleotide Excision Repair

The segment of DNA containing altered bases is recognised by enzymes that remove damaged bases, replaced with normal nucleotide using intact complementary strand as template.

Enzymes and their functions in Nucleotide excision repair

S.No.	Name of the enzyme	Function
1	Endonuclease	Cut the DNA close to the lesion
2	Exonuclease	Remove damaged segment
3	DNA polymerase	Produce new DNA segment
4	Ligase	Patch the gap with new DNA

If the extent of DNA damage is too excessive, ***p53*** can promote cellular apoptosis. Cells carrying mutated ***p53*** genes or cells infected with oncogenic DNA viruses that alter the function of ***p53***, do not arrest before entering the S phase of the cell cycle and cells cannot undergo apoptosis. Affected cells can continue to replicate with damaged DNA, and those that do not develop lethal genetic changes are at risk for acquiring additional genetic damage leading to neoplastic transformation.

Mutation in ***p53*** have been detected in canine neoplasms including thyroid carcinomas, osteosarcomas and mammary tumour.

Abnormal cellular distribution of ***p53***, indicative of mutant ***p53***, has been shown in canine colorectal tumours. Lack of expression of a gene, ***HOXA5*** may be primarily responsible for loss of expression of ***p53*** leading to breast tumour due to failure of apoptosis. The gene ***HOXH5*** alone, independent of ***p53*** can induce apoptosis by caspase 2 and 8 mediated cell death.

Regulators of Apoptosis

The genes ***Bcl-2*** *and* ***Bcl-x*** are antiapoptotic genes and expression of these genes block cell death pathways of cells that have sustained damage. Expression of ***Bcl-2*** in normal cells enables them to escape from apoptosis.

Bcl-2 controls apoptosis by regulating exit of cytochrome-c from mitochondria which activate proteolytic enzyme caspase-9. DNA damaged cells eluding apoptosis could multiply and are at risk to accumulate additional damage that can result in malignancy.

The gene ***p53*** is a proapoptotic and can promote cellular apoptosis if the extent of DNA damage is too excessive. When the DNA is damaged, **p53** arrest the cell at the G1 phase to allow time for repair.

However, if the DNA repair process fails, **p53** triggers apoptosis. ***p53*** stimulate the genes ***Bax*** and ***Bak*** which are also the members of ***Bcl*** family to produce proapoptotic proteins.

Along with ***Bax*** and ***Bak*** proteins, Apaf-1 (Apoptosis activating factor-1) protein stimulated by ***p53*** activate caspases and cause apoptosis. Other proapoptotic genes are ***Bim*** and ***Bid*** which are also ***Bcl*** family members involve in caspase activation to cause apoptosis in various situations.

The ***gag*** gene encodes for the capsid (internal) proteins. The ***pol*** gene encodes the Reverse transcriptase enzyme, and the ***env*** gene encodes the viral envelope proteins. Viral genes, like cellular genes, are expressed under the control of specific promoters. Retro viral gene expression is under the control of potent viral transcription regulators, termed ***long terminal repeats*** (LTRs) that flank the ends of the genome (upstream 5′ and downstream 3′). These regulatory regions determine the tissues in which the virus replicates and affect the pathogenicity of different viral strains.

The oncogenic capacity of retroviruses is facilitated by several features of their life cycle.

1. Infection is not cytolytic, enabling cells to survive and acquire additional genetic alterations that may be necessary for transformation.
2. Integration of the provirus damages the integrity of the host genome.
3. Integrated provirus can acquire intact or damaged cellular genes, usually at the expense of portions of viral genes, thereby incorporating portions of the cellular genome into the virus.
4. The function of cellular genes can by affected by retroviruses.

Oncogenic retroviruses can produce tumours by atleast two mechanisms and the viruses are divided into families based on how they cause infected cells to become neoplastic.

Acute Transforming Viruses (Type C / Transducing Retroviruses)

Transducing retroviruses are able to transform infected cells efficiently and rapidly. These viruses arise from the rare recombination of proviral DNA and host genetic material. They have a hybrid genome composed of portions of the original viral genome with the addition of a transduced cellular oncogene (v-***onc***).

Most of these viruses have lost some part of the viral genome during the incorporation of the oncogene, and as a result, the majority of these viruses cannot replicate on their own.

Rous sarcoma virus is an exception to this rule, it contains all the viral genes needed for replication as well as an oncogene. The oncogenes are expressed at high levels since they are under the control of potent viral promoters and infected cells are rapidly and efficiently transformed into neoplastic cells.

Feline sarcoma viruses (FeSVs) are a group of transducing retroviruses that are closely related to feline leukemia virus (FeLV). They contain a portion of the feline leukemia virus genome and one of several oncogenes, depending on the strain of FeSV. Each strain of FeSV is unique because each arises from a rare recombination between FeLV and cellular oncogenes (protooncogenes of host cell).

Thus, cats with FeSV induced fibrosarcoma are always infected with FeLV. FeSV cannot replicate independently, and horizontal transmission does not occur. Kitten injected with FeSV rapidly develop fibrosarcomas, often in a multicentric pattern, but an effective immune response by adults may eliminate the tumour.

Other tumour types, such as malignant melanomas, can be induced by some strains of FeSV. Avian and bovine leukemia viruses are also included in acutely transforming type C transducing retroviruses.

Acute Transforming Retroviral oncogenesis

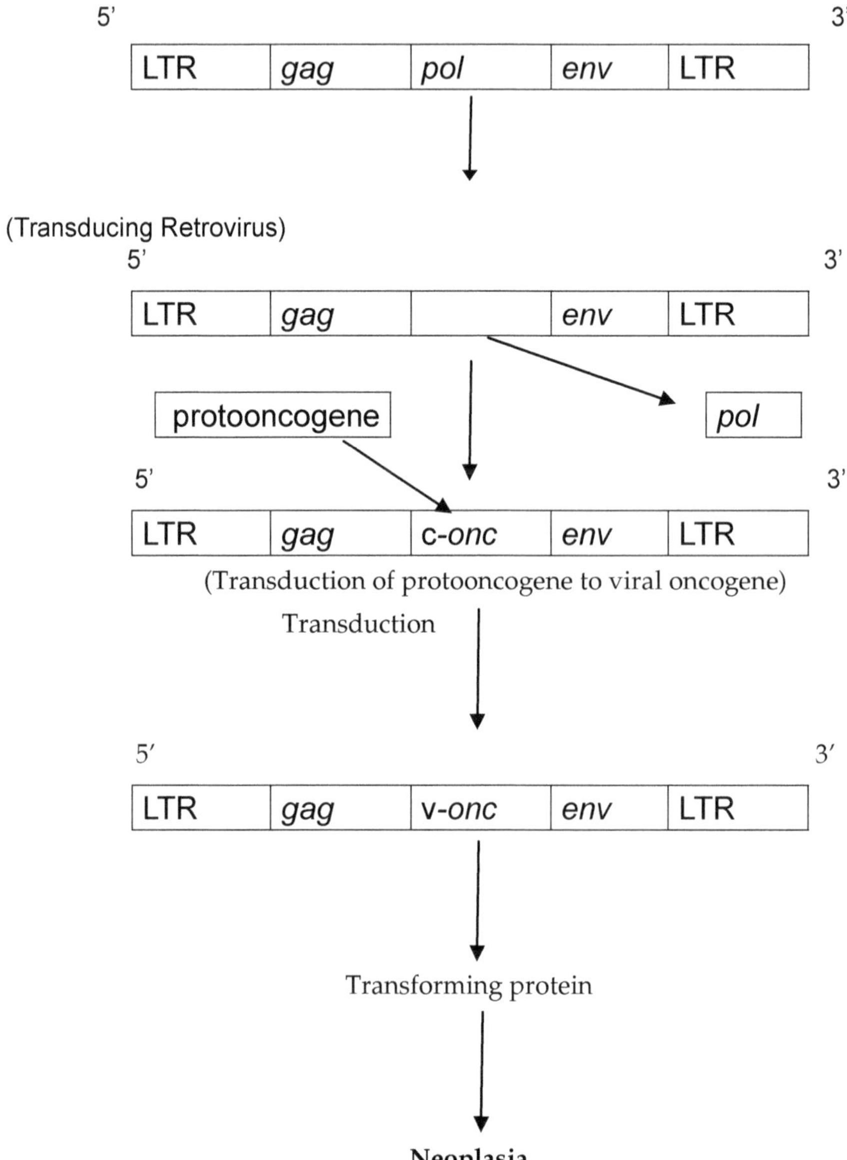

The ***pol*** gene of acute transforming retrovirus, which encodes for Reverse transcriptase enzyme, is lost during integration with host cell genome. The genetic information is lost which codes for multiplication of virus. So, the defective virus cannot replicate.

This is followed by insertion of new set of genes (protooncogenes) into the deleted whole genes (***pol***). These protooncogenes are transduced into viral oncogene by mutation (protooncogene ***fes*** is transduced into v-***fes***).

Approximately 20 viral oncogenes have been identified and named by three letter words like ***fes*** (feline sarcoma gene) and ***sis*** (simian sarcoma genes).

Thus the virus with transduced genes acquires ability to transform the host cell into cancer at the expense of ability to replicate.

Viral oncogenes are structurally different from protooncogenes from which they are transduced. The altered genes encodes for production of entirely different protein which inturn transform the host cell into cancer.

Slow Transforming Retroviruses (Type B Retroviruses)

These viruses don not contain an oncogene and they are replication competent. The mechanism of tumour production is **insertional mutagenesis** in which during integration of virus with host cell genome the slow transforming virus (eg. FeLV) insert proviral DNA (powerful viral transcription regulatory elements of the LTR region of virus) near the cellular protooncogenes and induce structural change in protooncogenes resulting in genetic damage and consequent over expression of protooncogenes ending in neoplastic transformation.

Tumours produced by these sort of viruses develop over a considerable period of time compared to those that develop from Transducing viruses.

FeLV is a slow transforming virus, approximately 20 percent of cats persistently infected with FeLV develop neoplasia and die.

Tumour development is considerably slower in FeLV infected cats than in cats infected with FeSV. Following experimental infection, there is a 1 to 23 months lag time (5.3-month average) before tumour develop. Mouse mammary tumour and leukemia in rodents are caused by slow transforming retroviruses.

Slow Transforming Retroviral oncogenesis

LTR	*gag*	*pol*	*Env*	LTR

(Slow transforming retrovirus)

↓ Insert proviral DNA (LTR)

Cellular promoter	Cellular genes	protooncogene

(Normal host cell)

↓

Cellular promoter	Cellular gene	protooncogene	LTR of virus

↓

Cellular promoter	Cellular gene	Altered protooncogene	LTR of virus

↓

Transforming protein

↓

Neoplasia

Human T-cell Leukemia Type 1 (HTLV-1)

HTLV-1 is associated with a form of T-cell leukemia / lymphoma that is endemic in certain parts of Japan and the Caribbean countries. Sporadic incidences have been recorded elsewhere, including the United States.

Like the Acquired Immuno Deficiency Syndrome (AIDS) virus, HTLV-1 has affinity for CD4+ T- cells and hence this subset of T-cells is the major target for neoplastic transformation.

Human infection requires transmission of infected T-cells via sexual intercourse, blood transfusion and breasts feeding. Leukemia develops in only about 1 % of infected individuals after a long latent period of 20 to 30 years.

Neither the HTLV-1 has v-***onc*** (viral oncogene) like the acute transforming virus nor the insertional mutagenesis occour like slow transforming virus, but it has a fourth gene ***tax***. The secret of its transforming activity is locked in the ***tax*** gene. The product of this gene is essential for viral replication.

The ***tax*** protein can also activate the transcription of several host cell genes, including gene encoding the cytokine interleukin 2 (IL-2) and its receptors, and the gene for the granulocyte-macrophage colony-stimulating factor (GM-CSF).

HTLV-1 infection stimulates proliferation of T- cells. This is brought about by autocrine as well as paracrine mechanisms. The gene ***tax*** turns on genes that encode a T-cell growth factor, IL-2, and the IL-2 receptor, settling up an autocrine system for proliferation (IL-2 acts on IL-2 receptors on the same CD4+ T- cell membrane).

At the same time, paracrine pathway is activated by the increased production of GM-CSF by CD4+ cells due to the action of tax gene.

This myeloid growth factor, by acting on neighboring macrophages, induces increased secretion of other T-cell mitogen such as interleukin-1 (IL-1) which inturn stimulate CD4+ cells proliferation with a ultimate result of T cell leukemia.

DNA Viral Oncogenesis

There are several families of oncogenic DNA viruses, including herpesviruses, PaPoVaviruses (papilloma and polyoma viruses), adenoviruses, hepadnaviruses, and poxviruses. DNA viruses, unlike retroviruses, transform infected cells by expressing genes of viral origin, and the genes of DNA viruses involved in oncogenesis are essential for the normal viral life cycle.

Oncogenic DNA viral action on permissive cells

Permissive cells allow the virus to complete its life cycle and viral progeny are released upon the lysis of infected host cell. Within the host cell, early and late viral genes are expressed. Early genes are responsible for subverting control of the cell to support viral replication.

Some early genes encode multifunctional proteins that bind critical cellular proteins encoded by ***Rb*** and ***p53*** genes and block the apoptosis pathway of cell death. Once viral progeny have matured, the infected cells are lysed and viral particle are released as a result of expression of late viral genes.

Because the infected cells are destroyed as part of the viral life cycle, the possibility of cell transformation is averted. In permissive cells, virus will not integrate with host cell genome, expression and encoding of early and late genes of virus in the cytoplasm of the host cell direct the genes of the host cell.

Oncogenic DNA Viral action on non-permissive cells

During aberrant infections of permissive cells or infections of non-permissive or semi permissive cells, usually only a part of the viral life cycle is completed and no viral progeny are produced. In these circumstances, unlike permissive cell, a portion of the viral genome can become integrated into the cellular DNA.

If the portion that is integrated contains the early genes the encoded proteins combine with proteins encoded by ***Rb*** and ***p53*** genes of host cell to prevent apoptosis. Because the viral late genes are not expressed, these cells are not lysed, and they survive with a high risk of developing into neoplastic cells.

DNA viruses are responsible for a variety of neoplasms in rodents, avian species, and to a lesser extent, nonhuman primates, but only papillomaviruses are a significant cause of neoplasia in domestic animals. Papillomavirus induced wart or viral papilloma is found in all domestic and wild animal species, including the cat.

Most virus-induced papillomas are self-limiting and are usually found in young animals. Like human papillomaviruses, certain strain of bovine papillomavirus (BPV) is more likely to be linked to neoplasms than others.

Infection with BPV-2 and BPT-4 has been associated with malignant neoplasms in cattle, and BPV-4 is associated with neoplasms of the digestive tract.

Herpes viruses cause cancer in human and several non-domestic animals. Herpesvirus saimiri is a virus of squirrel monkeys that produce oropharyngeal ulcerative lesions in the normal host, but infection of owl monkeys and New Zealand white rabbits with this virus can produce T-cell malignant lymphoma or lymphoid leukemia.

Marek's disease virus is a herpesvirus that infects chickens and produces malignant lymphoma. Hepadnaviruses, which include hepatitis B virus and squirrel hepatitis virus are responsible for an increased risk of liver cancer in their respective host from many other oncogenic DNA virus infections, because tumours are produced in the typical host and in cells that are normally infected.

However, it appears that, like other DNA oncogenic viruses, integration of viral genome into the cellular genome is necessary for tumour production. Another group of DNA viruses, the poxvirus, such as Shope fibroma virus of rabbits can cause myxomas and fibromas in their typical hosts.

9

Tumour Diagnosis

Cancer diagnosis aids in planning treatment and to assess prognosis. Early detection followed by removal or treatment can save most of the cancer-affected patients owing to the fact that all tumours are attaining malignancy and subsequent metastasis after certain stage of growth.

Various methods are employed for the diagnosis of tumours each with its own merits and demerits. Selection of method(s) depends on the type of tumours; anatomical location in the body, rate of growth and frequency of testing needed to assess the prognosis. The methods are ranging from cytology to microarrays, which are detailed below.

1. Cytology

Cytology is the examination of individual cells collected from lesions by scrapes, smears (cut surface of excised tissue collected for histopathology), swab smears, collected body fluids and exfoliated cells (Exfoliated cytology – Papanicolaou test).

Cytology can be used to make an initial evaluation of a lesion. Although cytology may not give a definitive diagnosis, it gives a broad classification of a lesion. Lesions may be broadly classified as inflammatory or non-inflammatory tissue cells. In non-inflammatory tissue cells, it is possible to distinguish benign from malignant neoplasia and cytology also helps to identify the cell of origin as round cell (lymphoid, mast cells, plasma cells, histiocytes), epithelial cell or mesenchymal cell (spindle cell). However, cytology can give definitive diagnosis of round cell tumours.

A) Fine Needle Aspiration Biopsy (FNAB)

The aim of this technique is to harvest individual cells or small clusters of cells with minimal haemodilution. A 23 or 25 gauge needle is used. Wider bore needles apart from haemorrhage, yield core of tissue rather than individual cells or small cell clusters. Core samples do not produce good smears, since the cells do not spread out adequately.

For skin mass, the area is clipped and swabed with surgical sprit. The mass is immobilized with one hand and the needle with 5 ml syringe inserted into the lesions. The needle is moved to and fro within the mass, whilst being redirected several times. Thus obtaining sample from different parts of the lesion. Maintain suction continuously throughout the sampling procedure.

Care should be taken not to advance the needle through the mass into the surrounding tissues, since there is a risk of metastasis or local dissemination along the needle tract. Release the suction slowly before removing the needle to prevent the material being aspirated back from the needle into the syringe.

Fill the syringe with air, connect the needle and depress the plunger briskly, expelling the contents of the needle on to the slide. Instead of air, drops of saline can be used to mix the aspirated cells within the needle; the saline drops can also be used to rinse the syringe so that the cells aspirated to the syringe can also be expelled.

The expelled cells onto a slide are spread by using another slide and the smear air-dried. Romanowsky stains (Leishman, Giemsa) can be used to study the nuclear and cytoplasmic details. Mast cell tumour and malignant melanomas need toluidine blue and Fontana stain respectively. Using a cover slip will enhance the clarity of microscope examination.

Fine needle aspirates can be obtained from the internal masses/organs also (liver, spleen, kidney, intra-abdominal mass). Insertion and progression of needle is monitored by ultrasonography, computed tomography, mammography and other computer controlled instruments.

B) Exfoliated cytology

Papanicolaou's (1928) technique of exfoliated cells examination is still being practiced to detect carcinoma of cervix and endometrium. This method can be applied to sputum, bronchial and nasal washings, pleural and sub-arachnoid fluids, discharges from nipples, prostatic secretions, urinary sediments, gastric washings and ethmoid tumours of cattle.

Smears are prepared with shed cells (collected as washings, brushings, swab) on to clear glass slides, air dried and stained with Romanowsky stains to observe microscopic details.

For better results, the smears are fixed with ether or ether-alcohol and stained with Harry's haematoxylin and orange O. Nucleus stains light purple and cytoplasm green orange or red.

2. Histopathology and Biopsy

Histopathology is the best way of tumour diagnosis wherever the piece of tissue is obtainable. It serves as a confirmative diagnosis and reveal the exact picture of neoplastic cells including mitotic index as well as non-neoplastic supportive mass exist in the tumour (amount of supportive tissue, blood vessels, extent of inflammation, necrosis, apoptotic cell populations *etc.*) to decide the degree of malignancy and fate of the tumour.

Ultrasonography and other imaging techniques are used to obtain biopsy samples from visceral tumours.

The demerits of this method include non-accessibility of tissue samples (biopsy) to all the tumours (visceral tumours) and non-applicability for continuous assessment, which warrant tissue sample each time. The delay in processing can be alleviated by frozen sections and the results of frozen sections agree with about 90 % of the results of paraffin sections.

3. Tumour Imaging

The diagnostic imaging techniques (DIT) used in veterinary medicine are

- ★ Radiography (X-ray)
- ★ Ultrasonography
- ★ Computed Tomography (CT)
- ★ Magnetic Resonance Imaging (MRI)
- ★ Scinctigraphy

These techniques are used for the following

- ★ To examine the nature and extent of the suspected primary lesions (Tumour / cyst / abscess)
- ★ To search for metastases
- ★ Continuous monitoring of lesions

Radiography and ultrasonography are primary diagnostic imaging techniques, which should be used as complementary with other tests owing to the fact that they cannot differentiate tumour from other swellings (cyst, abscess, hyperplasia). MRI and CT scans are producing cross-sectional images with more tissue details than the radiography and ultrasonography.

A) Radiography (X-ray)

Principle

An X-ray beam is produced by acceleration of electrons onto a tungsten target. An image is created on a film by the X-ray that penetrate an object placed in the path of that beam. The inability to penetrate tissue (*e.g.* Bone) cannot give the tissue details, only the outline can be seen.

Advantages

High quality radiographs are useful to detect abnormal masses especially in thoracic and abdominal cavities.

Disadvantages

- ★ It is non-specific, cannot differentiate tumour from cysts/abscess, granuloma or haematoma
- ★ It does not differentiate soft tissue and fluid, so no information about internal organ architecture
- ★ Non-applicable to bony details

B) Ultrasonography

Images are obtained by placing a hand-held scanner on the surface of animal and pulsing high frequency sound waves into an area of interest. Portions of these waves are returned to the scanner, where they are detected and processed electronically for viewing on a television screen. The interior of organs cannot be imaged, nor can anything beyond be seen.

Advantages

- ★ Since no ionizing radiation is involved, it is safe for both handlers and patients
- ★ It differentiates between fluid and soft tissue
- ★ Vascularity of a lesion can be assessed using colour flow Doppler ultrasonography
- ★ Ultrasound guided fine needle aspiration / biopsy is possible

Disadvantages

- ★ Nonspecific, cannot differentiate tumour from other swellings
- ★ Its use in skeletal disease is very limited

C. Computed Tomography Scans (CT-Scans)

Principle

CT-scanning is a cross-sectional radiography, producing images that represent slices of the body. The CT scanner is a ring like gantry containing X-ray emitting and detecting devices that encircle patient. The patient lies horizontally on a table, which is advanced in small increments between radiographic exposures, each of which produces a single slice image traverse to the long axis of the body.

As the X-ray beam passes through the body it is attenuated by the tissues in the same way as in conventional radiography, depending on their effective atomic number, specific gravity and thickness. Radiation emerging from the patient at each of many locations around the ring is detected and converted by a computer to a image. Very small differences between tissues, such as between brain parenchyma and CSF, can be detected that is not possible with conventional radiography. It is also sensitive for fine bony changes (osteolysis / calcification).

Advantages and Disadvantages

Tissue difference details within the swelling can be detected (fluid, soft / hard tissues), but cellular details to diagnose, as cancer cannot be investigated. Patients cannot be subjected to frequent CT-scans due to ionizing radiation hazards.

D. Magnetic Resonance Imaging (MRI)

Principle

It utilises the principle of chemical spectroscopy. It combines the energy of a magnetic field with radio frequency energy (RF) to produce and image that map out protons in hydrogen nuclei. Hydrogen is used because of its abundance in biological tissues and its protons are suitable for MR characteristics.

The scanner has a powerful magnet (0.2 – 1.5 Tesla) which magnetize the area of tissue under investigation, a painless and safe process. The area of the body is enclosed by a radio frequency coil (RF-coil). When the magnetic field is operated, the RF coil transmits pulses of RF energy at a predetermined frequency into the tissues, disorienting the protons of hydrogen nuclei and synchronizing their spins. Synchronized protons themselves emit a small RF signal that can be detected by the RF coil and transmitted to the computer for reconstruction as an image.

The MR images are cross sectional images and 3D images are also possible with special software which can be viewed from any angle on the computer screen.

Advantages

★ Mainly used to image the neoplasm of brain, spine, head and neck, dorsum and pelvis. It can be applied to other parts of the body also.

Disadvantages

★ Though it can be used to detect the fine tissue details of masses of brain and bones, it cannot give the exact picture of cellular details, so cannot be used to confirm cancer.

E. Scinctigraphy (Diagnostic nuclear medicine)

Principle

Radioactive pharmaceuticals (RAP) are introduced into the blood stream which will concentrate in particular tissue / organ by a variety of physiological processes including phagocytosis, active transport and passive adsorption producing **"hot spots"** of abnormal areas. RAPs specific to particular tissues / organs either alone or in combinations (eg. Bone seeking methylene diphosphonate, MDP in combination with ^{99m}technetium) are used.

After attaching with "hot spots" RAPs emit gamma rays which can be detected and quantified by gamma camera as small flashes of lights (scintillations) which are converted as greyscale / coloured dots by photo multiplier tubes corresponding to the severity of lesion and detected by using a computer to localize and quantify the lesions. In this technique information about organ function (pathophysiological processes) can be detected so that deviation of function is identified to localize each lesion. The anatomical resolution of Scinctigraphy images is very poor compared with radiographs.

This is helpful in detecting disease before it is visible with other imaging techniques, or in performing wide search of metastases. So this technique is useful to trace occult metastases after confirming primary tumour.

As with other imaging techniques it is not specific for the histological nature of the disease (In bone scanning it can indicate an area of increased bone turnover and will not differentiae neoplasm from other active lesions).

It is non-invasive, painless and may involve less radiation exposure than a series of radiographs. ^{99m}technetium is most commonly used RAP which is used as its pertechnetate form alone or bound to other RAP (bone-seeking MDP). The advantage of ^{99m}Technetium is its short half-life of only 6 hours. After administration of RAP via intravenous catheter, scanning is carried out within a few minutes for soft tissue studies, or after several hours for bone examinations.

Commonly used RAPs for tumour diagnosis

S.No.	Radiopharmaceuticals	Tumours identified
01	^{99m}Tc-MDP	Skeletal system, especially metastases from osteosarcoma to lymph nodes and soft tissues
02	^{131}I (Iodine)	Thyroid tumours (best for metastases from thyroid adenocarcinoma), also used for treatment
03	^{123}I(Iodine)	Thyroid tumours
04	^{99m}Tc-methoxy-isobutyl-isonitrite (sestamibi)	Lymphoma; Parathyroid adenomas
05	^{111}In (Indium) pentetreotide	Insulinoma
06	67Ga (gallium)	Soft tissue sarcomas
07	^{123}IMetaiodobenzylguanidine (MIBG)	Phaeochromocytoma
08	^{99m}Tc-labelled erythrocytes	Gastrointestinal bleeding
09	^{99m}Tc-glucoheptonate	Focal brain lesions
10	^{99m}Tc-ciproflaxacin	Differentiate bone infection from neoplasia

By using RAP conjugated specific monoclonal antibodies against the surface antigens of particular tumour accuracy of detection can be enhanced and inclusion of therapeutic agent to this RAP-Mab complex can serve as a therapy to that particular tumour. A Geiger counter should be used to check that the animal is no longer emitting significant amount of radiation before being discharged back to the owner, with ^{99m}Tc it is 24 hours.

Advantage

★ Early detection of metastases

Disadvantages

Though tumour kind can be detected by using specific RAPs and Mabs, histological difference to confirm benign / malignant types and overall picture of neoplastic and non-neoplastic supportive tissues cannot be assessed.

4. Electron Microscopy (EM)

Electron microscopy is helpful to decide the histologic nature of cells in highly anaplastic tumours. It is used to differentiate closely resembling tumours (eg. lymphoma Vs small cell carcinoma). Surface ultrastuctural studies with scnning EM are helpful in recognizing early neoplastic changes of cells (low grade bladder tumour cells are identified by studying the polymorphism of their surface microvilli).

Ultra thinness of section cannot reveal the clear picture of histopathological changes.

5. Immuno Peroxidase Test (IPT)

Several tumours are expressing cell surface specific antigens against which Mabs are produced and supplied commercially. Mabs conjugated with enzyme-substrate (Horse Radish Peroxidase-H_2O_2) combine specifically to the surface tumour antigens, if present on the tumour cells of tissue HP sections and biopsies. This specific combination is detected by colour development by using a chromogen (ABTS-Green; OPD- brown). Fine needle aspirated cells can also be subjected to this test.

Tumour specific Mabs

S.No.	Mab	Tumour	Remarks
01	2D1,Leu, M1	Lymphoma	Differentiate benign and malignant lymphomas based on increased expression of tumour cells.
02	CEA, B 72.3, LEUMI	Mesothelioma	Differentiate benign and malignant types

Mabs against cytokeratin, vimentin, CEA, S-100, Epithelial membrane antigen are used to detect and type large varieties of tumours.

Equine pulmonary tumours can be detected by using Mabs against vimentin and S-100 proteins of cancer cells. CD-44 present within the benign and malignant melanomas, but the expression is more intense in malignant tumours. Immunohistochemical (IHC) detection of more CD-44 cells by using specific Mab against it can be utilised to detect malignant type of melanomas.

CD-44 and CD-24 cells have been identified as stem cells in breast cancers and more number of these stem cells indicate malignancy and metastatic tumours are established due to these stem cells when they are detached and seeded in other locations. Indefinite propagation of these stem cells both *invitro* and *invivo* has been proved. IHC detection of these CD-44 and CD-24 stem cells of breast tissue indicates highly proliferating tumour with possible metastases.

Disadvantages

- Very high prices of Mabs
- Mabs are not available to all tumours

6. Flow cytometry

The fluorescence detection cytometer developed by Marvin Van Dila in the year 1969 has attained several modifications to have the today's shape of Flow cytometer. It quantitates the total DNA content of a cell population.

Principle

A single cell suspension is prepared from a sample of tissue and the method involves dissolving the cell membrane lipids with a nonionic detergent eliminating the cell cytoskeleton and nuclear proteins with trypsin, digesting the cellular RNA with an enzyme, and stabilizing the nuclear chromatin with spermine.

Fluorescent dye Propidium Iodide (PI) is bound to the clean, isolated nuclei which are then run on a flow cytometer in which LASER beam is passed on them. PI stained nuclei emit fluorescent light between 580 and 650 nm which are analyzed by detectors and converted into DNA histogram by computer. Nuclei are allowed to run at the rate of 5000 / second.

The resulting fluorescence histograms are analyzed and compared with normal tissue histogram of the same kind. DNA Index (DI) and cell cycle percentages can be derived from DNA histograms.

$$\text{DI (Ploidy)} = \frac{G_0/G_1\text{peak channel of the tumour suspect}}{G_0/G_1\text{peak channel of a diploid standard of the tissue/organ}}$$

A DI of 1.0 is said to be diploid. Normal cells containing two copies of each chromosome are said to be diploid. If the resulting ratio is not equal to 1.0 (> or < 1.0), the sample is defined as being aneuploid indicating tumour cells.

Flow cytometry in tumour cell surface antigen identification

By using fluorescent dye (PI / FITC) conjugated specific Mabs against tumour cell surface antigens (CD-44, CD-24 *etc.*), it is possible to identify percentage of tumour cells per 5000 / 10000 cells promptly by using flow cytometer which is time consuming by IHC method.

Presence of more than one tumour antigens in the same cell can also be detected by using different Mabs conjugated with different dyes due to the fact that flow cytometry is a multiparametric device which can analyze more than one antigen at the speed of more than 5000 cells / second which is practically impossible in other methods.

7. Polymerase Chain Reaction (PCR)

In tumour diagnosis, PCR is employed as a *in situ* PCR to detect the bacteria or virus within the tumour cells. Human papilloma virus, Bovine papilloma virus and *Helicobacter pylori* are traced in tumours to confirm the etiological factors by using specific primers against the conserved regions of these infectious agents.

With the use of a specialized thermal cycler block, PCR can be performed directly on slides containing fixed, thin tissue section.

This method reduces the sample contaminations; which can lead to fake positive results in PCR. Positive signal is localized to specific areas within the cell, which are identified by using detecting agents.

It also provides enormous amount of information relative to the histological distribution of the amplified PCR product. As on date PCR is not used to detect a swelling as a tumour, only the infectious agents of tumours are identified.

8. *In situ* hybridization (ISH)

For certain tumours like leukemia, lymphoma, breast tumour, testis tumour and urological tumour, cancer cell DNA alterations at specific restricted sites have been identified.

ISH is carried out by using labeled specific probe to a particular tumour. If the cells under investigation have the changed conserved DNA sequence, which will be hybridized and detected by using detecting agents.

The following points are essential for ISH

- ★ Selection of specific probes and modification of probe by non-isotopic, enzymatic or chemical labeling for direct observation on slides avoiding autoradiography
- ★ Pretreatment of tissue material on the slide for ISH
- ★ Specific hybridization of the modified probe with denatured target DNA
- ★ Immuno cyto chemical detection of the hybridized probe by using antibodies against the probe used.

Fresh tumour materials obtained as biopsy / FNAB is used. Proteolytic enzymes like proteinase-k and pepsin are applied in ISH tissue to accomplish good penetration of the DNA probes and subsequently for the antibodies. The major disadvantages are non-availability of probes to all sorts of tumours and inability to analyze the histological details.

9. Southern Blotting

DNA is extracted from suspected tissue cells as per the standard procedures and fragmented by using restriction enzymes (Endonucleases: BamH-K, EcoR-I, Hind III) and the fragments are separated according to their size by Agar gel electrophoresis. These DNA fragments are transferred by capillary action and deposited on a blotting material-Nylon.

Tumour specific radioactive labeled DNA (probe) with a buffer is treated on DNA fragments transferred to Nylon membrane, if the membrane contain the DNA sequence complimentary to the specific probe used it will hybridize it and this hybridization is detected by suing a photographic film placed against the nylon membrane (Autoradiography).

Hybridized band registered on the photographic film indicates the presence of required DNA sequence to diagnose it as a specific tumour. The disadvantages of this technique are non-availability of probes to all sorts of tumours and inability to reveal histological details of the tumour under investigation.

10. Tumour markers

Tumour markers are biochemical indicators of the presence of tumour, which includes cell surface antigens, cytoplasmic proteins, cell adhesion molecules, enzymes and hormones.

These markers can detect only well established or metastasizing cancers. These markers cannot be considered as sole criteria for the diagnosis of cancer. Their main utility is to support the tumour diagnosis. Some markers serve as yardstick to indicate response to therapy and recurrence during follow-up period.

Salient features of Tumour markers

- ★ Tumour markers are biochemical substances produced by normal cells as well as cancer cells
- ★ They are higher than normal level in cancer cells and it is either due to the cause or effect of malignant process
- ★ They are detected mainly by Radioimmunoassay (RIA) and immunohistochemical (IHC) techniques
- ★ They serve as a yardstick to assess the cancer's response to treatment and to check for recurrence
- ★ Proliferation markers are primarily used for population screening, detection, diagnosis, staging and prognosis or follow-up of malignant status

Characteristics of an ideal tumour marker

- ★ It should be highly sensitive and should have low false negativity
- ★ It should be highly specific and should have low false positivity
- ★ It should have high positive and negative predictive values
- ★ It should have 100% accuracy in differentiating between healthy individuals and tumour patients
- ★ It should be able to differentiate between neoplastic and non-neoplastic disease and show positive correlation with tumour volume and extent
- ★ It should predict early recurrence and have prognostic value
- ★ It should be clinically sensitive *i.e.*, detectable at early stage of cancer
- ★ Its level should be preceding the neoplastic process, so that it should be useful for screening early cancer
- ★ It should be either a universal marker for all types of malignancies or specific to one type of malignancy
- ★ It should be easily assayable and be able to indicate all changes in cancer patient receiving treatment

Classification of tumour marker

I. General markers (For all malignancies)

- ★ Argyrophilic Nucleolar Organizing Region (**AgNOR**)
- ★ Ki – 67
- ★ Proliferating Cell Nuclear Antigen (**PCNA**)
- ★ Thymidine labelling index
- ★ Bromodeoxyuridine labelling index
- ★ Mitotic Index (MI)
- ★ P^{53}

II. Specific markers (for specific tumours)

a. Colon cancer	-	Carcinoembryonic antigen.
b. Breast cancer	-	Estrogen receptor, Progesterone receptor
c. Prostate cancer	-	Prostate specific antigen
d. ovarian cancer	-	CA – 125.
e. Thyroid cancer	-	Thyroglobulin, calcitonin
f. Testicular cancer	-	Human chorionic gonadotrophin
g. Melanoma	-	Tyrosinase
h. Adrenal carcinoma	-	Steroids, catecholamines
i. Lymphoma	-	CD25, CD44
J. Hepatic carcinoma	-	α - fetoprotein.

The cell cycle

It is a ubiquitous complex process involved in the growth and proliferation of cells and regulation of DNA damage repair as responses to injury and disease such as cancer.

Cyclin dependant kinases (Cdks) and **the cyclins** are two regulatory proteins that regulate cell's progression through the stages of the cell cycle referred to as G_o, G_1, S, G_2 and M phases.

The cell cycle can be subdivided into 'interphase' and stages of 'M' (mitotic) phase, which include prophase, metaphase, anaphase and telophase. 'Interphase' encompasses G_0, G_1, S and G_2. The G_1 and G_2 phases of cell cycle represented the 'gaps' in the cell cycle that occur between the two obvious landmarks, DNA synthesis and mitosis.

In the first gap - $\mathbf{G_1}$, cell is preparing for DNA synthesis, 'S' phase cells are synthesizing DNA and therefore cells have an aneuploid DNA content between 2n and 4n. $\mathbf{G_2}$ is the second gap phase in the cell cycle during which the cell prepares for mitosis or 'M' phase. In $\mathbf{G_0}$ the cells are not actively cycling. It was originally used to indicate cells not in the cycle but with potential for division such as hepatocytes.

Mitosis - cellular events and stages of cell cycle

S.No.	Cell cycle phases	Events	Period
1.	G_0 phase	Quiescent stage after mitotic division	Vary
2.	G_1 phase	RNA and proteins are synthesized, but not DNA	6 –12 hours
3.	S phase	Synthesis of DNA (diploid to tetraploid chromosome)	3-8 hours
4.	G_2 phase	Chromosomes divide as two diploid sets	3 – 4 hours
5.	M phase	Nucleus divides into two daughter nuclei	Vary

G – Growth, M – Mitotic phase

Cell cycle regulators

- ⋆ Cyclin – dependant kinases (Cdks)
- ⋆ Cyclins

Cell cycle regulators involved in different phases of cell cycle

G_1 -	Cdk -H, 6
	Cyclin D
S -	Cdk - 2
	Cyclin E
G_2 -	Cdk - 2
	Cyclin A
M -	Cdk -1
	Cyclin B

Cyclin is necessary for the activation of Cdks. After binding with appropriate cyclin the Cdks is activated and it phosphorylate a variety of substances thereby catalyzing the cell progression.

Check points (Pause)

- ⋆ G_1/S check point
- ⋆ G_2/ M check point

When cell sustain injury by radiation or other chemical carcinogens, cell cycle is halted between G1 and S phase. During this phase, DNA that has been damaged can be repaired before mutations are passed on to the genomes of daughter cells. A similar check point is present at the transition between G1 and the M phase of cell cycle. In cells in which tumour suppressor genes (p^{53} and Rb gene) are absent or not functioning properly, genetic damage is left unrepaired and often leads to genetic instability and additional oncogenic events.

Rb gene and p53 encode nuclear phosphoproteins that regulate cell cycle progression. P53 can detect cell that sustain genetic damage and arrest the entry of the cell into the 'S' phase from the G1 phase to allow time for repair of cellular DNA damage. It also induces DNA repair enzymes to aid in eliminations of mutations.

Nucleotide Excision Repair

The segment of DNA containing altered bases is recognized by enzymes that remove damaged bases, replaced with normal nucleotide using intact complementary strand as template.

If the extent of damage is too excessive, p^{53} can promote cellular apoptosis. Cells carrying mutated p^{53} genes or cells infected with oncogenic DNA viruses that alter the function of p^{53}, do not arrest before entering the S phase of cell cycle and cells cannot undergo apoptosis. Affected cell can continue to replicate with damaged DNA, and those that do not develop lethal genetic changes are at risk for acquiring additional genetic damage leading to neoplastic transformation.

Enzymes and their functions in NER

S.No.	Name of the enzyme	Function
1.	Endonuclease	Cut the DNA close to the lesion
2.	Exonuclease	Remove damaged segment
3.	DNA polymerase	Produce new DNA segment
4.	Ligase	Patch the gap with new DNA

Abnormalities of cancer cells

i. Increase in Nuclear: Cytoplasmic ratio

ii. Increase in Nucleolus: Nuclear ratio

iii. Chromosomal and DNA ploidy get increased *i.e.,* 2n - 4n become, 4n – 8n and 8n –12n.

Tumour growth depends on the ratio of cellular proliferation and cell death. Cell proliferations are regarded as one of the most important biological mechanism in oncogenesis and are considered as a principal determinant of tumour progression and prognosis. In recent years, measurement of tumour proliferation has shown a good correlation with biological behaviour in certain tumours in man providing valuable additional prognostic information.

Determination of cell proliferation in tumours recently has been focused on demonstration of proliferation antigens by means of the following:

General Tumour Markers to detect all Malignancies

A. Argyrophilic Nucleolar Organizing Region (AgNOR)

★ Nucleolar Organizing Regions (NORs) are loops of ribosomal RNA

★ (r RNA) occurring in all nucleoli of cells and is directly related to the proliferative activity of the cell due to the transcription of ribosomal RNA needed for the assembly of ribosomes.

★ Decondensation of the r RNA loops during higher transcription activity leads to segregation of the associated proteins. This can be demonstrated at the optical level by an increased number and area of silver stainable intranuclear and intranucleolar particles.

★ Ribosomal RNA genes play an important role in protein synthesis, cell growth, cell differentiation and malignant transformation.

★ In domestic dog, NORs were exclusively found on telomeric regions of chromosomes 7,8,27 and sometimes in 38.

★ NORs can be readily demonstrated in formalin fixed tissues because of their close association with proteins containing a large number of disulphide bonds which bind to silver ions. Silver stained NORs are referred as AgNORs.

★ AgNORs appear as black dots in the nucleus

- ★ AgNOR quantity increases progressively when a resting cell enters mitotic cycle (from G1 to S phase)
- ★ AgNOR quantity is strictly related to the rapidity of cell proliferation and higher the AgNOR quantity, the faster will be the cell proliferation and neoplastic mass expansion.
- ★ More recently it has been suggested that ***the numbers of AgNORs in nuclei may reflect their state of activation or, indeed malignancy.***
- ★ Quantitative analysis of interphase NORs has proved to be valuable in tumour pathology for distinguishing malignant from benign lesions of the same origin

AgNOR staining

Stock solutions

1. Formic acid - gelatin solution

- ★ 530 mg of gelatin to be dissolved in 26.1ml of distilled water at 37°C and then add 300µl of 1% formic acid solution.
- ★ The solutions should be freshly prepared before use.

2. 50 % silver nitrate solution

3. Add one part of solution 1 to two parts of solution 2

Procedure

- ★ Deparaffinize the tissue sections and rehydrate it with distilled water and wash three changes in triple distilled water
- ★ Keep the slides in coplin jars, fully immersed in 10 mM of sodium citrate buffer (pH – 6) and autoclave at 120°C for 20 min
- ★ Cool down the slides to room temperature
- ★ Mix the working solutions thoroughly and pour it on the slide so as to cover the section
- ★ For ideal staining, slides should be kept in dark place for 15 min
- ★ Wash the slides in three changes of distilled water
- ★ Sections are then dehydrated in graded alcohol and then cleared in xylene
- ★ Mount the slides using DPX

AgNOR index

- ★ The number of clearly defined silver stained black dots in 100 neoplastic cells per specimen is counted under oil immersion objective and expressed as mean value per cell.
- ★ The AgNOR dots both intra and extra nucleolar should be counted

$$\text{AgNOR index} = \frac{\text{No.of AgNOR dots}}{\text{No. of nuclei counted}}$$

★ The NORs in stained sections appears as dark brown or black coloured dots or specks distributed within the nucleolus or dispersed in the nucleoplasm

Based on morphological and distribution pattern within the nucleus, NORs are classified into three types:

Type	Description
I	Round and solitary NORs varying in size, found anywhere in the nucleus It is seen in resting cells of tumours and small lymphocytes
II	NORs restricted to the nucleolus with dispression of 2 or more NORs within nucleolus contributing to an enlarged and irregular shape It is observed in proliferating cells irrespective of being neoplasia or hyperplastic
III	NORs which are dispersed as small dots throughout the nucleoplasm, seen in malignant cells

The AgNOR index range

a. Neoplastic cells - 2.05 - 6.40 / nucleus

b. Malignant cells - 6.21 - 10.08 / nucleus

c. Benign cells - 2.71 ± 0.08 / nucleus

AgNOR index for various tumours

S.No	Tumour type/sp	AgNOR index
1	Myeloma / mouse	6.35± 1.39
2.	Venereal sarcoma / dog	5.61 ± 1.91
3.	Basal cell carcinoma / human	5.58 ± 1.86
4.	Squamous cell carcinoma / horse	4.58 ± 1.39
5.	Epidermoid carcinoma / hourse	4.73 ± 1.16
6.	Sertoli Cell tumor / dog	5.71 ± 1.66
7.	Fibroadenoma (Breast) / human	4.25 ± 1.44
8	Cutaneous papilloma / buffaloe	8.24 ± 1.27
9.	Mammary tumour / human	3.16 ± 2.35
10	Perianal gland adenoma	3.09 ± 1.50
	Control tissue	
1	Esophagus / goat	2.36 ± 1.07
2.	Salivary gland / goat	2.00 ± 0.99
3.	Spleen lymphocytes / mouse	1.53 ± 0.63

B. Ki – 67

★ Ki – 67 antigen is a nuclear protein expressed during all active stages of cell cycle (G, S, G_2 and M phases) but absent in resting, non-cycling cells (G_0)

- ★ It is a part of chromosomal DNA matrix and possibly play a role in break down of the nuclear envelope during cell division
- ★ Ki - 67 is expressed 24-36 hours after cell stimulation in the G_1 phase and remains immunohistologically detectable throughout the interphase of the cell cycle, reaching its maximum level during mitosis
- ★ It contributes to the condensation of chromosome
- ★ It is an excellent marker for determining growth fraction or proliferation of a given cell population
- ★ Recently a mouse monoclonal antibody Ki-67 (clone MIB-1) against Ki- 67 antigen is being used in many human neoplasms
- ★ Evaluation of growth fraction by the Ki - 67 proliferations index is highly predictive of biological behaviour of various canine neoplasm

Procedure

Materials required

1. Immunochemicals
   - i. Primary antibody - Anti human / dog ki-67, Clone MIB –1 raised in mice
   - ii. Anti mice antibody IgG is raised in goat conjugated with HRPO (used at dilution of 1:100; it should be stored at 2 – 8 °C)
2. Adhesive - 3 Aminopropyl triethoxysilane (APES)
3. H_2O_2 in methanol (3%)
4. 0.01M citrate buffer (pH- 6)
5. Substrate - 3, 3-diamine benzidine tetrahydrochloride (DAB, it should be prepared freshly).
6. 0.01M PBS (pH – 7.4)
7. Harris haematoxylin for nuclear staining

Method

- i. Clean grease free glass slides are immersed in 2% solution of APES for 5 - 15 min. Then the slides are rinsed in acetone and then two changes of distilled water and dried at 37° C for 3 hours.
- ii. Tissue sections are mounted on APES coated slides and then they are dried at 37°C for 3 hours.
- iii. Tissue sections are deparaffinized and rehydrated.
- iv. Endogenous peroxidase is blocked by covering the section with 3% H_2O_2 in methanol. Incubate at room temperature for 15 min. Wash the slides thrice in 0.01M PBS.
- v. **Antigen retrieval by heat:** It is carried out by immersing tissue sections in a cooker containing citrate buffer (pH – 6.0) and cooked for 2 min,

after maximum pressure is obtained, sections are allowed to cool down to room temperature for approximately 20 –30 min.

vi. Addition of primary antibody: Mouse anti-human / dog ki-67 clone MIB – 1, ready to use is added to cover the section. Subsequently the section is incubated at 37 °C in humid chamber for one hour and washed with 0.01 M PBS thrice.

vii. **Addition of secondary antibody:** (Anti goat conjugated with HRPO)The whole section is covered with secondary antibody and incubated at 37 °C in humid chamber for 1 hour and washed with 0.01M PBS thrice.

viii. **Addition of substrate**: Freshly prepared DAB with 3% H_2O_2 is poured to cover the section. Incubate it for 5 –10 min or until the desired colour is developed at room temperature and sections were washed with PBS thrice.

ix. Stain the nucleus with Harry's haematxylin for 3 min.

x. Calculate Ki - 67 Proliferation index

- ★ The positive reaction for Ki - 67 proliferation antigen is observed as dark brown coloured granular material restricted to the nucleus of proliferating cell.
- ★ Ki - 67 expressions is mainly assessed at the periphery of the tumour where the active proliferation is likely to be higher than in other areas
- ★ To determine Ki - 67 per tumour section, approximately 1000 neoplastic cells should be counted in 10 representation fields. The number of positive cells per 1000 cells is expressed as percentage (%)
- ★ $$\textbf{Ki} - \textbf{67 Proliferation index} \frac{\textbf{Number of Positive cells}}{\textbf{Total no. of cells counted}} \times \textbf{100}$$
- ★ **Ki - 67 index ranges from**

a. Benign 8.57 ± 0.97

b. Malignant 23.26 ± 1.33

C. Proliferating Cell Nuclear Antigen (PCNA)

- ★ Proliferating cell nuclear antigen is a 36 KD acidic auxiliary nuclear protein of DNA polymerase expressed in dividing cells during G1 phase of cell division.
- ★ PCNA increases in late G1, peaks in S- phase and decline during G2 and M phase
- ★ Its level correlates directly with rates of cellular proliferation and DNA synthesis
- ★ PCNA may act as an auxiliary protein of DNA polymerase delta to play a fundamental role in the initiation of cell proliferation.

★ It is therefore a potentially useful proliferation marker but has been shown to stain non-proliferating cells in some circumstances because this enzyme is most likely involving in the catalysis of DNA strand synthesis DNA repair during the G0 or G1 phase of cell cycle

★ Two population of PCNA are seen. The first is expressed exclusively during S-phase and the second one is a non-specific, mainly associated with cytoskeletal elements during metaphase

• The monoclonal antibody PC-10 recognizes PCNA and is effective in formalin fixed, paraffin wax embedded tissues

Protocol for PCNA immunohistochemistry

Mount 3 – 4 μm thick paraffin section on slides coated with poly- L-lysine and dry at 56°C overnight

↓

Deparaffinize in xylene and wash with isopropyl alcohol

↓

Wash in running tap water - 10 min

↓

Place the slides in microwaveable plastic jars filled with 250 ml of 0.01 M citrate buffer (pH - 6) for antigen retrieval

↓

Heat the jar in pressure cooker for 2 min

↓

Keep the jar in 30 min at room temperature

↓

Wash with PBS (15 min)

↓

Overlay the slides with peroxide block solution for 10 min

↓

Wash with PBS (5min x 2)

↓

Incubate slides with primary antibody (PC-10) for 1 hour

↓

Wash with PBS (5 min)

↓

Incubate the slides with secondary antibody (Anti-antibody for 30 min)

↓

Wash with PBS (5 min)
↓
Treat with DAB and buffer substrate (5-8 min)
↓
Wash with PBS (5 min)
↓
Wash with tap water
↓
Counter stain with haematoxylin
↓
Wash with water and then alcohol and clear in xylene
↓
Examine under microscope

Evaluation of immunostaining

Positive cells are identified by the presence of brick red colour in the nucleus and cytoplasm. Expression is seen as

I. Non-mitotic cells - Expression of PCNA is restricted to nucleus

II. Mitotic cells - Nuclear and cytoplasmic

III. $$\text{PCNA index} = \frac{\text{No. of positive cell / labelled nuclei}}{\text{Total no. of cells}} = 100$$

IV. There are two types of PCNA index noticed:

(a) **Strongly Positive (SP)** – PCNA index, which is calculated by means of strongly labelled nuclei

$$\text{SP- PCNA index} = \frac{\text{Strongly labelled nuclei}}{\text{Total no. of cells}}\ 100$$

(b) **Total Positive** – PCNA index, which is calculated by means of all the stained nuclei

$$\text{TP PCNA index} = \frac{\text{All the labelled nuclei}}{\text{Total no. of cells}}\ 100$$

PCNA Values

PCNA	Benign (%)	Malignant (%)
SP – PCNA	2.55 ± 2.32	9.53 ± 5.94
TP – PCNA	10.48 ± 8.53	38.94 ± 20.78

- ★ The score of the strong PCNA positive nuclei alone is suggested as confirmatory diagnosis by some authors, because, the cells in which they occur are undoubtedly in the G1/S phases of the cell cycle

D. Thymidine labelling index (TLI)

It is a measure of the percentage of tumour cells in the 'S' phase (DNA synthetic phase) of the cell cycle.

Method

- ★ TLI is measured in vitro by incubating freshly excised tumour tissue in a medium containing tritiated thymidine which is incorporated in to the DNA of the cells which are in 'S' phase
- ★ The microscopic slides are prepared by usual processing methods
- ★ Then photographic film is placed over the slides which have tumour cells and this arrangement is kept as such for several days (Autoradiography)
- ★ The film will record the radiation and auto radiographs are prepared on the film. The thymidine labelled cells are counted and compared with non labelled interphase population
- ★ Thymidine labelling is useful in the diagnosis of Breast tumour, Fibroadenoma, plasma cell tumour and familial colonic carcinoma
- ★ $\text{Thymidine labelling index} = \frac{\text{Thymidine labelled cells}}{\text{Total no. of cells}} \; 100$

Limitations

- ★ It requires viable cells
- ★ It involves *in vivo* administration of radiolabelled thymidine
- ★ Before fixation the biopsy materials must be incubated with tritiated thymidine for sometime.
- ★ Autoradiography associated radiation hazard is also a untoward effect

E. Bromodeoxyuridine (BrDU) labelling index

- ★ This is a 'S' phase labelling index
- ★ BrDU is incorporated into the cells during 'S' phase specific and antibody against the BrDU is used and the combination is detected by using enzyme and chromogen technique
- ★ It is mainly used in gastric carinoma

Method

Take thin slices of cold, freshly exised tumour tissue

↓

Incubate with 1 µl of BrDU for 2 hours at 37 °C

↓

Wash with PBS

↓

Place it in a buffered formalin

↓

Carry out IPT with anti – BrDU - Mab

$$\text{BrDU labelling index} = \frac{\text{No. labelled cells}}{\text{Total no .of cells}} \quad 100$$

Limitations

- *In vitro* incubation or *in vivo* administration of BrDU
- It requires fresh samples
- Applicable to limited number of tumour

F. Mitotic Index (MI)

Mitotic index

- It is an indirect measure of cell proliferation based on the quantification of mitotic figures (cells in different stages of cellcycle) in a histopathologic specimen
- It is easier to perform than AgNOR, PCNA and Ki-67 assessment, which require additional staining technique and automated image analyzer that is not currently widely available
- It has been demonstrated that MI is a strong predictor of outcome of a variety of human and canine cancers, including thyroid carcinoma, breast carcinoma and sarcoma *etc*

Evaluation of MI

It can be evaluated by examining the histopathological sections under high power field (HPF) and the number of mitotic figures is counted in 10 HPF to express the MI of that particular tumour. In benign tumours, it is less than ten, whereas in malignant varieties it exceeds ten. Mitotic index is used to evaluate a particular tumour as benign or malignant.

Demerits

- It is arbitrary and differ from one pathologist to another
- Intensity may vary from one part of the slide from another
- Pyknotic nuclei may be mistaken for mitotic figures
- The quality of microscope is also a important factor for this count

G. P ^{53}:

- P^{53} is a tumour suppressor gene which is most frequently mutated in human cancer

- ★ It is named as p^{53} due to its molecular weight of 53,000 Kilo Dalton.
- ★ P^{53} seems to be an important growth regulator in a wide variety of cell types
- ★ P^{53} genes are frequently mutated in colon, lung, breast, esophageal, liver and brain tumours, as well as in leukemia
- ★ Point mutations create oncogenic alleles of p^{53}, such mutations occurs with great frequency of these alleles of P^{53} appreciated in tumours
- ★ P^{53} protein accumulates within the malignant cells where it can be readily detected by IHC
- ★ P^{53} protein is present in low concentration in normal cells but elevated levels of mutant p^{53} (allele) have been found in many common cancer.
- ★ An anti –antibody BP^{53}- 12- 1 is used in IHC techniques to detect brown colour dots in nuclear area in positive cases

Specific Tumour Marker to evaluate Breast / Mammary tissue Cancer

Estrogen Receptor (ER – α)

- ★ Estrogen receptor (ER-α) and progesterone receptor (PR) have become accepted and useful tools in prognosis and prediction of hormonal therapy response in human breast cancer. ER- α and PR are present in more than 50 % of mammary neoplasms in dogs
- ★ The initial biochemical methods such as dextran coated chracoal (DCC), have been replaced in the last decades byusing IPT ith the receptor, which needs less tissue and is less expensive
- ★ IPT is a more accurate technique and these receptors are preferentially located within the nuclear compartment. Several monoclonal antibodies against human ER have been developed to avoid the disadvantages of biochemical methods

Immunoperoxidase Test to evaluate Estrogen Receptors

(Streptavidin, biotin and peroxidase complex method)

Mount the 4 μm paraffin embedded section over clean glass slide

↓

Boil in a pressure cooker containing 2L of 10mM sodium citrate buffer and incubate for 2 min after attaning the higher pressure

↓

Cool the slides and then wash it with tris base saline buffer (0.1 m tris base, 0.9% NaCl)

↓

Block endogenous peroxidase activity by treating with 1.5ml H_2O_2/100 ml of methanol for 15 min

↓

Incubate the slides with an anti – ER α antibody at 37º C (1:40, anti mouse biotinlated secondary antibody and stoptavidin conjugated with peroxidase) in a humid chamber

↓

Dilutions were made in TBS

↓

Incubate the slides with 3, 3 DAB and 0.01 % H_2O_2 in TBS

↓

Wash the slides and counterstain with Haematoxylin for 45 min

↓

Wash in tap water and dehydrate with alcohol

↓

Clear it in Xylol

↓

Examine under microscope

↓

Positive slides show golden-brown nuclei

Interpretation

i. Normal and hyperplastic cells - Homogenous and uniform staining

ii. Benign and Malignant - Variable heterogeneous staining with golden-brown nuclei

11. Microarray Tumour Diagnosis

Microarray is a small device that allows genomic explorations with speed and precision. Glass chips containing tens of thousands of genes are used to examine fluorescent samples prepared by labeling messenger RNA (mRNA) from cells, tissues and other biological sources.

Procedure

mRNA is isolated from cells, labeled with fluorescent tags, and hybridized to a glass chip containing a microarray gene sequences. Each spot on the chip binds specifically to fluorescent mRNA molecule in solution, carrying the spot to glow with intensities proportional to the expression level each gene that encoded the message to the mRNA.

Quantitative gene expression data are obtained by determining the fluorescence intensity at each microarray location. Microarrays are used for early diagnosis and continuous assessment of tumours. Several hundred tumours have been analyzed and the susceptible genes identified which can be spotted by Microarray methods.

Cancers and susceptible genes

S.No	Cancer tissues	Susceptible genes
01	Colon	MCH-1, MSH-2, MSH-6
02	Breast	BRCA-1, BRCA-2
03	Prostate	HPC-1
04	Pancreas	DPC-4 (Smad-4)

12. Telomerase biology in tumour diagnosis

Telomeres are specialised nucleoprotein structure at the eukaryotic chromosome ends that are essential for stable chromosome maintenance. These telomeres are simple repeated sequences (Human - TTAGGG)n of many kilobases (human telomeres length varies from 5 –15 kilobases) bound by protein.

Telomeres capping the chromosome termini are essential to prevent aberrant recombination and end to end fusions. The telomeric DNA is lost at each cell division due to the inability of the DNA in this place to replicate. Telomeres length is shorten with each cell division and a critically shortened telomere may arrest the cell division.

Telomerase is the enzyme if present in the cell will not allow the shortening of telomere. Telomerase activity is absent in all body cells except male germ cells, lymphocytes and certain stem cells.

Cancer cells are expressing telomerase activity and the length of telomeres is not shortened. So by estimating the telomerase activity and or measuring the length of telomeres caner cells can be identified.

Length of telomeres and telomerase expression for most of the human tumours are predetermined and the results of sample are compared to decide benign and malignant types.

Detection techniques for telomerase activity and telomeres length

S.No.	Criteria	Techniques
01	Telomerase gene expression	Northern blot for telomerase RNA
		RT-PCR for telomerase RNA
		(telo-RNA length: 450 Base pairs)
		3. ISH
02	Telomere length	Southern blot
		ISH
		Flow cytometry

Out of all the methods discussed, Histopathology is the best confirming method for tumour diagnosis. Early detection is also possible, if the tissue is available. All other methods can serve either as initial diagnostic tools to suspect tumours or as continuous assessment aids after histopathological confirmation of tumours.

Suitable method(s) should be selected for a particular tumour as pre and post confirmative assessment, but the confirmation warrants Histopathology due to the fact that it can reveal a clear picture of neoplastic cell type, grade as well as non-neoplastic supporting cell mass, blood vessels, necrotic and apoptotic severity which is not possible by other diagnostic methods.

More than one method should be combined for preliminary screening and clinical assessments depending upon the type of tumour, anatomical location, frequency of usage and cost. Care should be taken while handling radioactive substances and proper time interval should be given for repeated usage of such substances. It must be ensured that the animal is no longer emitting radiation before discharge.

Tumour Diagnostic methods in Veterinary Oncology

S.No.	Purpose	Tumour Diagnostic methods
01.	Preliminary screening	Cytology A) FNAB B) Exfoliated cytology Imaging Techniques A) X-rays B) Ultrasonography C) CT-Scans D) MRI-Scans
02.	Confirmation	Histopathology
03.	Screening of sub-clones (Identification of metastasizing cells, Growth fractions, Cellular antigens)	Electron Microscopy Immunoperoxidase Test Flow cytometry Southern Blotting
04.	Metastatic search	Scinctigraphy
05.	Infectious etiology search	*In situ* PCR *In situ* Hybridization
06.	Clinical Assessment	Tumour Markers Telomerase Biology
07.	Preliminary Screening and Clinical Assessment	Microarrays

Recent study reveals that controlling the level of telomerase can prevent cancer metastasis. In a human or animal, when a protein called NME2 (Non-metastasis-2) level is high; the tendency of tumour metastasis is low. This NME2 protein binds to the telomerase promoter DNA, G-quadrauplex. This complex facilitates the expression of tumour suppressor gene called REST Complex to produce REST Complex tumour suppressor protein, which combine with the telomerase promoter gene and controls the telomerase production. This has been proved by a Proteomics study (study of protein – protein interaction). Laboratory production of NME2 protein and targeting the G-quadrauplex may reduce the metastasis and this can be attempted to suppress the tumour cell life span by reducing the telomere length.

10

Biology of Tumour Growth

- ★ Etiological agents like UV-B, chemical carcinogens and oncogenic viruses transform normal cell into neoplastic cell by causing genetic damage
- ★ Transformed neoplastic cells attain monoclonal proliferation into several cells to become a detectable tumour mass
- ★ Sub populations of tumour cells occur with different characteristics due to additional spontaneous mutations and genetic instability of tumour cells
- ★ Some of these sub populations are attaining the ability of migration and establish secondary tumours

Kinetics of Tumour Growth

- ★ Mitotic cell division that occurs in normal tissues is also happen in tumours. But the difference is more than 80 % of the tumour cells are in G-o or prolonged G-1 sub phases of interphase without involving in proliferation (resting cells)
- ★ Only 20 % of the neoplastic cells are entering into regular proliferation cycle
- ★ This 20 % of the cells are called as growth fractions. Abrupt proliferations of resting cells have also been reported. Though blood vessels are forming, most of them are tortuous and cannot keep all the cells alive. This factor along with poor lymphatics leads to necrosis and loss of tumour cells. So the difference between cell proliferation and loss decides the rate of tumour growth

Tumour Angiogenesis and Stroma Formation

- ★ Proliferating tumour cells are secreting fibroblast growth factors which has two fold action:
  - i. It is chemotactic and mitogenic sprouting endothelial cells.
  - ii. It also possesses proteolytic enzymatic property, which allows penetration of blood vessels. Along with the action of fibroblasts growth factor, the products of activated macrophages like transforming

growth factor alpha and epidermal growth factor are also involving in the blood vessels formation and ramification

- ★ The newly formed blood vessels are leaking the blood fibrin to the proliferating tumour cells. This fibrin is acting as a scaffold for the fibroblast migration and settlement. In the initial stage, thin walled blood vessels are dominating the fibroblast which almost resemble the granulation tissue, but in the later stages the products of fibroblasts like collagen, fibrin, fibrinonectin and proteoglycans will dominate the blood vessels, which restrict the tumour growth

Tumour Progression and Heterogenecity

- ★ Monoclonally expanded neoplastic cells after certain stage attain spontaneous mutation and genetic instability, which leads to the formation of sub population within the same tumour. These sub populations are having different abilities like:
  - Invasiveness
  - Active proliferation
  - Secretion of hormone or hormone like products
  - Metastatic ability
- ★ Spontaneous mutation are restricted to protooncogenes and tumour suppressor genes.

11

Tumour Spread

- ⋆ Malignant tumours often spread to other areas by means of metastasis
- ⋆ Metastasis is an inefficient multi step process. All the neoplastic cells present in the malignant tumour are not metastazing, only a sub clone of population among the neoplastic cells are attaining the ability of metastasis
- ⋆ Neoplastic cells are attaining metastatic ability through the process of tumour progression

Process of Metastasis

- ⋆ Sub clones of neoplastic cells, which are having metastatic ability become loosen by increasing inter cellular gap. Loss of epithelial adhesion by impaired activity of cell adhesion factors such as E-catherins precedes invasion by epithelial tumours
- ⋆ When a tumour is transformed into carcinoma from non-invasive *insitu* carcinoma, breakage of basement membrane is observed
- ⋆ The tumour cells attach to the basement membrane and subsequently they secrete proteolytic enzymes that degrade the basement membrane
- ⋆ Tumour cells are now degrading the matrix connective tissue and reach the capillaries to further degrade inter epithelial cellular connective tissue to make entry into the blood
- ⋆ The tumour cells thus carry out this process by their moving ability and producing collaginase
- ⋆ The tumour cells, which mix with the blood stream are evading the host immunological mechanisms of NK and CTL activity by adhering with fibrin of blood and thrombocytic pools
- ⋆ By the sweeping effect of venous blood flow, tumour cells are washed away and filtered by lung and liver blood capillary buds (general circulation and portal blood are filtered by lung and liver respectively). So, lung and liver are acting as primary soils for the metastasis

- ★ From these primary metastatic areas, in turn, tumour cells are mixed with blood stream and circulate to find their respective soil of tissue for secondary metastasis
- ★ The extent of growth in the seeded tissue depends on the tissue affected. Loose structured tissues like the muscle and parenchymatous organs are easily infiltrated. Tough tissues like the fibrous tissue, cartilage, bone and tendon resist infiltration, but finally these structure may also be infiltrated.

Seed - Soil Hypothesis

- ★ Tumour cells in the circulation are expressing ligands on their surfaces seeking their respective receptors on the endothelial cells of particular tissue or organ. When ligand and receptor are uniting, the tumour cells can enter into the tissue and establish their growth
- ★ Cytokines produced by the activated macrophages and their tissue cells are also attracting tumour cells to establish metastatic tumours
- ★ The primary and secondary metastatic foci should also withstand the action of host immune mechanism for their establishments.

Pathways of Metastasis

Lymphatic metastasis

- ★ This pathway is preferred mostly by carcinomas. Lymphatic vessels offer little resistance to the penetration by tumour cells, because they lack basement membrane
- ★ After mixing with the lymphatics, they are trapped in the first lymph node that encounters these cells and they are removed by immunological mechanisms
- ★ This stage is hyperplastic stage in which nodes are not converted into neoplastic growths. If the tumour cells overcome the immunological reactions, then the node can serve as a primary metastatic foci
- ★ Initially, tumour cells are found in the sub capsular region, some tumour cells can bye-pass the activity of lymph node to establish distant metastasis called as skip-metastasis.

Haematogenous metastasis

- ★ Sarcomas prefer this route, carcinomas may also utilise this route due to the fact that lymph is mixing with blood through venous tributaries
- ★ Primary tumours spread along the venacava or along the portal vein route. Arteries cannot be invaded due to their thick wall and more elastin content (tumour cells are not secreting elastase to degrade elastin). Veins are serving for the transport of tumour cells due to the flow of blood towards heart and increasing their lumen size towards heart
- ★ Melanoma and prostatic carcinoma of dog and human are preferring brain and bone as their secondary soils respectively.

Transcoelomic Metastasis

- ★ This route is preferred by the primary tumours of cavities (thoracic, abdominal and pelvic) hollow organs and surface tumours
- ★ Peritoneal or pleural carcinomas in dogs are often associated with primary tumours of ovarian and pulmonary carcinomas
- ★ Primary tumours on the mesothelial surface of lung, liver, spleen and pancreas are disseminating tumour cells as seeds, which can fall and grow in the respective cavities
- ★ Tumours of hollow organs like intestine, trachea and cervix can supply the tumour cells, which can be implanted in other locations of the same organ.

12

Tumour Immunity

- ★ Tumour immunity means the state of resistance against tumour. It is a result of interactions among varies cells of the immune system and tumour cells
- ★ The occurrence of spontaneous regression, although extremely rare and the presence of lymphoid infiltrates in and around tumour indicates that immunological mechanism may interfere with the development of tumours

Tumour Antigens

Tumour cells can be recognised by the immune system. They often bear unique tumour specific antigens. These tumour specific antigens arise from mutations of cellular genes that give rise to abnormal proteins that are expressed on the cell surface.

Tumour cells may differ antigenically from normal in that they gain or lose cell membrane molecules. Some tumours of the intestine and colon carcinomas may lose the ability to produce mucus.

In other cases, tumour cells gain antigens and some naturally occurring tumours of adult animals are characterised by the production of proteins normally found only in the fetus.

Antigens

1. Tumours of gastro intestinal tract may produce a glycoprotein known as carcino embryonic antigen (CEA), which is usually found only in fetal intestine. Presence of CEA indicates colon / rectal adenocarcinoma.
2. The generation of fetal antigens by tumour cells (oncofetal antigens) includes production of alpha-feto protein by hepatoma cells. (Alpha feto protein is normally found only in fetal liver). The oncofetal antigens are poor immunogens and do not provoke protective immunity, perhaps because they are not recognized by CD4+ and CD8+ cells.
3. Tumour induced by oncogenic viruses tends to gain new antigens. Marek's tumour specific antigens are found on Marek's disease tumour cells in chickens.

4. Chemically induced tumours differ from virus induced variety by carrying surface antigens unique to the tumour and not to the inducing chemical. Tumours induced by a single chemical in different animals of the same species may be antigenically quite unrelated. Even within a single chemically induced tumour mass, antigenically distinct sub population of cell exist. As a result, resistance to one chemically induced tumour does not prevent growth of a secondary tumour induced by the same chemical.

Classification of Tumour Antigens

1. Tumour specific antigen
2. Tumour associated antigen
3. Oncofetal antigens

Tumour specific antigens

They are observed only on tumour cells (normal cells are devoid of these). It has been shown most clearly in chemically induced tumours. The chemically induced tumours express private or unique antigens not shared by histologically identical tumours induced by the same chemical, even in the same animal.

During cancer transformation, several mutations occur and it affects genes that encode normal cytoplasmic proteins and therefore altered forms of these normal proteins are generated. The peptide-class I complex assembled from each mutant protein is non-self, just as a complex derived from a viral protein is treated as foreign. Thus each mutant protein forms a distinct tumour antigen in association with MHC – I protein.

Tumour associated antigens (TAAs)

They are noticed on tumour cells and also on some normal cells. These tumour antigens are not unique to the individual tumours; they are shared by similar tumour in the other hosts. Two categories are identified:

1. Oncofetal antigens
2. Differentiation specific antigen

Because TAAs are normal cell proteins, they do not evoke an immune response and are not important in tumour rejection. However they are of value in the diagnosis of certain tumours, antibodies raised against them and it can be useful for immunotherapy.

Oncofetal antigens

These are embryonic antigens and are not normally expressed by adult tissues, because they are pertaining to developing embryonic tissue. Two examples of these oncofetal antigens are

1. Alpha feto protein
2. Carcino embryonic antigen

They are of value in the diagnosis of certain tumours like colon or rectal adenocarcinoma and hepatoma.

Differentiation specific antigens

These antigens serve as useful differentiation markers in the diagnosis of lymphoid and prostatic cancers in humans.

Different Tumours and its Differentiation Markers

MARKER	MOST COMMON TUMOUR TYPE
Alpha feto protein	Primary liver and gonad
Bence jones protein in unine	Multiple myeloma
CA 15	Breast tumour
CA 19	Pancreas,
CA 72	Gastro intestinal malignancies
CA 125	Ovary
Calcitonin	Medullary thyroid carcinoma
CEA	Colon
Prostatic specific antigen	Prostate
Thyroglobulin	Thyroid carcinoma
Immunoglobulin in EPP	Testes

Their main use (*i.e.* marker) is in monitoring the treatment progress in established tumours.

Anti-tumour Effector Mechanism

Both cell mediated and humoral immunity have anti tumour activity. The cellular effectors include tumour infiltrating lymphocytes (TILs), which includes

1. Natural killer cells
2. Helper and cytotoxic lymphocytes
3. Macrophages
4. B - lymphocytes

Tumour infiltrating lymphocytes

In many cases TILs are viewed as inflammatory cells mediating non-specific action rather than tumour specific interaction. T-lymphocytes and macrophages are the main component of TILs in solid tumours. B - cells are rarely found with the exception of melanoma. NK cells are observed relatively in small numbers.

T-lymphocyte mediated immunity

It is occasionally possible to detect a cell mediated immune response to tumour antigens either by skin testing or by the use of an *in vitro* test such as macrophage migration inhibition. Lymphocytes from some tumour bearing animals may exert a cytotoxic effect on tumour cells. Nevertheless, anti tumour responses by T cells are probably only significant in the control of virus induced tumours.

Macrophage mediated immunity

- ★ In some experimental tumour systems, macrophage may exert an anti tumour effect. Macrophages are activated by exposure to interferon gamma. These activated macrophages may act in either a specific or a non specific fashion. They release cytotoxic factors such as arginase and reactive oxygen metabolites
- ★ Non specific activation of macrophages by BCG / propionin / bacterium result in enhanced production of interleukin -I and tumour necrosis factor alpha and subsequent activation of helper T cell activity

Interleukin -1 cytostatic activity

- ★ Unfortunately, malignant tumours may release a factor that inhibits macrophage activation, and the macrophage of tumour bearing animal may show defective mobilisation and chemotaxis

Natural killer cells

- ★ About 15 % of peripheral blood lymphocytes are neither T nor B cells, but form a distinct third population of Natural killer cells. They are characterised by the ability to kill tumour, virus infected and some normal cells in the absence of previous sensitisation

Surface markers

- ★ NK cells have characteristic surface markers and they include CD 56 in humans as well as CD2, CD16 and CD95 in animals m

Mechanism of anticancer activity

- ★ NK cells selectively kills target cells that fail to express or express much reduced amount of MHC-I molecules. Many viruses use repression of MHC –I expression as a strategy to hide within the infected cells and metastatic tumour cells often don't express MHC –I. NK cell killing is mediated like T cells through perforins and cytotoxins (TNF-α ,TNFβ) as well as through CD95

Immune Surveillance

There are immune cells that can recognise cancer cells and remove them. In the absence of this surveillance, there would be many more tumours in animals and human being. Patients with suppressed T cell response to viral infections are at increased risk of virally induced cancers. So, HIV patients tend to get lymphoma and squamous cell carcinoma.

Humoral immunity

It occurs by means of two ways

1. Activation of complement.
2. Antibody dependant cell mediated cytotoxicity (ADCC).

13

Tumour Effects

The effects of a tumour on the body depends on its

1. Size
2. Location
3. Tissue from which it is derived
4. Presence of malignancy
5. Presence of infection
6. Haemorrhage

Both benign and malignant neoplasms cause problems due to

1. Location and pressure on adjacent structures
2. Functional activities such as hormone synthesis
3. Bleeding and secondary infections when they ulcerate through adjacent natural surfaces

The following are the major effects of tumour

1. Pressure atrophy
2. Mechanical obstruction
3. Exudation
4. Destruction
5. Infection
6. Cachexia
7. Anaemia
8. Hormonal effects
9. Death

Pressure Atrophy

Pressure atrophy of the surrounding tissue occurs when the neoplasm expands. The cells suffer as fluid exchanges are interfered with. Pressure on blood and lymph vessels may also interfere with nutrients of the cells.

Mechanical Obstruction

The lumen of the hollow organs may be obstructed either by the tumour projecting from the wall of an organ into its lumen or the tumour may press from outside. The narrowing or obliteration of the lumen interferes with the passage of contents.

The following are the examples of complications caused by mechanical obstruction of hallow organs by tumours

1. Intestine - intussusception
2. Urinary tract - hydronephrosis
3. Portal vein - ascites
4. Bronchus - collapse of lung
5. Biliary tract - obstructive jaundice

Exudation

Tumour cells deposited on serous membranes cause inflammatory exudates with high protein content. *e.g.*, malignant ascites.

Destruction

Invading cells destroy the tissues producing functional loss. For eg.,

1. Destruction of hepatic tissue by cancer of liver resulting in fatal hepatic failure
2. Anaemia may develop when much of haemopoietic tissue is replaced by cells of leukemia
3. Invasion of nerves is followed by their degeneration and destruction

Infection

Surface tumours may be ulcerated and subsequently infected by contamination with infectious agents.

Cachexia

Many cancer patients suffer progressive loss of body fat accompanied by severe weakness, anorexia and anaemia. Animal suffering from malignant tumours become emaciated and weak due to starvation when the gastro intestinal tract is affected.

Factors responsible for Cachexia

It may due to complications like frequent haemorrhages, septicaemia and toxaemia due to infections. The neoplasm may utilise for themselves many essential amino acids and vitamins and so the body become deficient of these, resulting in cachexia. Some of the catabolic products of the cancer cells such as large quantities of lactic acid may be injurious to the host cells. The circulating factors like TNF- and IL-1, released from activated macrophages cause depressed appetite and inhibit the action of lipase, thereby inhibiting the release of free fatty acids from lipoproteins.

Anaemia

Malignant neoplasia causes a progressive anaemia, which may be due to

1. Malnutrition (Eg. tumour of gastro intestinal tract interferes with proper digestion and assimilation causing nutritional anaemia)
2. Recurrent haemorrhages causing haemarrhagic anaemia
3. Depression of the marrow caused by:

   (a) Long standing infections: Toxins may injure the haemopoietic tissue and may cause aplastic anaemia.

   (b) Secondary (metastatic tumours): Neoplasms may invade the bone marrow and cause atrophy of the haemopoietic tissue.

Hormonal Effects

★ Tumour of the endocrine glands may produce increased hormones resulting in various pathological conditions

★ Tumour of anterior pituitary causes gigantism

★ Tumour of parathyroid results in osteoporosis and 'Big head disease' in horses

★ Tumour of sertoli cells cause feminisation

★ Arrhenoblastoma in the female (hen) causes masculinisation

★ Tumour of adrenal gland causes Cushing's syndrome in dogs

Death

A malignant neoplasm ultimately causes death of the host.

14

Paraneoplastic Syndrome

Symptoms observed in cancer patients due to elaboration of hormones or hormone like substances or other chemically active substances, which are not indigenous to the tissue from which the tumour arise are known as paraneoplastic syndromes.

Paraneoplastic syndromes are important to recognise, because they may represent the earliest manifestation of an occult neoplasm. In cancer affected patients, they may represent significant clinical problems and may even be lethal. They may resemble metastatic diseases and therefore do not respond to treatments.

Classification of Paraneoplastic Syndrome

Endocrinopathies

These are frequently encountered paraneoplastic syndrome. The native cells that give rise to cancer are not of endocrine origin, the functional activity is referred to as ectopic hormone production. *e.g.*, Cushing syndrome.

Approximately 50 % of the patients with this endocrinopathies have carcinoma of the lung, chiefly the small cell type. This cancer produces adrenocorticotrophic hormone (ACTH) or ACTH like peptides.

Hypercalcaemia

Hypocalcaemia occur due to the production of calcaemic humoral substances by extra osseous neoplasms.

Neuromyopathies

It may be in the form of peripheral neuropathies, cortical cerebellar degeneration, a polymyopathy resembling polymyositis and a myasthenia syndrome.

Some neural antigens are ectopically expressed by visceral cancers, in such cases the immune system recognises these antigens as foreign and mount an immune response.

Hypertrophic Osteo-Arthropathy

It is encountered in 1-10 % of the patients with bronchogenic carcinomas. This disorder is characterised by

1. Periosteal new bone formation
2. Arthritis of adjacent joints
3. Clubbing of the digits.

Commonly noticed Paraneoplastic Syndromes

Clinical syndrome	Major forms of cancer	Mechanism
Cushing syndrome	Small cell carcinoma of lung Pancreatic carcinoma Neural tumours	ACTH or ACTH like substance production
Hypercalcemia	SqCC of lung Breast carcinoma Renal carcinoma Adult T-cell leukemia or lymphoma Ovarian carcinoma	Parathyroid hormone-related peptide, TNF-α, TGF-α and IL-I production
Hypoglycemia	Fibrosarcoma Other mesenchymal sarcomas, Hepatocellular carcinoma	Insulin or insulin like substance production
Carcinoid syndrome	Bronchial adenoma Pancreatic carcinoma Gastric carcinoma	Serotonin, Bradykinin and Histamine production
Polycythemia	Renal carcinoma Cerebellar haemangioma Hepato cellular carcinoma	Erythropoietin production
Nerve and muscle Syndrome		
Myasthenia		
Disorder of central and peripheral nervous system	Bronchogenic Carcinoma	Immunologic reaction
	Breast carcinoma	Immunologic reaction
Dermatological Disorder		
Acanthosis nigricans		
	Gastric carcinoma, lung and uterine carcinoma	Immunologic reaction or secretion of epidermal growth factor (EGF)
Dermatomyositis	Bronchogenic carcinoma Breast carcinoma	Immunologic reaction

Clinical syndrome	Major forms of cancer	Mechanism
Vascular Disorder		
Venous thrombosis	Pancreatic carcinoma	Tumour product (mucin) that activate clotting
	Advanced cancers	Hypercoagulopathy
2.Non bacterial thrombotic endocardial	Thymic neoplasia	Unknown
Others		
Nephritic syndrome	cancers	Tumour antigens production and immune complexes formation

Part II
Special Oncology
(Specific Neoplasms)

1

Connective Tissue (Mesenchymal) Tumours Fibroma and Fibrosarcoma

Incidence and Site

Fibroma is a benign tumour that affects all animals. It is common in horses and dogs. In dogs, Terrier breed is more affected. This tumour is commonly seen in the dermis or subcutis and may arise from all tissues or organs from fibrous connective tissue.

Gross appearance

- ★ These tumours are well circumscribed, firm or rubbery or rarely soft in consistency, round or ovoid in shape, often pedunculated with grayish white cut surface
- ★ Ulcerated and infected tumours may show yellow to red colour
- ★ The weight varies from one gm to several kgs and the size from 1mm to several cm in diameter

Histological features

- ★ Interlacing bundles of fibroblasts and collagen fibres running in all directions (Haphazard arrangement) can be observed
- ★ Fusiform or stellate shaped neoplastic fibroblasts with large pale ovoid to elongated nuclei and multiple nucleoli are noticed
- ★ The collagen fibres are dense (hard fibroma with more fibres and less cells-fibroma duram) or loose (soft fibroma with more cells and less fibres-fibroma molle)
- ★ Edema or mucinous ground substance and variable degrees of vascularisation are observed

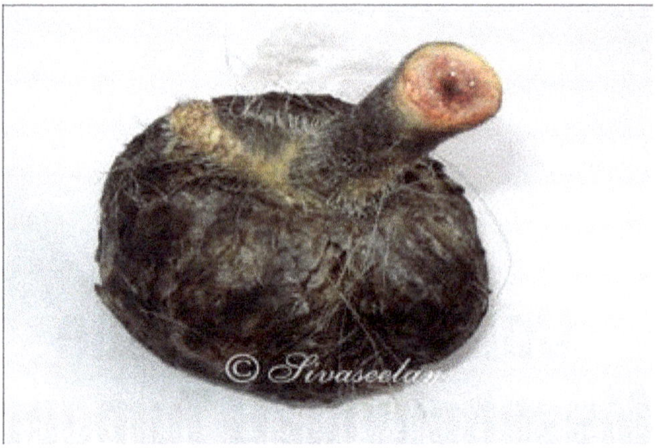

Fig. 1. A round solitary fibroma amputated from tip of the tail of a dog

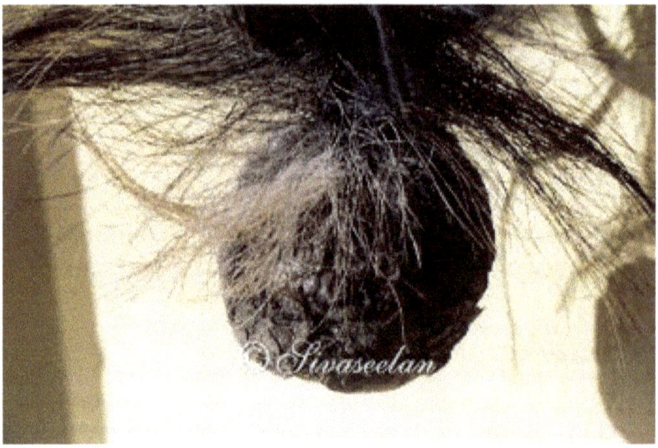

Fig. 2. A fibroma arising from the tail of a cow

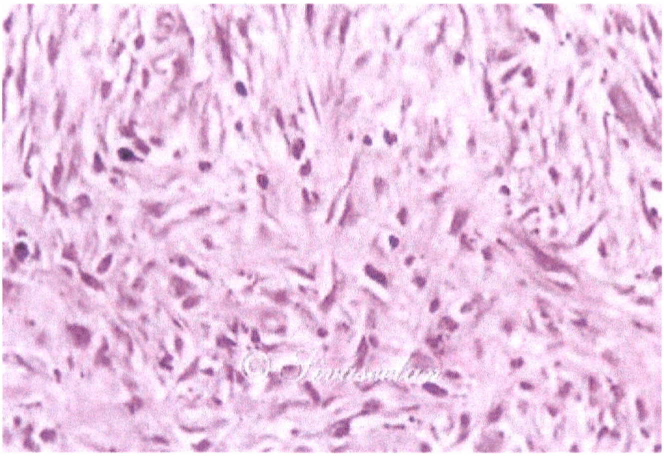

Fig. 3. Histological appearance of the fibroma shown in fig. 1 & 2 revealing loosely arranged fibroblasts and fibres.

Nodular fasciitis / Aggressive fibromatosis / Pseudosarcomatous fibromatosis

This type of growth is not a true fibroma, but it is a mixture of fibroblast proliferation and inflammation reported in some dogs. Few mm to cm firm, poorly circumscribed, nodular growth is seen on the skin, subcutis, and de'eper fascia of muscles of head, face and eyelids.

Histological features

- ⋆ Fusiform or plump fibroblasts are haphazardly arranged in a matrix of variable amount of collagen and reticulum fibres or in whorls around well formed capillaries
- ⋆ Hyperchromatic nuclei and mitotic figures can be seen in few of the fibroblasts, but these cells are well differentiated in contrast to anaplastic cells of fibrosarcoma
- ⋆ Scattered foci of inflammatory cells consisting of lymphocytes, plasma cells and macrophages can be seen
- ⋆ Multinucleated giant cells may be seen in some areas
- ⋆ This growth rarely recur after excision

Fibroma v_s Granulation tissue

Granulation tissue has parallel bundles of fibroblasts and collagen fibres with proliferating capillaries running at right angles. Fibroma lacks this definite order.

Neurofibromata

- ⋆ This arises from fibroblasts of the connective tissue of the nerve sheaths
- ⋆ The neoplastic fibroblasts are farming nodules along the course of the nerve
- ⋆ They are multiple and firm in consistency
- ⋆ They are located subcutaneously, in man it is called as Recklinghausen's disease (cells are arranged as whorls to produce nodules subcutaneously)
- ⋆ A viral etiology is suspected

Fibrosarcoma

Incidence

- ⋆ Dog and cat are affected mostly, but they do occur in all species. Breed, age and sex predisposition have not been reported. Metastasis is not the feature, but recurs quickly after removal

Gross appearance

- ⋆ They are irregular and nodular in shape, poorly demarcated and non encapsulated
- ⋆ The consistency is firm or soft
- ⋆ On cut surface, it is lobulated and reddish white in color

★ Reddish brown areas of haemorrhage and yellow areas of necrosis are common characteristics

★ Topical tumours when ulcerated emit foul odour

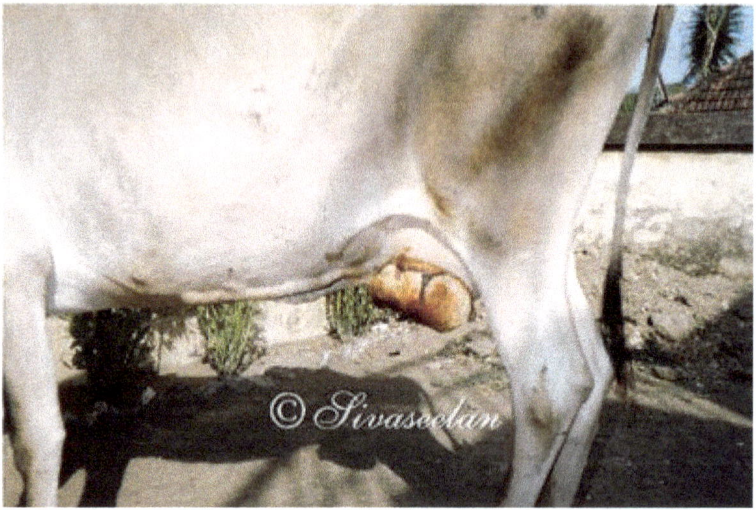

Fig. 4. An ulcerated fibrosarcoma of the udder of a cow

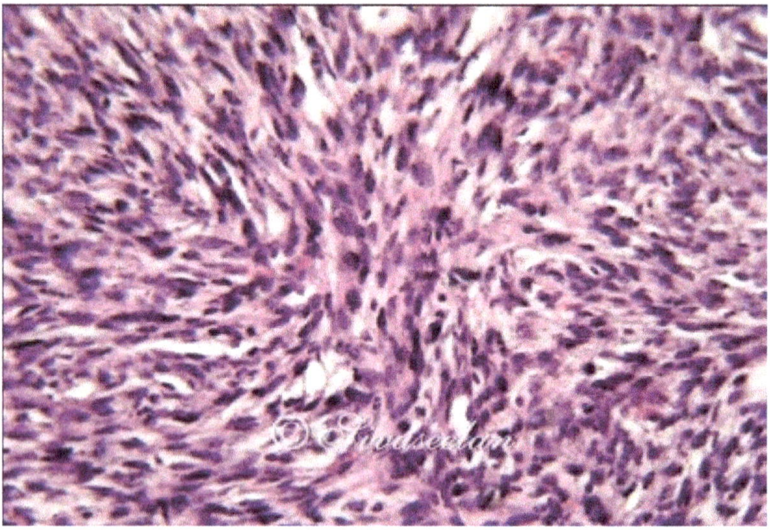

Fig. 5. Fibrosarcoma shown in fig. 4 histologically revealing criss-cross pattern of fibroblasts with hyperchromatic nuclei and fibres.

Histological feature

★ Neoplastic fibroblasts dominate the collagen fibres

★ This tumour is more cellular than fibroma

★ Fusiform or ovoid or stellate shape cells with anisokaryotic nuclei are seen

- ★ Undifferentiated tumours may have multinucleated giant cells
- ★ The hyperchromatic nuclei may have 2-5 nucleoli and mitotic figures are common
- ★ It is highly vascular and bleeds easily

Cells are arranged in the following patterns

- ★ Interlacing bundles of fibroblasts and collagen
- ★ Criss cross pattern
- ★ Interlocking pattern
- ★ Storiform pattern
- ★ Haphazard or mixed pattern

Malignant fibrous histiocytoma / Undifferentiated sarcoma

This tumour arises from pluripotent Mesenchymal cells that differentiate into either fibroblasts or histiocytes, so that the neoplastic cells of this category resemble the morphology of both of these cells. Several cases have been reported in aged cats and most of the cases were limited to skin and subcutis. Grossly, this tumour resembles fibroma.

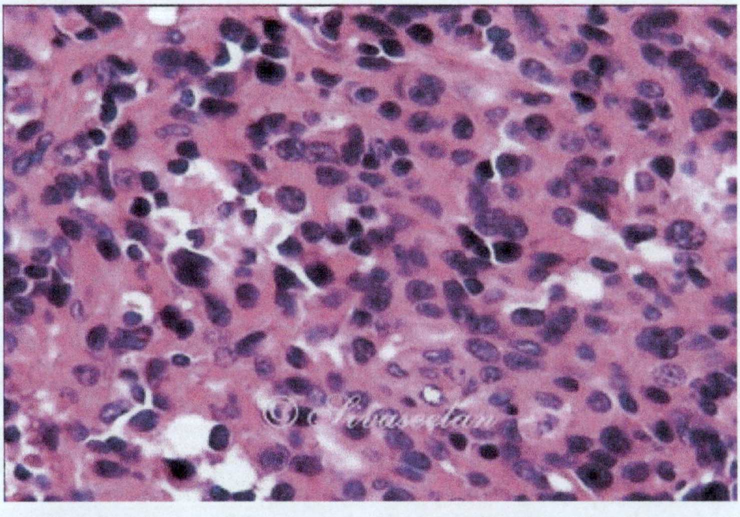

Fig. 6. A malignant fibrous histiocytoma of a cat depicting bizarre cells resembling fibroblast as well as histiocytes with atypical mitotic figures

Histological features

- Neoplastic cells resemble both fibroblasts and histiocytes
- Giant cells, foam cells and inflammatory cells can be seen occasionally
- Most of the cells show atypical mitotic figures
- Highly proliferating tumour may reveal anaplastic round cells with prominent nucleoli

Metastasis

This tumour grows rapidly infiltrating into adjacent tissues. Though recurrence has been reported after surgical removal, metastasis has not been proved.

Equine Sarcoid

It is locally aggressive, recurs after excision, but seldom metastasizes. A viral etiology is suspected to cause this fibrosarcoma like tumour, but with less malignancy.

Incidence

Horses, mules and donkeys are affected. No predisposition of age, breeds, sex and coat colour is reported. Skin of the leg, ventral trunk, ears and commissures of the mouth are the common sites of occurrence.

Gross appearance

Grossly, three types are seen. About 30% of the affected horses have multiple lesions.

1. Verrucous type (warty type)
2. Fibroblastic type (proud flesh)
3. Mixed type

Verrucous type

It is small (less than 6 cm in diameter), sessile or pedunculated, horny and cauliflower like in appearance.

Fibroblastic type

It is larger (some masses exceed 25 cm in diameter), discrete nodule like in appearance and situated within the dermis and subcutis. This type has often ulcerated surfaces that bleed easily.

Mixed type

Occur when the Verrucous type progress into Fibroblastic type.

Histological feature

★ Spindle shaped fibroblasts with varying amount of collagen fibres are arranged as bundles and as whorls (resembling neurofibroma)

★ Epidermal and dermal components are often seen

★ Epithelial hyperplasia with epithelial rete pegs extending deep into the underlying tissue is the characteristic feature

★ Few mitotic figures, which are lesser than fibrosarcoma and mononuclear cellular infiltration with or without eosinophils are the other features

★ Rapidly growing type will depict numerous mitotic figures

★ Epidermis over the tumour, if not ulcerated reveals acanthosis and hyperkeratosis

Metastasis

They are locally invasive, do not metastasize, but recurrence is often noticed after surgical removal. Most of the sarcoids regress spontaneously, but this will take several years.

Difference between Fibrosarcoma, Sarcoid and Keloid

Fibrosarcoma	Sarcoid	Keloid
More number of mitotic figures and anaplasia can be observed in highly progressive type	Cells resemble fibroblasts, but with lesser number of mitotic figures	Inflammatory in origin so, its collagen content, number of inflammatory cells and blood vessels are numerous
Mitotic index of more than 10 is observed	Mitotic index of less than 10 is the feature	-

Shope Fibroma (Infectious Myxomatosis)

In 1932, Shope a scientist described subcutaneous fibroma of wild rabbits caused by virus. This tumour may occur as a single or multiple tumours subcutaneously. Mosquitoes can mechanically transmit the virus to produce this tumour.

2

Lipoma and Liposarcoma

They are neoplasm of well differentiated lipocytes and lipoblasts, the later is rare in animals.

Incidence

This tumour is commonly reported in dogs and less frequently in other animals. Aged dogs above 5 years show more incidences. No breed predisposition has been reported. Incidence is more in overweighing female dogs than males.

Site of occurrence

- ★ Single or multiple tumours (lipomatosis) are found in the subcutaneous tissue, sub-mucosa, sub-serosa and mesentery
- ★ Lipomas in the intestine of horse can cause strangulation of the organ
- ★ Lipomatosis are rarely seen when compared to lipoma

Gross appearance

- ★ Lipomas vary in size from one gram to 50 kgs, they are round or ovoid in shape, may be lobulated and encapsulated with thin fibrous tissue
- ★ They are sessile or pedunculated in attachment
- ★ Soft or hard in consistency is depending on the variable amount of connective tissue present in that tumour
- ★ Capsule is not seen and the tumour may merge with the normal fat tissue
- ★ On section, oily substance ooze out
- ★ Calcification and metaplastic bone formation can also be seen
- ★ Needle aspiration will reveal oily material with few intact fat cells
- ★ Areas of fat necrosis within the tumour will reveal chalky white colour
- ★ The tumour will float in formalin fixatives
- ★ Liposarcomas are neither encapsulated nor circumscribed and firmer than lipomas

Histological features

- ★ Closely packed fat cells farming several lobules divided by fibrous septa can be seen
- ★ Fibrous septa act as a scaffold for blood supply
- ★ If septa dominate it is called as **fibro-lipoma**
- ★ It is difficult to differentiate lipoma from normal adipose tissue. Fibrous septa within and capsule around the mass will be helpful to identify a lipoma
- ★ Liposarcomas are more cellular and consist of anaplastic cells in some of the tumours
- ★ Abundant infiltration of inflammatory cells differentiates fat necrosis from lipoma
- ★ In lipoma, the fat cells are round or polyhedral and nuclei are flattened due to pushing to a side by lipid vacuoles

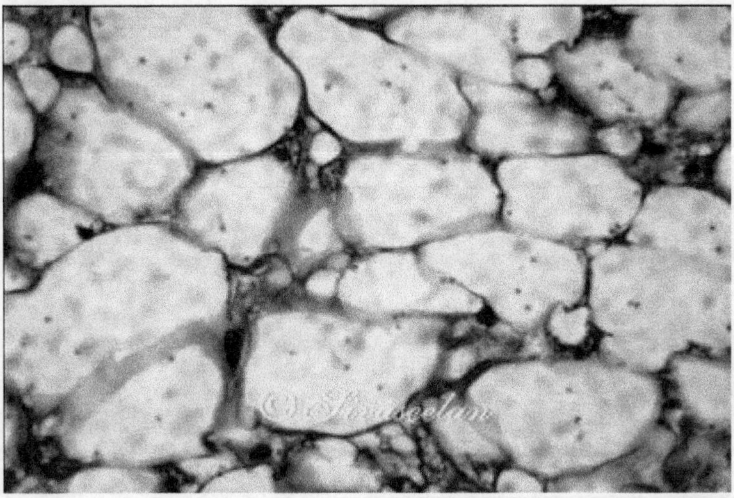

Fig. 7. A lipoma of subcutis of dog revealing lipocytes with large lipid vacuoles

- ★ In malignant type, more number of cells can be seen. Neoplastic lipocytes show many lipid vacuoles as against single large vacuole found in lipoma. Nuclei are round or ovoid, located in the centre of the cell and show prominent nucleoli. Multinucleated cells can also be seen
- ★ Anisokaryosis, poikilokaryosis and mitotic figures can also be seen in the malignant type

Growth and metastasis

Do not recur after removal, but rarely metastasizes to lung.

Myelolipoma

- ★ This is a combined tumour of lipoma with myeloid tumour
- ★ It is found commonly in the liver of cat

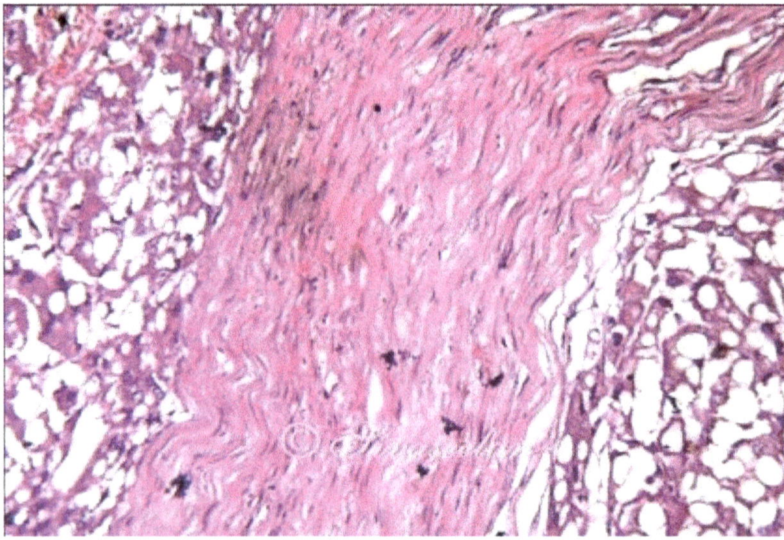

Fig. 8. A fibro-lipoma of skin of a dog showing neoplastic lipocytes divided by thick fibrous septa

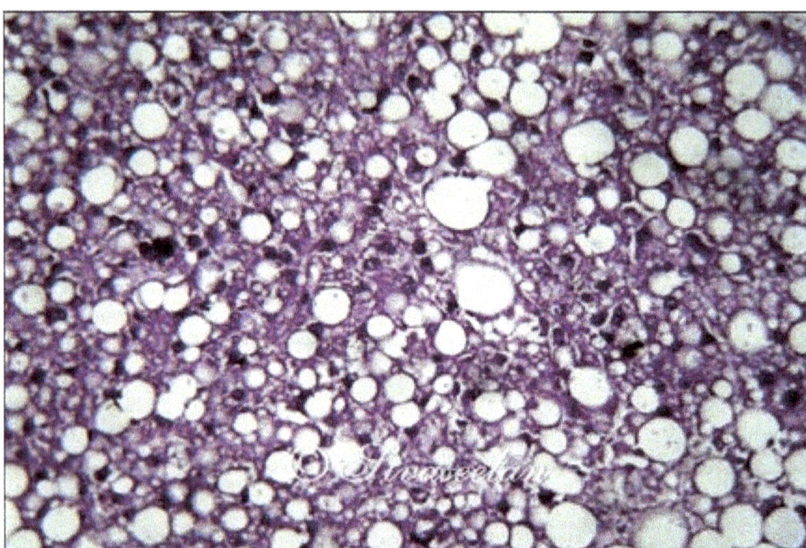

Fig. 9. Liposarcoma of skin of a dog depicting pleomorphic lipocytes with hyperchromatic nuclei and variably sized cytoplasmic vacuoles

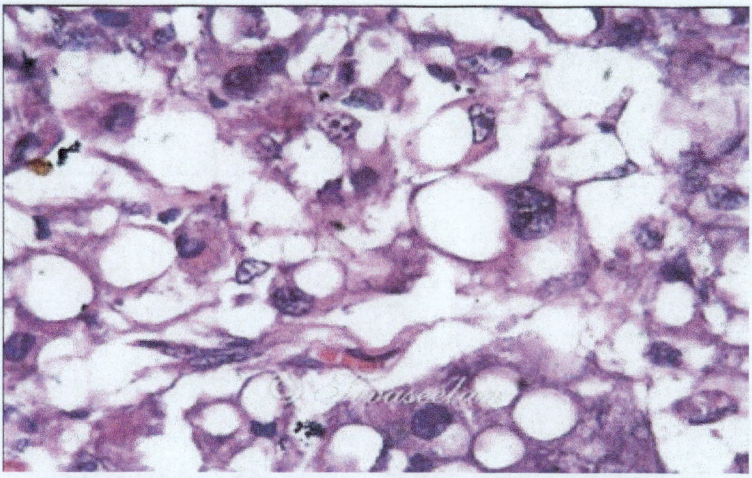

Fig. 10. Liposarcoma of skin of a dog showing lipocytes with multiple nucleoli within the anisokaryotic and poikilokaryotic nuclei

Infiltrative Lipoma / Atypical lipoma / non-encapsulated lipoma

This tumour is commonly reported in human, but in animals it has been reported in the dog, the horse and the cat. It occurs in large muscles like thigh and shoulder muscles. Rarely the incidence has been reported in abdominal muscles and myocardial muscle.

Histological features

- ★ Lipocytes are infiltrating into the muscle bundles; neoplastic fat cells are arranged often as single or double rows between atrophic muscle fibre
- ★ Low fibrous septa and absence of encapsulation are other features
- ★ Assessment of recurrence and metastasis has not been fully carried out

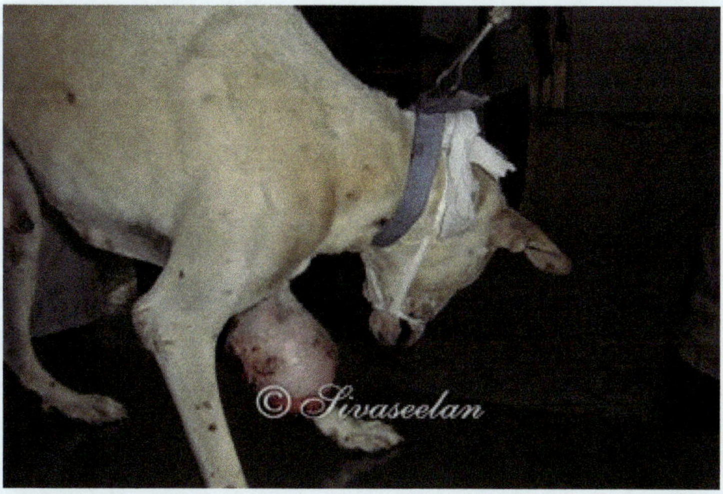

Fig. 11. A large infiltrative lipoma of the skin of a dog showing ulceration

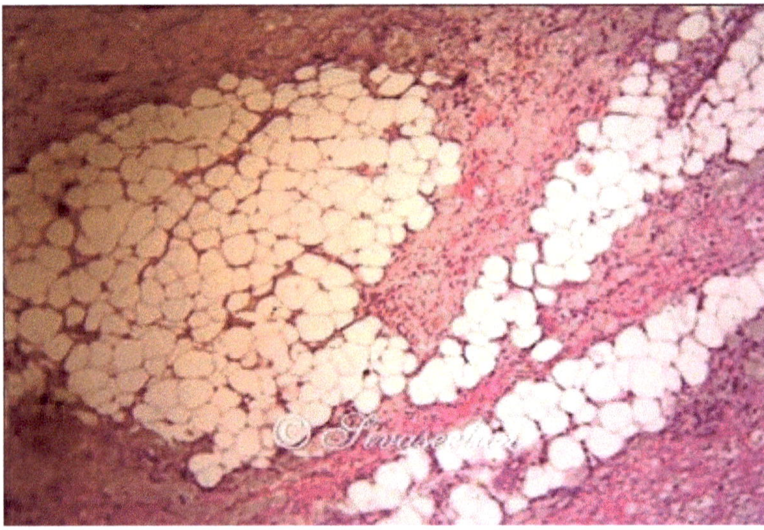

Fig. 12. Infiltrative lipoma of the skin of a dog showing lipocytes infiltrating between and atrophying the muscle fibres.

3

Myxoma and Myxosarcoma

A special type of fibroblasts produces mucin in embryos. In adults, they remain as dormant cells. Under certain circumstances, due to metaplasia these fibroblasts are modified as anaplastic embryonic cells (myxoblastic cells) with capability to produce mucin. When such cells proliferate myxoma and myxosarcoma will be the result.

It may be associated with other tumours to form lipomyxoma, chondromyxoma and fibromyxoma. Mucin in the intercellular matrix is the chief feature that distinguishes myxoma and myxosarcoma from fibroma and fibrosarcoma.

Incidence and Site

They are rarely seen in animals and more cases have been reported in aged animals than young ones. There is no breed or sex predisposition reported. It can arise from any site where there are fibroblasts. In dog, the skin is the most common site. They have also been recorded in unusual locations such as heart and liver of dogs and uterus of cow.

Gross appearance

- No definite shape is attributed
- They are soft in consistency, slimy (due to mucin) and non encapsulated
- Cut surface reveals grayish white color with viscid clear mucin

Histological features

★ Spindle or stellate shaped cells with round or ovoid or elongated nuclei that appear singly or in small clusters lying in the basophilic mucinous matrix can be seen

★ If the cell content is more, they appear as either whorls or lobules. Connective tissue septa divide the lobules

★ Myxosarcoma exhibit moderate numbers of mitotic figures and the nuclei are more hyperchromatic than in the benign type

* Myxosarcoma cannot be removed completely due to its infiltrating nature. So recurrence is commonly observed
* It rarely metastasizes to lung. Myxoma can be differentiated from other spindle cell tumours by appreciating blue (acid mucin) or magenta (neutral mucin) colour with alcian blue stain.

Myxomatosis of rabbits

* Both domestic and wild rabbits are susceptible
* It is caused by a pox virus
* It can cause total mortality of the affected flock within 10 days of occurrence
* Phlebaroconjunctivitis is almost always seen in affected cases
* Edema of lung and bronchopneumonia are noticed in some affected rabbits
* The lesions are found on the lips, nose, eyelids and other parts of the skin
* Soft, white or pink colour tumours (nodules) reveal clear serous fluid on section
* Some of the tumours may show ulcer on the surface due to blood circulation arrest
* Mosquitoes and flies are suspected as a mechanical carrier of the virus
* Surviving rabbits develop immunity.

Histological feature

* Fibroblasts, reticulo-endothelial cells and histiocytes can be seen
* Serous fluid rich in hyaluronic acid can be seen within the connective tissue spaces
* Neutrophils and eosinophils infiltration is commonly seen
* Histiocytes are hypertrophied, which appear as stellate myxoma cells that contain intracytoplasmic acidophilic inclusions
* Vacuolar degeneration and lysis of histiocytes and leucocytes can also be seen
* Overlying epithelium may show vacuolar degeneration and some of them may contain intracytoplasmic inclusions.

4

Chondroma and Chondrosarcoma

Cartilage is formed by chondrocytes which are derived from fibroblasts of perichondrium of existing cartilage. These fibroblasts are differentiated into cartilage cells, which are reverted back to fibroblasts like cells in anaplastic Chondroma. Cartilage cells are having limited proliferating ability to produce iso-groups of 2 or 4 or 8 cells.

Incidence

Chondrosarcoma are common than chondroma. In aged dogs and sheep, they have been reported. In mixed mammary tumour of bitches, this type of tumour is commonly observed. No breed or sex prevalence is attributed.

Gross appearance

★ Size varies, they are firm and covered by capsule

★ Cut surface reveal whitish multilobular structure

★ Flat bones are more affected than long bones

★ Affected bones are deformed

★ In dogs, mammary gland is the common site in which it is often reported in mixed mammary tumour

★ The costo-chondral junction, trachea, larynx and epiphysis of long bones are the common sites of occurrence.

Ecchondroma (Periosteal chondroma/Juxtra cortical chondroma)

Chondroma that develops from periosteum or surface of the cartilage is called as ecchondroma. This is seldom reported in animals.

Enchondroma

Chondroma that originates within the medullary region of cartilage of bone is called as enchondroma.

Histological feature

- ★ Sheet of round or ovoid cells in a bluish matrix are arranged as lobules separated by strands of fibrous tissue
- ★ The cells appear as individual cell in contrast to group of cells (2/4/8) noticed in normal cartilage
- ★ Dedifferentiation of cartilage cells into spindle shaped cells are observed in the peripheral zone of chondrosarcoma, but the central zone may have fully differentiated round or ovoid tumour cells
- ★ Connective tissue which divides the tumour into different lobule contains thin walled blood vessels which is not seen within cartilage cells
- ★ Poor blood supply within neoplastic cells may cause necrosis of central areas in large sized tumour
- ★ Mitotic figures and anaplasia are other features of malignant variety
- ★ Metastasis may occur to the lung

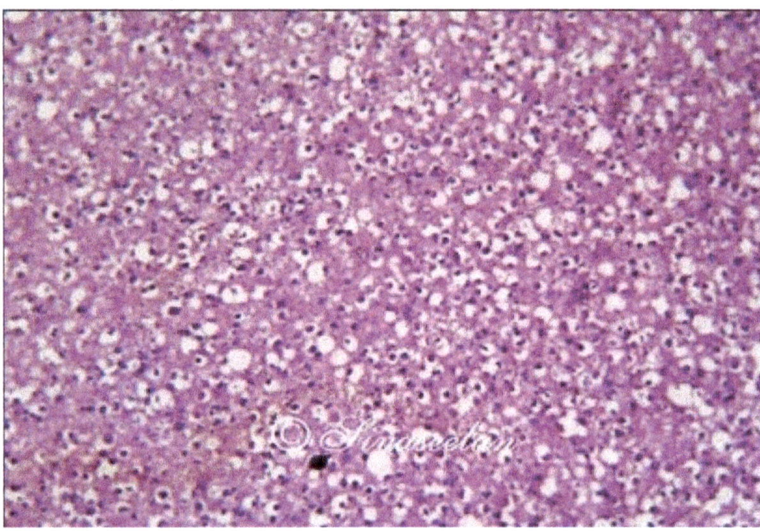

Fig. 13. Chondrosarcoma of mammary tissue of a dog showing pleomorphic individual chondrocytes arranged as sheet

5

Osteoma and Osteosarcoma

These tumours occur as a bony outgrowth and they are hard in consistency.

Osteoma eburnum /compact osteoma/sclerotic osteoma

It is harder and found in flat bones (skull, scapula, pelvic bones).

Osteoma spongiosum/spongy osteoma

It is less harder and larger than the former type, found near the ends of long bones (humerus, femur *etc*).

Incidence

They have been reported in cattle, horses, and dogs. Age, breed, sex predisposition is not encountered. Head of dogs are the most commonly observed site.

Gross appearance

- ★ Solitary bony growth covered by capsule can be seen
- ★ Osteomas are hard and need saw for cutting
- ★ They blend with normal bone but demarcation can be observed

Histological feature

- ★ Trabeculae (bone spicules) in which packing of osteocytes (condensation of osteocytes) can be seen
- ★ Normal bone has evenly distributed osteocytes
- ★ Inter trabecular soft areas contain one or more thin walled blood vessels, spindle shaped osteoblasts and fibroblasts
- ★ The matrix of nasal osteoma may reveal the mucoid appearance
- ★ Anisocytosis, anisokaryosis and presence of moderate number of mitotic figures differentiate osteocytoma from exostosis (arise from periosteum of bone extremities due to inflammation and degeneration), and metastatic bone formation in muscles, heart and larynx from fibroblasts

Osteosarcoma

Gross appearance

Round or ovoid shaped mass, which occupies and replaces the normal bone including marrow cavity. Osteosarcoma of flat bone show diffuse swelling.

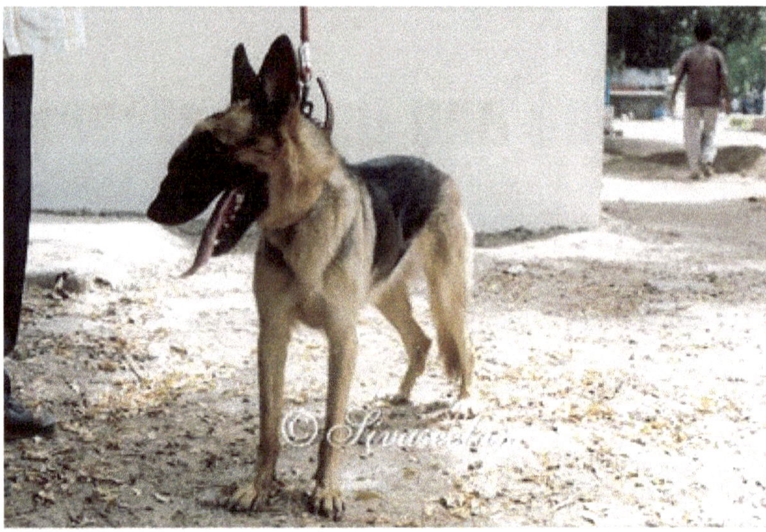

Fig. 14. Osteosarcoma of facial bone of a dog causing disfigurement of face

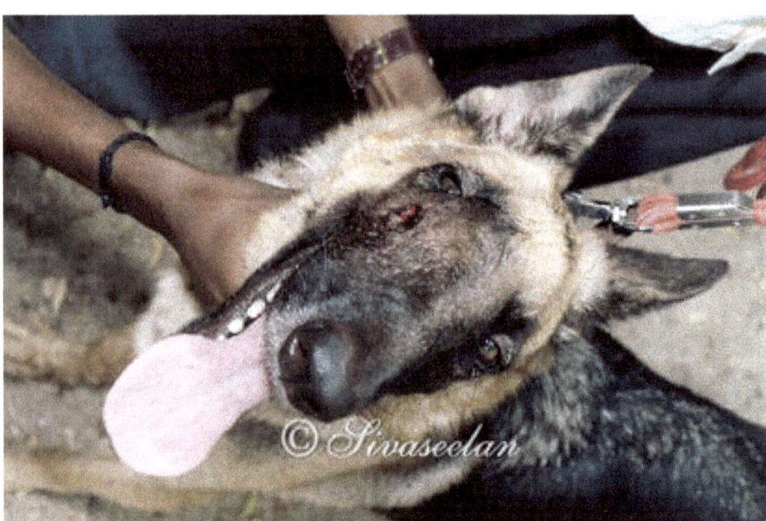

Fig. 15. Osteosarcoma shown in fig. 14 revealing ulcer on the tumour

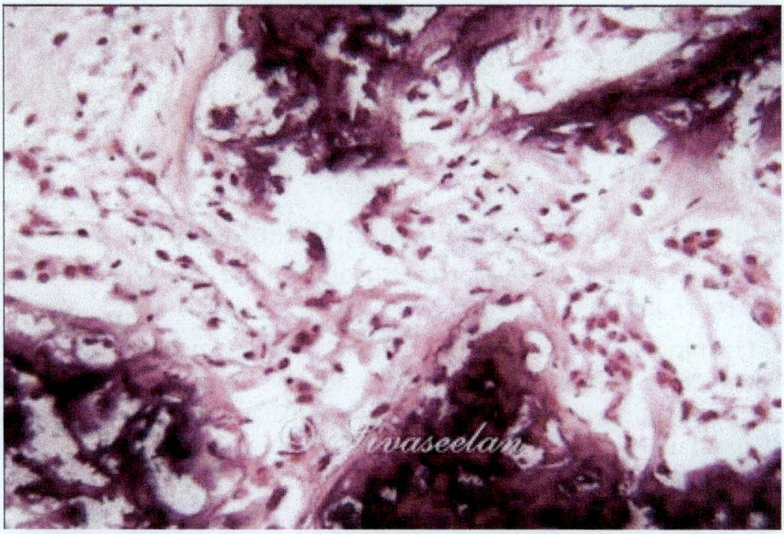

Fig. 16. Osteosarcoma revealing neoplastic osteocytes arranged as sheet without lacunae

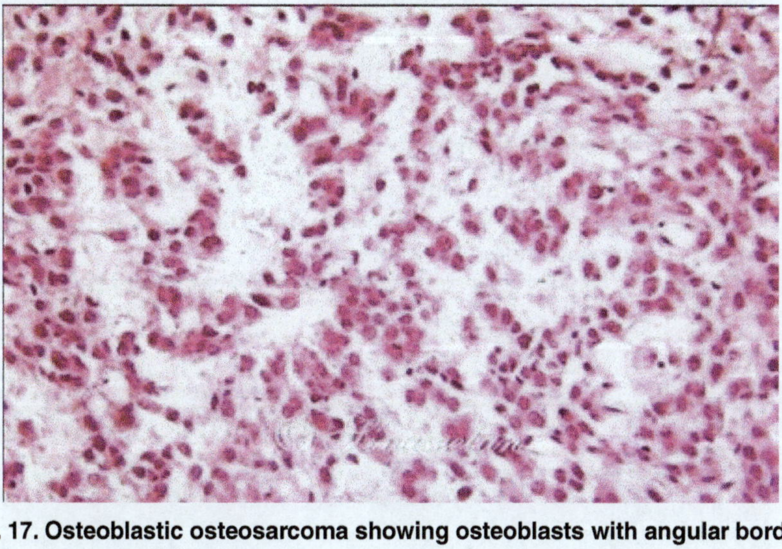

Fig. 17. Osteoblastic osteosarcoma showing osteoblasts with angular borders

Histological features

- ★ Highly cellular, round or spindle or polyhedral cells show pleomorphism and arranged as a compact masses
- ★ Anisokaryosis, anisocytosis with hyperchromicity can be commonly seen
- ★ Few tumour giant cells and more mitotic figures can be seen
- ★ Metastasis to lung has been recorded
- ★ Neoplastic osteocytes more than one can be seen within the lacunae (normal bone has only one cell in a lacunae)

- ⋆ Poorly differentiated type show no lacunae arrangement
- ⋆ The spindle shaped cells are arranged as a sheet in osteoblastic osteosarcoma in which the cells will have angular borders and form irregular islands on osseous matrix

Fibrous Osteoma

(Osteofibroma, Osteogenic fibroma, Osteoid fibroma)

- ⋆ This is a fibrous tissue mixed osteoid tumour like growth found in the jaws of animals
- ⋆ Histologically, fibroosseous stroma shows irregular spicules rimmed with spindle shaped isomorphic and isochromic fibroblasts, which are transforming into osteoblasts (spindle cells are becoming plumpy and angular)
- ⋆ Isomorphic cells differentiate this type with osteosarcoma

Giant Cell Tumour / Osteoclastoma

- ⋆ This is a slowly growing tumour that seldom occur in animals, which are arising from osteoclasts.(multinucleated modified macrophages of bone)
- ⋆ Growing tumour occupy the compact bone and destroy it leaving thin outer layer, which make egg shell crackling sensation upon palpation in advanced condition
- ⋆ Metastasis is seldom found
- ⋆ Histologically, numerous multinucleated giant cells can be seen. Large sized super giant cells are produced by the dividing osteoclasts in which nuclei are arranged as solid sheets

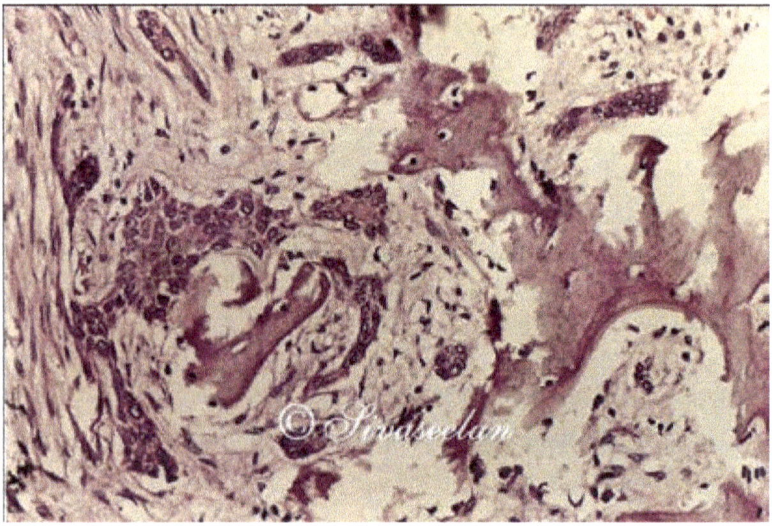

Fig. 18. Osteoclastoma depicting variably sized giant cells

6

Leiomyoma and Leiomyosarcoma

It arises from smooth muscles of hollow organs (uterus, vagina, intestine, stomach, urinary bladder and esophagus), spleen, kidney and broad ligament of oviduct of birds. Cattle, cat, sheep, goat and fowl are often affected.

Gross appearance

- ★ They are solitary, pedunculated and non- encapsulated tumours
- ★ It may protrude in or out of the hollow viscera within the wall with intact mucosal and serosal surfaces
- ★ Cut surface reveal white to pink mass, some are lobulated

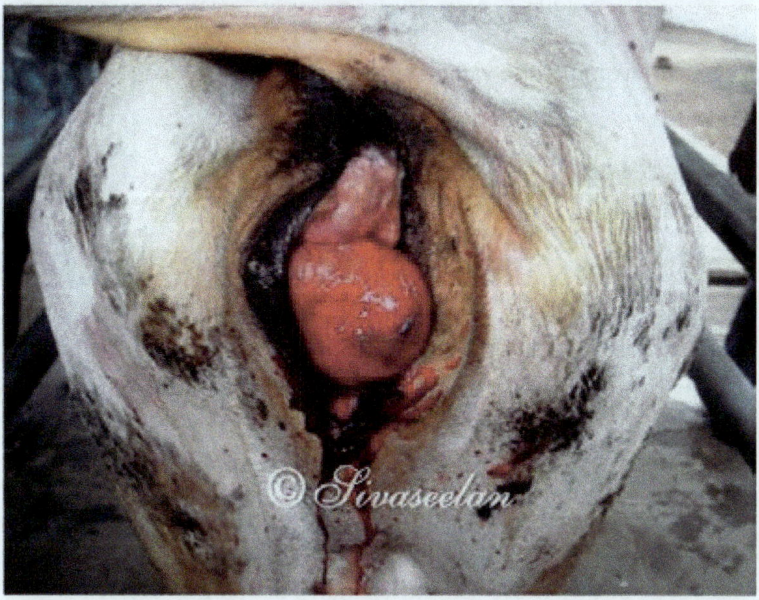

Fig. 19. A solitary pedunculated Leiomyoma protruding from the vagina of a cow.

Histological feature

- ★ Interlacing bundles of spindle shaped cells divided as lobules by fibrous tissue, which bear blood vessel can be seen
- ★ In cross section, round oval shaped centrally placed nuclei and in longitudinal section, cigar shaped (elongated nuclei with rounded ends) can be seen
- ★ Haphazard arrangement (run in all the directions) of bundles differentiates it from normal smooth muscle

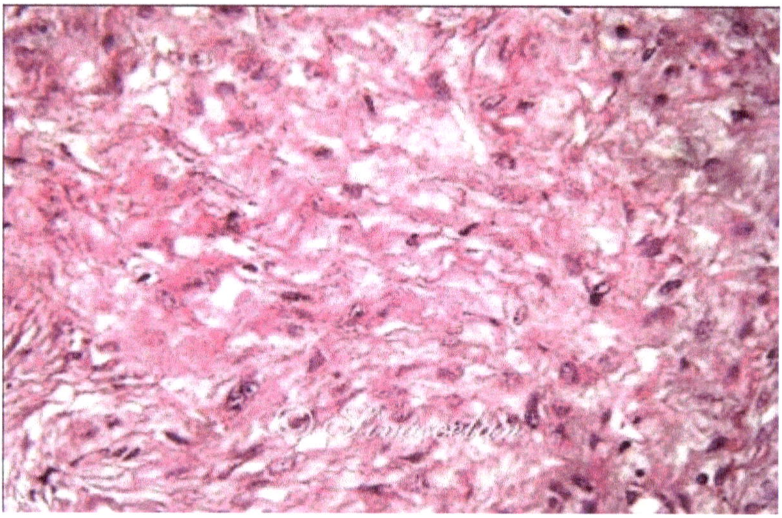

Fig. 20. Leiomyoma of the vagina of cow revealing elongated muscle fibres and scattered neoplastic leiomyocytes.

Leiomyosarcoma

Incidence

Cat is more affected. Apart from the sites of leiomyoma, leiomyosarcoma have also been reported from ovary.

Gross appearance

- ★ It may protrude out of the hollow organs and spilling of tumour cells may serve as seeds for transcoelomic spread of tumour
- ★ Often occur as multiple entity in bladder and uterus, whereas in kidney it occurs as a solitary mass

Histological feature

- ★ This type shows more cellularity than the benign variety
- ★ Fastly growing tumours destroy the adjacent tissues due to invasion
- ★ Pleomorphism and anisokaryosis with more number of mitotic figures can be seen

- ★ In anaplastic type, shorter and plumper cells can be observed
- ★ Differentiation from fibrosarcoma and rhabdomyosarcoma should be done carefully
- ★ Masons trichrome stain is useful to distinguish it from fibrosarcoma (blue colour collagen can be seen in fibrosarcoma), but for the differentiation from rhabdomyosarcoma, iron haematoxylin should be used to demonstrate the striations in striated muscles
- ★ Electron microscopy can be used to demonstrate the attachment plagues, pinocytic vesicles and dense bodies with or without filament in leiomyosarcoma
- ★ Immunohistochemical techniques can also be used to demonstrate these bodies
- ★ Metastasis to distant organs, especially to the lung is commonly observed.

7

Rhabdomyoma and Rhabdomyosarcoma

This tumour arises from skeletal and cardiac muscles. Cardiac tumours are common than the other.

Incidence

Cardiac tumour in human occurs as a congenital tumour. Among animals, cardiac tumour has been reported in pig, cow, dog and sheep.

Gross appearance

- ★ Cardiac rhabdomyoma may be solitary or multiple as in pigs
- ★ These tumours may either be pedunculated or completely embedded in the heart muscles
- ★ Inter-ventricular septum is the common site in the heart
- ★ This can be differentiated by its different colour from normal myocardium
- ★ The tumour is not well demarcated from normal myocardium
- ★ Very rarely encapsulation is seen

Histological features

- ★ Pleomorphic large sized cells with single or multinuclei with abundant granular vacuolated cytoplasm can be seen. These cells are called as **spider cells**
- ★ Round or oval nuclei with prominent nucleoli can be observed
- ★ Fibrillar cross striations can be demonstrated by using iron haematoxylin
- ★ Vacuoles within the cytoplasm represents glycogen which can be demonstrated by using PAS
- ★ High glycogen content is the diagnostic significance of this tumour
- ★ Electron microscopic features of intercalated discs and glycogen granules are useful to distinguish cardiac muscle tumour from other skeletal muscle tumours

Rhabdomyosarcoma

Incidence and clinical significance

This tumour has been very rarely reported in animals. Cow, sheep, dog, cat and horse are the reported animals and limbs, tongue, cheek, pharynx, esophagus, thorax, brisket, uterus, bladder and ovary are the reported areas.

Tumour in legs causes irregular swelling and lameness. Digestive disorders are noticed when it occurs in gastro-intestinal tract. Uterine and bladder obstruction may be caused when the tumour grows in these places. Since rhabdomyosarcoma metastasize early to a variety of tissues, prognosis will be often unfavorable. Tumour that grow in skeletal muscle cannot be surgically removed due to the irregular border, which warrants amputation of the affected organ in many cases.

Gross appearance

- Pinkish nodular growth without encapsulation can be seen in tissues
- Multiple nodular, metastatic rhabdomyosarcoma that protrude from mucus membrane of hollow organs like bladder and uterus are called as "**botryoid**"
- Metastasis may occur to lung and other tissues

Histological feature

Embryonal type

- ★ This type reveals irregularly lobulated sheets of cells showing anisocytosis and marked anisokaryosis. Spider cells and cytoplasmic cross striations are the important features
- ★ Cells may be round or oval or racket shaped. Myofibrils can be appreciated by specail stain as mentioned in rhabdomyoma
- ★ **"Strap cells"**, the long myoblast without myofibrillar striations can also be seen

Alveolar type

- ★ This type of rhabdomyosarcoma reveals acinar pattern with round or oval shaped cells, which seldom show cross striations

Pleomorphic type

- ★ Cells arranged in sheets show high degree of size and shape variations
- ★ Elongated cells (ribbon cells) with central ovoid nuclei and spider cells with cytoplasmic vacuoles can be observed in some areas
- ★ Angular cells with anisokaryotic nuclei dominate other cell type (small cells, spider cells and ribbon cells)
- ★ Giant cells with multiple nuclei are another feature of this tumour

8

Epulis (Gingival Enlargement)

Incidence

Most of the cases have been described in dogs, rarely in cattle and very rarely in other domestic animals.

Types

Based on the dominating tissue type, Epulis has been classified under three types

- ★ Fibromatous type
- ★ Ossifying type
- ★ Acanthomatous type

Gross appearance

- ★ Possibility of occurrence in the descending order is molar, premolar, canine, and incisors
- ★ They may occur as a round elongated solitary mass or as a small multiple foci (0.5-2 cm in diameter)
- ★ They arise from periodontal region and covered by epithelium
- ★ The surface may be ulcerated or infected
- ★ The consistency depends on the amount of bony tissue present
- ★ It may be so firm, if the bony tissue is more

Histological feature

- ★ The picture will depict a mixture of fibroma, papilloma, and osteoma with the infiltration of lymphocytes and plasma cells
- ★ Overlying epithelium runs downwards, branching and reuniting to produce cords
- ★ Similar to bovine fibropapilloma, the cords have peripheral palisading of columnar cells

- ★ Below the epithelium, masses of keratinocytes with the intercellular bridges without keratin pearls and occasional cysts lined by stratified squamous epithelium can be seen
- ★ Below which fibroma like appearance constituting closely packed collagen fibres with moderate number of fibroblast can be observed
- ★ The deeper layer shows osteoma like appearance of spicule formation with osteocytes and some of the matrix may be calcified
- ★ Rare mitotic figures and more number of blood vessels can be appreciated
- ★ An Epulis may have epithelium, fibrous tissue and bony tissue. Depending upon the dominating tissue, the name fibromatous (fibrous tissue), ossifying (bony tissue) and acanthomatous (epithelium) is assigned.

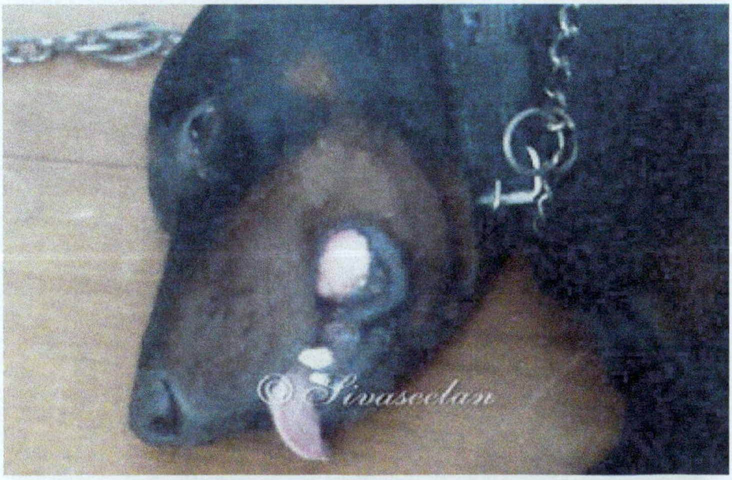

Fig. 21. Ossifying solitary mandibular Epulis of a dog.

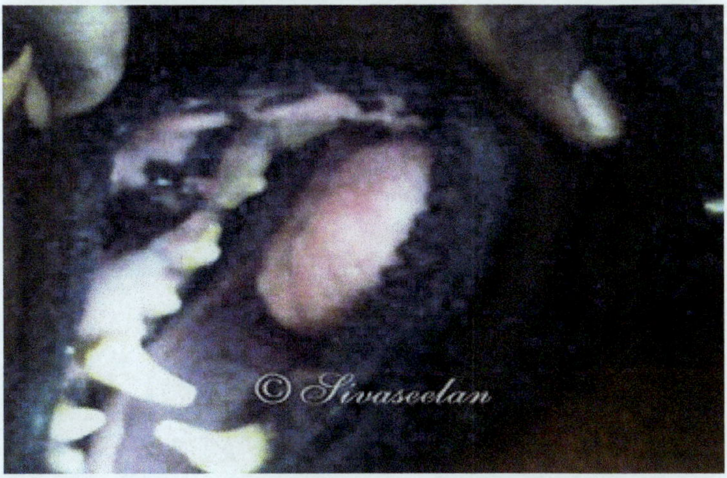

Fig. 22. Closure view of the Epulis shown in fig. 21 revealing a solitary mass occupying about 5 cm in length on the mandibular gum.

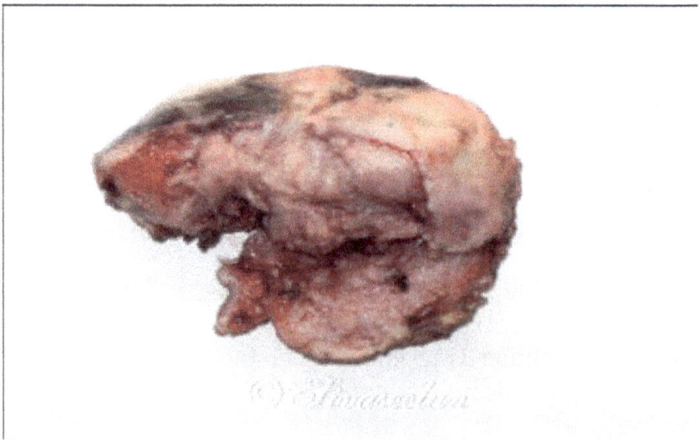

Fig. 23. Removed Epulis mass shown in fig.22 revealing lobulations.

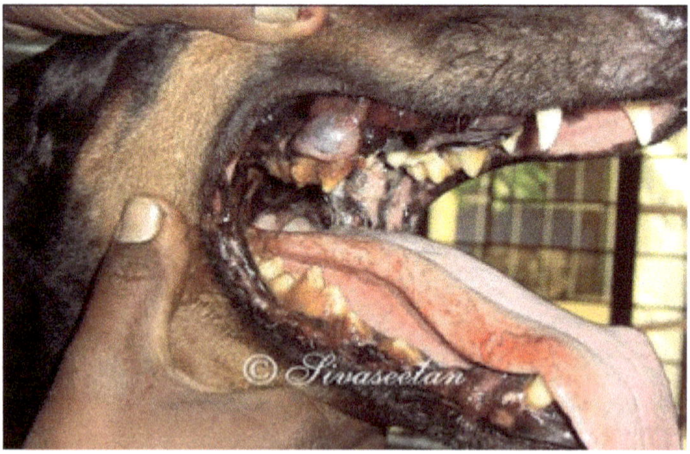

Fig. 24. An Epulis on the maxillary molar gum region of a dog.

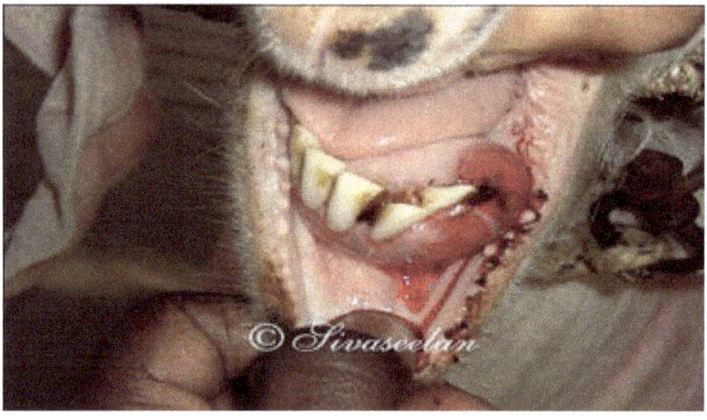

Fig. 25. An Epulis on the mandibular premolar gum region of a goat revealing disruption of orientation of teeth.

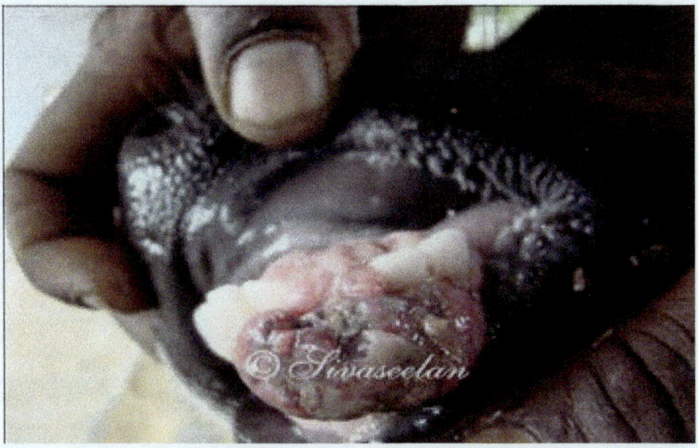

Fig. 26. An ulcerated large acanthomatous Epulis growing inside as well as outside of the incisor region of a cow.

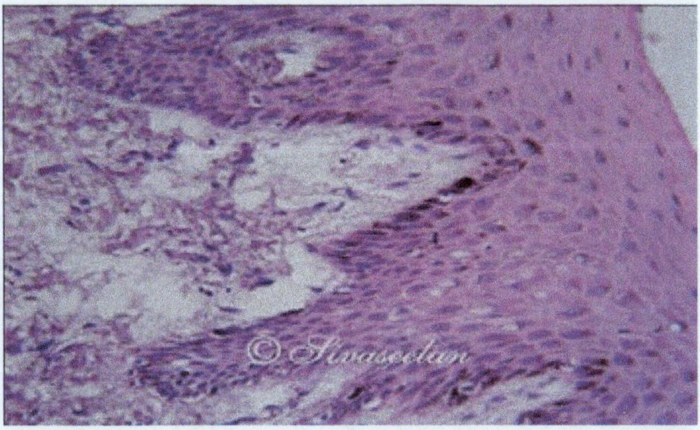

Fig. 27. Ossifying Epulis shown in fig. 22 revealing rete pegs of proliferating surface epithelium bordered by palisading arrangement of the cells.

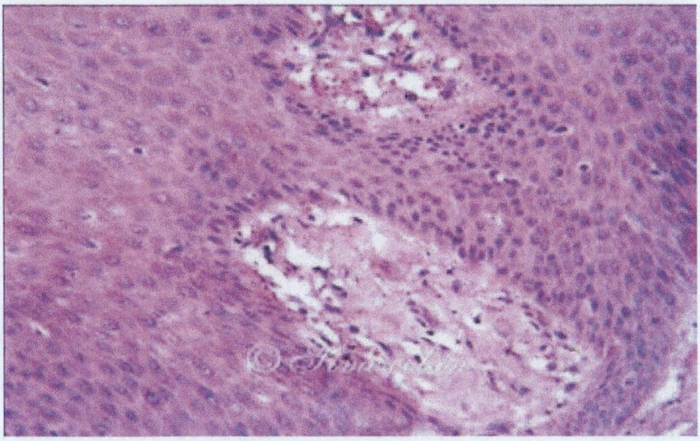

Fig. 28. Ossifying Epulis shown in fig. 22 depicting pseudo cyst formation Among proliferating epithelial cells.

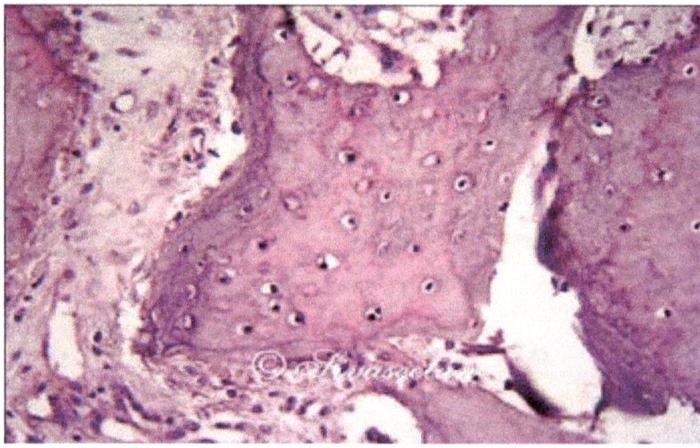

Fig. 29. Ossifying Epulis shown in fig. 22 revealing ossifying regions in the deeper areas.

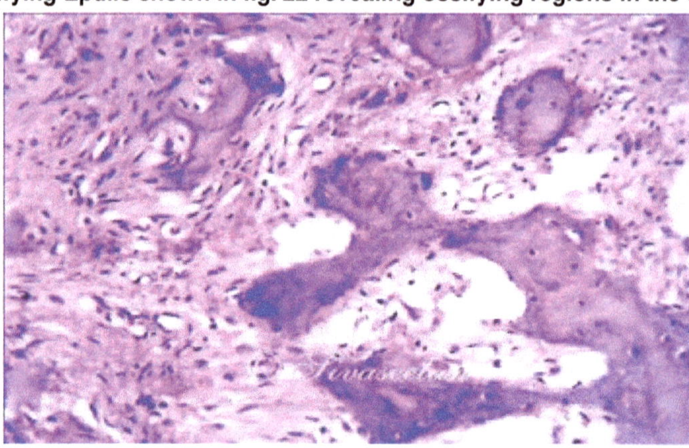

Fig. 30. Ossifying Epulis shown in fig. 22 revealing proliferation of fibroblasts and ossification in the deeper areas of the mass.

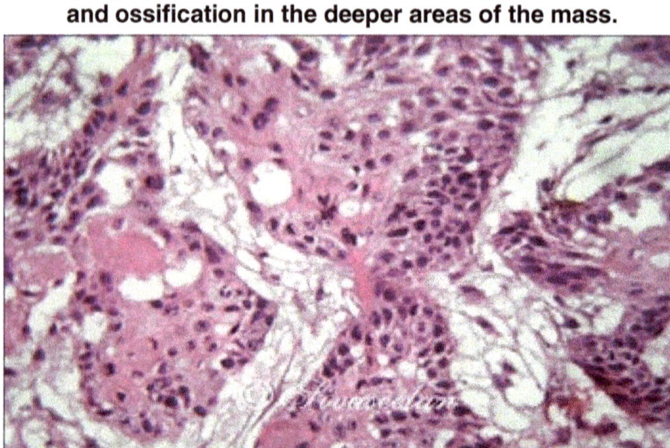

Fig. 31. Acanthomatous type of Epulis shown in fig. 26 revealing island arrangement of keratinocytes that depict anisocytosis, anisokaryosis, hyperchromatic nuclei with variable number of nucleoli and rare mitotic figures.

A rare case of mandibular ossifying epulis was recorded in a seven years old male Doberman dog by **Sivaseelan** *et al.* (IJVP, 2010, 40-1: 74 – 76). Histopathologically, the mass revealed rete pegs of proliferating overlying epithelium, deep seated bony trabeculae and nuclear remnants, and scattered fibrous tissue. Since the bone tissue occurs in the ossifying epulis, the origin of this tumour might be from the odontogenic epithelial cells (cell rests of Malassez) of periodontal membrane.

Growth and metastasis

Epulis arises from gingival tissue and do not invade the underlying bone (acanthomatous type is exceptional). Though recurrence is seen in all these three types, acanthomatous type often recur when compared to other two types. Metastasis is seldom noticed.

9

Angioma and Angiosarcoma (Tumours of Blood and Lymph Vessels)

Haemangioma and haemangiosarcoma are the benign and malignant tumours of blood vessels respectively. Lymphangioma and lymphangiosarcoma are benign and malignant tumours of lymph vessels respectively.

Haemangioma

Incidence

They have been reported in dog, cattle, horse, small ruminants, swine and fowl.

Gross appearance

- ★ Size varies from 0.5 to 2 cm in benign type and up to 10 cm in malignant variety
- ★ Solitary tumour is commonly seen when compared to multiple occurrence
- ★ Due to endothelial cells and RBCs, the colour varies from dark red to purple
- ★ Due to more blood content the consistency will be soft in most of the cases and bleed easily when punctured

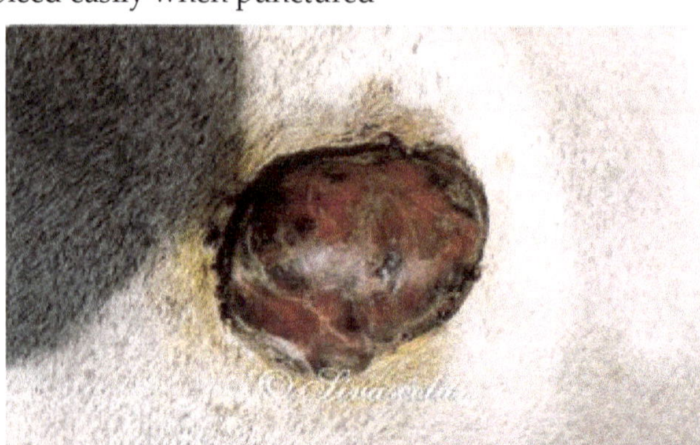

Fig. 32. A subcutaneous haemangioma of cattle revealing dark red colour

Histological feature

Depending on the vascular space size and degree of cellularity, these endothelial cell tumours are grouped as haemangioma hypertropicum (solid haemangioma), haemangioma cavernosum (cavernous type) and haemangioma simplex (capillary type).

Haemangioma hypertropicum (Solid haemangioma)

- ★ It is considered as the conversion stage to malignant type with the features of tightly packed neoplastic endothelial cells that mimic the parent cells (elongated cell with oval nucleus)
- ★ After the malignant conversion, the cells are becoming short and plumpy (round to oval cells with round nucleus) with many mitotic figures
- ★ Haemangioma hypertropicum and haemangiosarcoma should be differentiated from other spindle cells tumours by appreciating atleast few blood spaces with RBCs in the former

Haemangioma cavernosum (Cavernous type)

- ★ Irregular sized blood spaces are lined by one or many layers of endothelial cells. Bood spaces contain accumulated RBCs

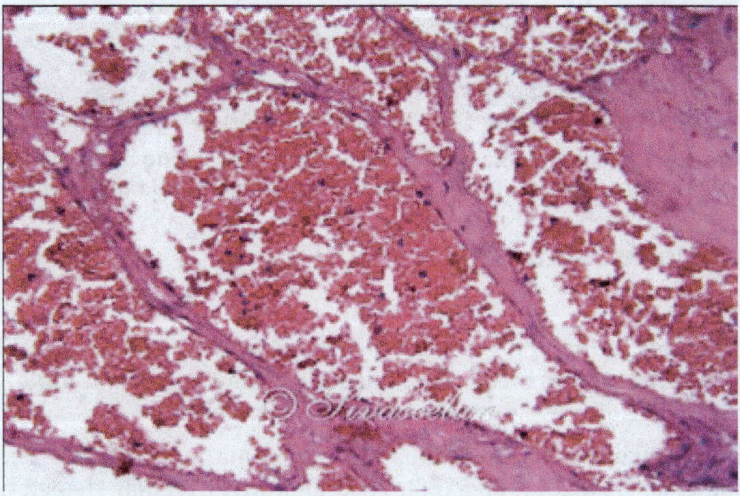

Fig. 33. Cavernous haemangioma of the subcutis of cattle shown in fig. 32 revealing irregular spaces filled with blood cells and separated by fibrous bands.

Haemangioma simplex (Capillary type)

- ★ Proliferating endothelial cells are attempting to form capillaries
- ★ More or less uniform sized capillaries with accumulated few RBCs lined by one or several layers of cells can be observed
- ★ Acute inflammatory conditions and highly vascularised other tumours must be differentiated from haemangioma. Inflammation is characterised

by exudate accumulation and infiltration of cells. Other tumours reveal along with delicate capillaries, the parent tissue involving neoplasia

- ★ Hamartoma of subcutis of white leghorn birds and telangiectasis of liver may also mimic haemangioma, but the spaces will be lined by matured elongated single layer of endothelial cells without RBC accumulation.

Metastasis and Recurrence

No proper evidence has been recorded in these aspects.

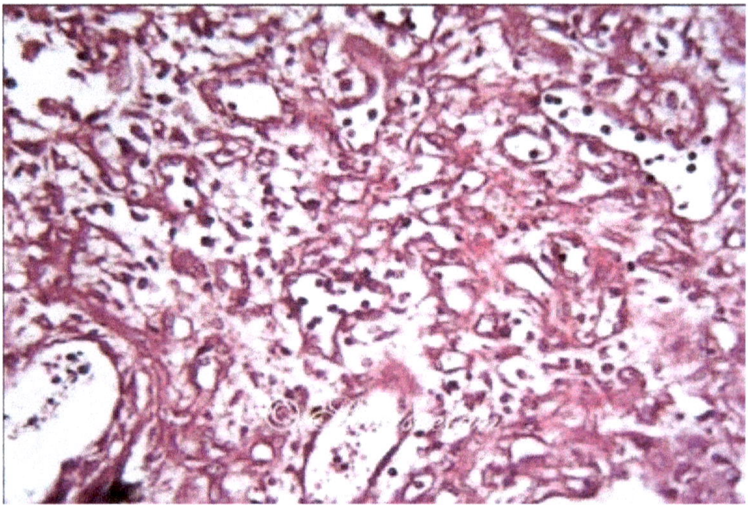

Fig. 34. Capillary haemangioma of subcutis of a dog depicting numerous capillaries lined by endothelial cells and few capillaries reveal blood cells.

Haemangiosarcoma

Incidence

This tumour is commonly noticed in aged male dogs. German shepherd is the most commonly reported breed. Occur as solitary, but may be multiple. They can arise from any tissue but skin tumours are more common.

A multiple cutaneous cavernous haemangioma in a dog was reported by **Sivaseelan** *et al.* (IVJ, 2011, 88-5: 66). Histologically, irregular shaped and sized cavernous spaces containing RBCs were noticed. The cavernous spaces were lined by single or double layer of endothelial cells. The neoplastic endothelium was supported by fibrous stroma, in which occasional aggregates of inflammatory cells, primarily lymphoid cells and macrophages were scattered. Occasionally, thrombi filled lumina were also noticed.

Gross appearance

- ★ Size varies from few to several centimeter
- ★ These tumours are well circumscribed and reveal round to oval shape
- ★ Moderately firm in consistency and appear reddish black in colour

★ Cut surface reveal reddish mass that should not be confused with brownish melanomas

Histological feature

★ These tumour reveal immature endothelial cells that form small cavernous canals/islands

★ The cells are anaplastic, pleomorphic and packed into masses

★ Some of the cavernous spaces show thrombi formation

★ Highly cellular type shows solid sheet arrangement, which resemble fibro sarcoma, but the presence of at least few blood spaces with RBCs distinguish the former

★ Haemosiderin laden macrophages, and neutrophilic infiltration can also be seen in a highly proliferating type of haemangiosarcoma

★ Cavernous lumen may be filled completely with endothelial cells

★ The cells are oval, polyhedral or spindle shaped with large oval nuclei and clear bluish cytoplasm

Metastasis and Recurrence

Haemangiosarcoma often metastasize to other organs, especially to the lung and recurrence after removal is also commonly observed.

Haemangiopericytoma

Incidence

Older female dogs are commonly affected. Subcutaneous area, especially the extremities is the common site of occurrence.

Gross appearance

★ This tumour may attain up to 25 cm in diameter

★ They are firm in consistency and nodular in appearance and easily movable

★ Cut surface may reveal lobulations

Histological feature

★ Characteristic appearance is formation of whorls, around blood vessels resembling fingerprints

★ Some tumours may reveal few/no whorl formation. These tumours show interlacing bundles or pallisading arrangement

★ Cells are spindle shaped with cytoplasmic processes and ovoid nuclei

★ Round/avoid cells with pink staining cytoplasm can also be seen

10

Round Cell Tumours

Tumours that show discrete round cells histologically are called as Round Cell Tumours. They are

1. Histiocytoma
2. Transmissible Venereal Tumour
3. Lymphoma
4. Plasma Cell Tumour
5. Mast Cell Tumour

Histiocytoma and Histiocyticsarcoma

Incidence

Younger dogs are mostly affected. Skin of the ear neck, limbs, trunk and tail are the common sites affected.

Gross appearance

- ★ They occur as solitary or multiple tumours
- ★ Size varies from 2-5 cm in diameter
- ★ They reveal dome or button like in appearance
- ★ Most of the tumours are non encapsulated

Histological feature

- ★ Monotonous sheet arrangement of discrete round cells can be seen
- ★ Dense to loosely packed round to oval shaped cells with ovoid or bean shaped nuclei are the feature
- ★ In the skin, the cells infiltrate heavily into the deeper layers of dermis and loosely into the dermis
- ★ High mitotic figure, pleomorphic nuclei and prominent multiple nucleoli are the characteristic feature

- ★ Cytoplasm is abundant and pale in appearance
- ★ Malignant type will depict more giant cells

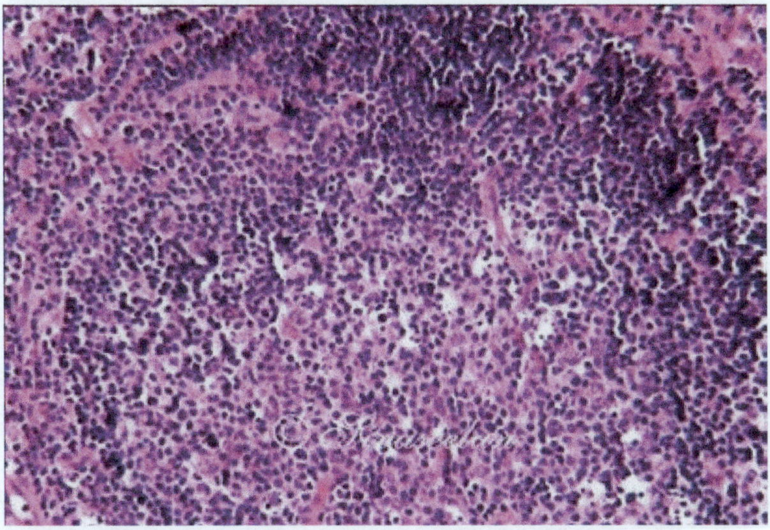

Fig. 35. Histiocytoma of the skin of a dog revealing densely populated cells in the dermis and loosely arranged cells in the epidermis.

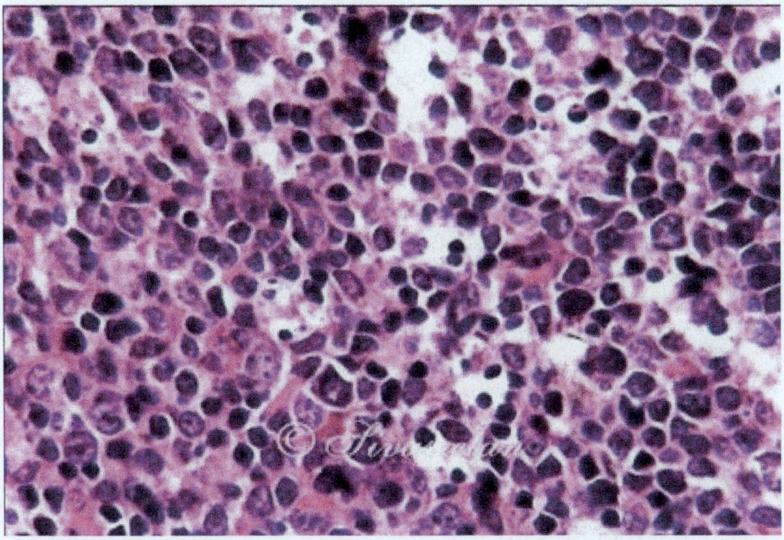

Fig. 36. Higher magnification of the fig. 35 depicting cellular as well as nuclear pleomorphism with prominent multiple nucleoli in the loosely packed cells.

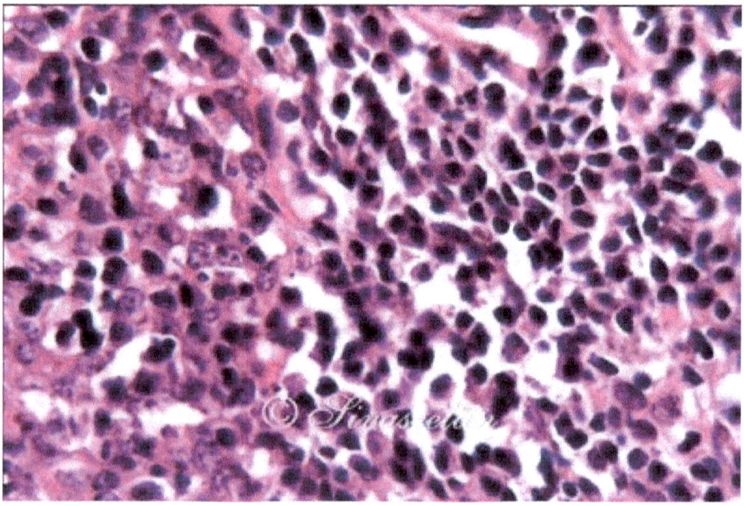

Fig. 37. Histiocytoma of the skin of a cow revealing mixture of round, ovoid and polygonal cells with pleomorphic nuclei.

Transmissible Venereal Tumour (TVT, Sticker tumour, Transmissible sarcoma, Lymphosarcoma)

Incidence

They occur commonly in dogs, readily transmitted through coitus, but transplanted tumour cells need an abraded mucosa or skin for their implantation and growth. Extra-genital TVT that occur in other non-genital areas are due to licking and transfer of genital TVT cells.

Gross appearance

- ★ They occur as nodular or papillary or multilobulated growths
- ★ Size ranges from 0.5 mm -10 cm in diameter
- ★ They appear as solitary or multiple growths
- ★ They are noticed almost always on the external genitalia, but may occur in oral, nasal and conjunctival mucosa, and skin (extra-genital TVT)

Histological feature

- ★ Origin of cell may be lymphocytes or histiocytes or R.E cells
- ★ Resemble histiocytoma, but the cytoplasm reveal punctuate vacuoles, at least in few of the cells
- ★ TVT is such a type of tumour, which can progress within the shortest period into a big mass, may stand still or may regress
- ★ Highly progressing tumour shows more mitotic figures (mitotic index >20)

★ Regressive tumours show more cells with punctuate vacuoles

★ Punctate vacuolated cells are undergoing apoptosis in which the vacuoles indicate digested lipid by increased lipase activity in apoptotic cells

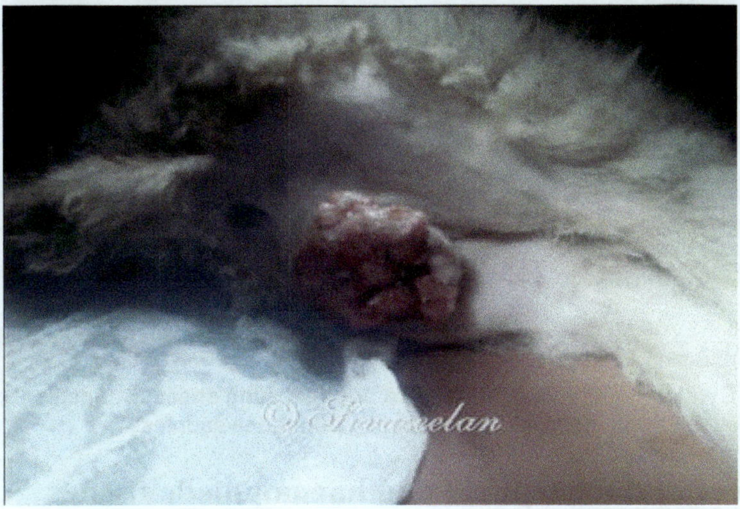

Fig. 38. Multilobulated TVT protruding from the vagina of a dog.

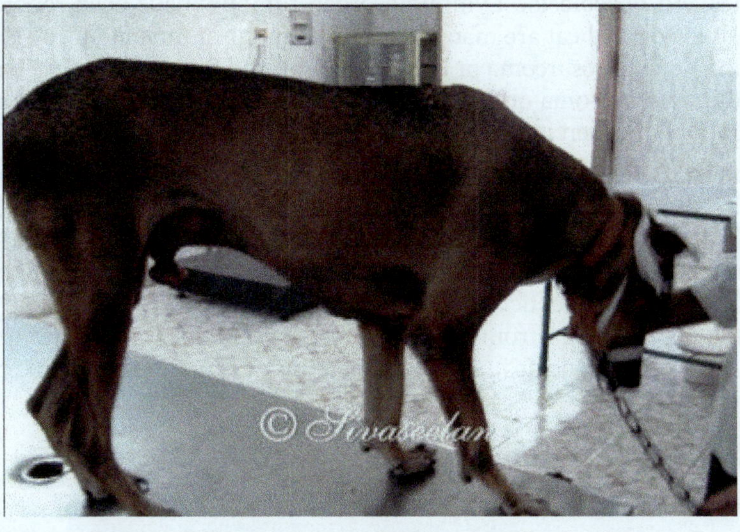

Fig. 39. TVT arising from the glans-penis of a dog.

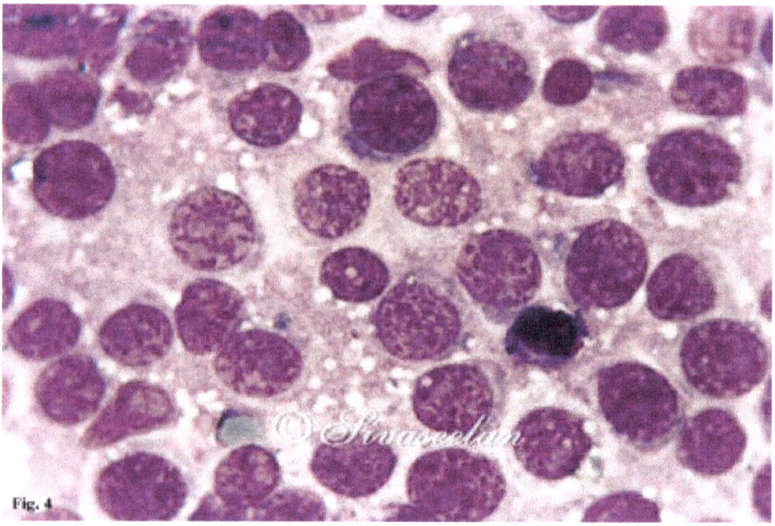

Fig. 40. Cytology of the vaginal TVT of a dog revealing sheet arrangement of round cells with cytoplasmic punctate vacuoles.

Tumours of the lymphoid and haemopoietic tissues

Tumour of lymphoid organs like lymphnodes, thymus and spleen may involve neoplastic condition of functional cells of these organs (lymphocyte) alone or also with supporting cells of the sinus of lymphoid organs (reticulum cells/ histiocytes and fibroblasts). Lymphoid organ tumours have been reported in all animals, but dog and cat are many in them. Tumour of functional cell is called as lymphoma / Lymphosarcoma or lymphocytoma and the supporting cell is termed as reticulum cell sarcoma or histiocytic tumour. If the tumour arises from both of these components, then it is called as Hodgkin's disease.

Bone marrow is the major haemopoietic tissue from which Red blood corpuscles, White blood corpuscles and Thrombocytes are produced. All these components either alone or in combination may involve in neoplasia called as Leukemia. Erythrocyte and Thrombocyte neoplasms are called as Erythrocytic leukemia and Thrombocytic leukemia respectively. From WBCs Myeloid tumours (Myelogenous leukemia from granulocytes), lymphoid tumours (Lymphocytic leukemia from lymphocytes) and Reticular tumours (Monocytic leukemia from monocytes) may arise.

Lymphoma / Lymphosarcoma

Incidence

- ★ Older cattle, cat and pigs are commonly affected, and horse and sheep are seldom affected
- ★ Some of the lymphomas are caused by corona virus
- ★ In lymphoma, rapid enlargement of lymph nodes occur (up to ten times of the normal)

- ★ Both peripheral and visceral lymphnodes, spleen, diffuse lymphoid populations like skin, stomach and intestine are affected
- ★ In cattle, fore-stomach mucosa is often affected
- ★ All lymphoid organs are affected in multicentric lymphoma
- ★ Most often bilateral and symmetrical enlargement of lymphnodes are seen
- ★ The affected animal or human seldom experiences pain
- ★ In lymphosarcoma, metastasis often occurs to almost all organs, no organ is immune (*e.g.* Marek's disease of birds)

Types of Lymphoma (depending on the site of occurrence)

Cutaneous lymphoma

- ★ This often occur as a solitary mass, multiple occurrence has also been reported. Edema may be seen in multicentric type

Thymic lymphoma

- ★ Thymus and the regional lymph nodes are involved.

Multicentric lymphoma

- ★ Wide spread multiple occurrence of tumours are noticed
- ★ Involvement of lymph nodes and a variety of organs are affected (liver, spleen, kidney, lungs, heart, G.I. tract with or without bone marrow)
- ★ In this type, the affected animal die soon

Alimentary lymphoma

- ★ This type only affects G.I tract lymphoid areas (Peyer's patches, caecal tonsils, loose and dense lymphoid cellular areas). This is also a highly fatal type in which chronic diarrhoea is often experienced
- ★ If bone marrow is not involved, animals with other organ lymphomas exhibit either normal haematology or slight neutrophilia
- ★ Lymphocytic leukemia with massive lymphocytosis may occur without any solid tumour growth of organs which indicate the bone marrow origination of tumour

Gross appearance

- ★ Great enlargement of lymphoid organs and lymph nodes are seen
- ★ Lymphnodes are firm and non adherent to the surrounding tissue
- ★ Freely movable mesenteric lymphnodes are often fused together
- ★ Cortex and medullary distinction of lymph node is lost
- ★ Liver and spleen often show multiple foci of masses or occasional diffused enlargement of whole organs

- ★ Gastro intestinal tract may have multiple nodular or diffuse growth in many locations
- ★ Affected lymphoid organs and other metastatic organs are bulky, soft and friable due to the replacement of original cells by neoplastic lymphocytes
- ★ In multicentric lymphoma all peripheral as well as visceral lymph nodes are enlarged in a symmetrical manner

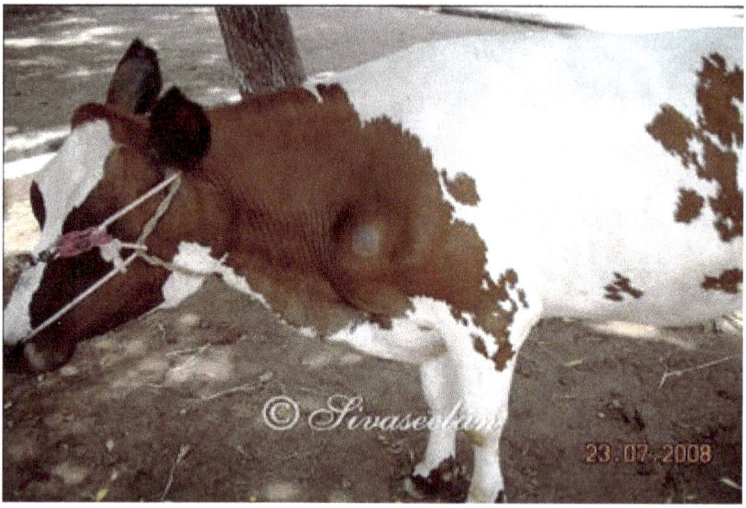

Fig. 41. Prescapular lymph node lymphoma of a cow.

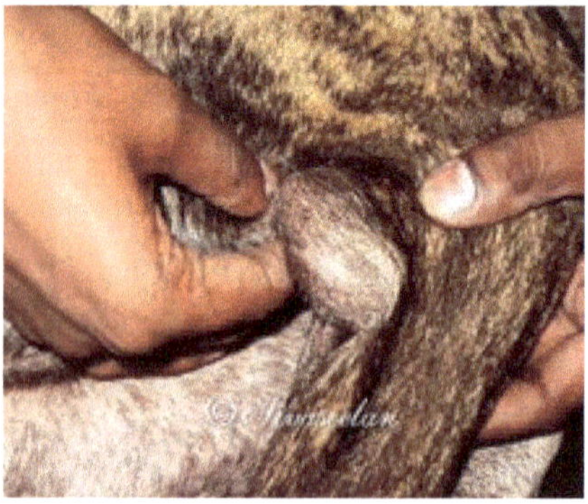

Fig. 42. Pre-crural lymph node.

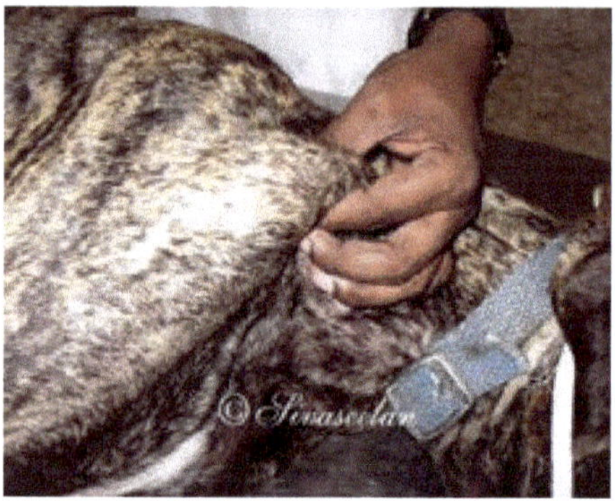

Fig. 43. Pre-scapular lymph node.

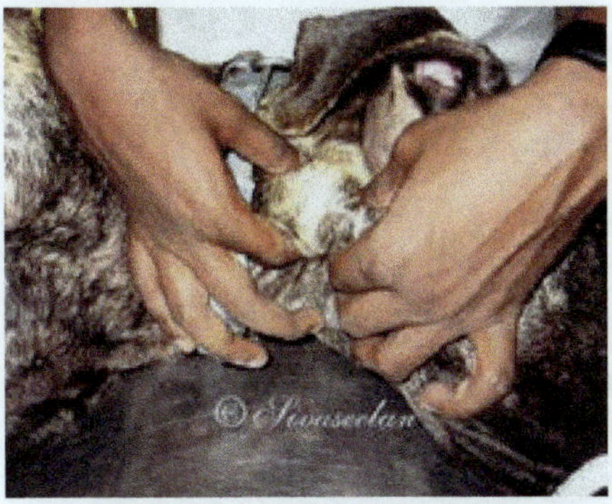

Fig, 44. Sub-mandibular lymph node.

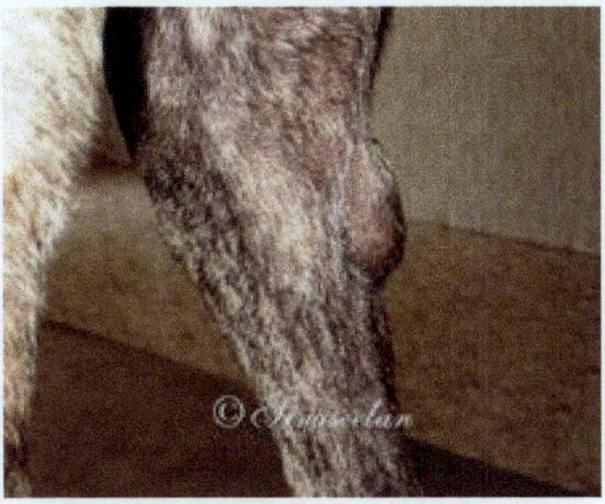

45. Popliteal lymph node.

Fig. 42 – 45. Multicentric lymphoma of a dog.

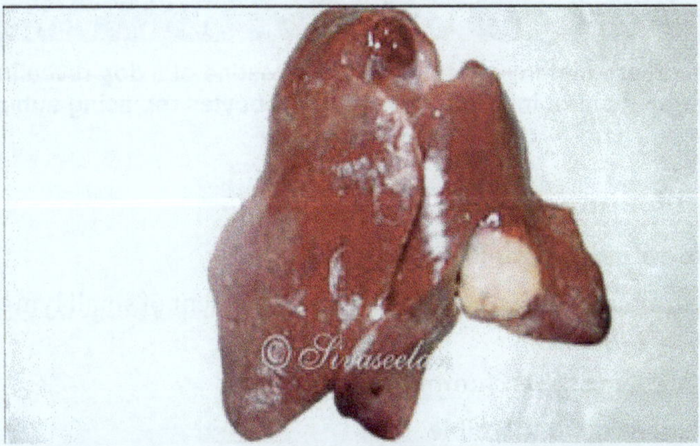

Fig. 46. Solitary lymphoma of the liver of a fowl.

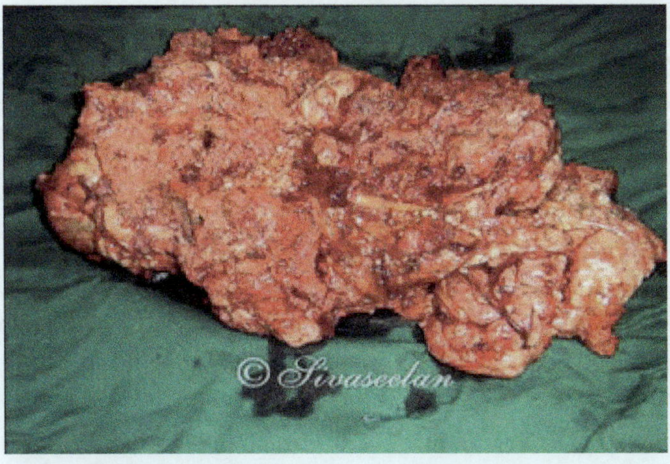

Fig. 47. Multicentric lymphoma of the mesentery of a dog revealing fusion of lymphnodes causing concretion of intestine.

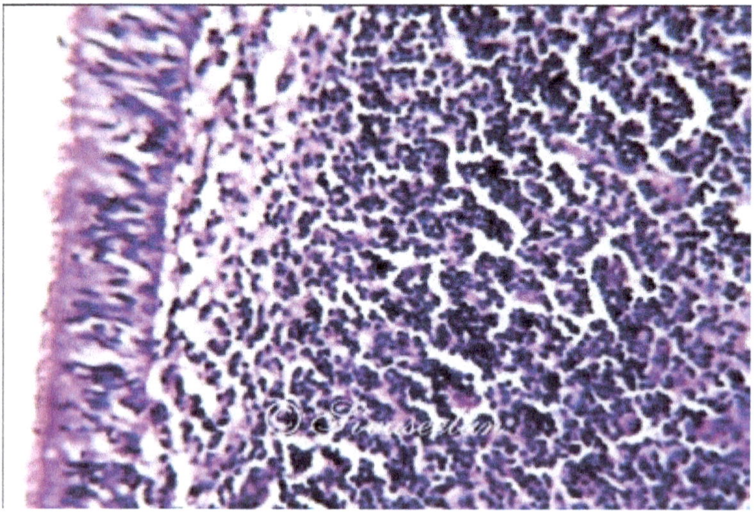

Fig. 48. Well differentiated lymphoma of the intestine of a dog revealing uniform sheet arrangement of infiltrating small lymphocytes replacing sub-mucosal structures.

Histological features

1. Well differentiated lymphoma

- ★ This tumour shows uniform sheet arrangement of small lymphocyte with scanty cytoplasm
- ★ Nuclei often shows clumping of chromatin
- ★ Nucleoli is not discernible
- ★ Few histiocytes with intended nuclei and pale cytoplasm can also be seen

2. Poorly differentiated lymphoma

- ★ Most of the cells are lymphoblasts (immature lymphocytes which is large and ovoid in shape with large nucleus placed eccentrically) often show pleomorphism
- ★ Mitotic figures are commonly noticed
- ★ Few irregular anaplastic cells with variable shape and size can be seen that show multiple angular nucleoli
- ★ Lymphoblast should be differentiated from anaplastic cell. Lymphoblast and its nucleus will maintain its ovoid shape, where as the anaplastic cell will not
- ★ Some of the lymphocytes are phagocytosed by interspersed histiocytes to produce "stary sky" appearance

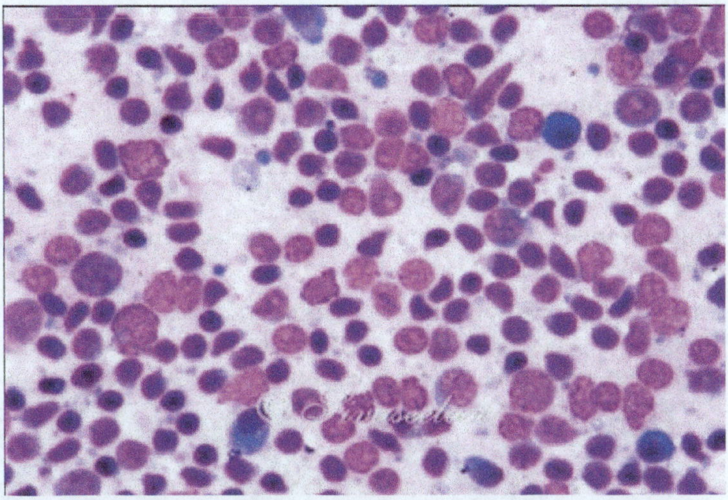

Fig. 49. Poorly differentiated lymphoma of prescapular lymph node of a cow revealing more number of lymphoblasts and few irregular anaplastic cells with multiple angular nucleoli.

3. Intermediate lymphoma

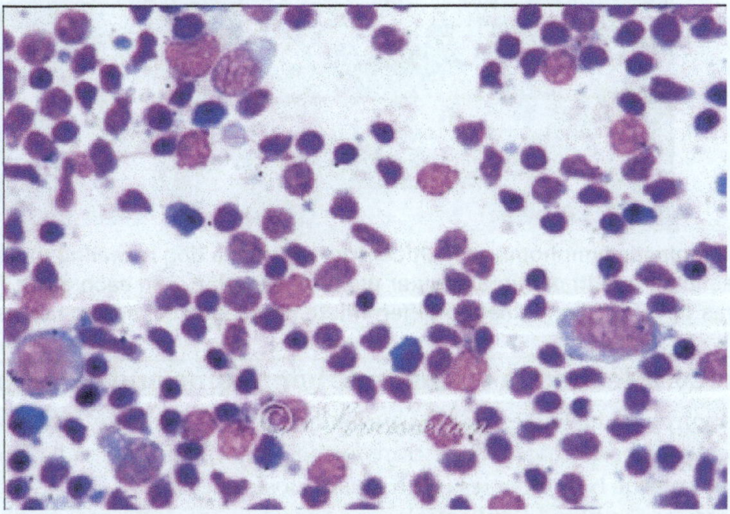

Fig. 50. Intermediate lymphoma of prescapular lymph node of a cow revealing more number of small lymphocytes, few lymphoblasts and rare irregular anaplastic cells with multiple angular nucleoli.

- ★ It is in between well and poorly differentiated lymphomas, and most of the animal lymphomas are of these type
- ★ Uniform sheets containing lymphocytes of various sizes (small, intermediate, large lymphocytes) can be seen

★ Small cells dominate other cell types
★ Few lymphoblasts and rare anaplastic cells can also be observed

4. Anaplastic lymphoma

★ Anaplastic type shows more number of irregular cells
★ Anaplastic cells adhere with each other in most of these type of tumour
★ Multiple nuclei can be seen within the nucleus that are angular is shape in most of the cells
★ Anaplastic lymphosarcomas can be differentiated from other round cell tumours by cytochemical stains and electron microscopy and the same techniques are also useful to differentiate B &T cell lymphomas

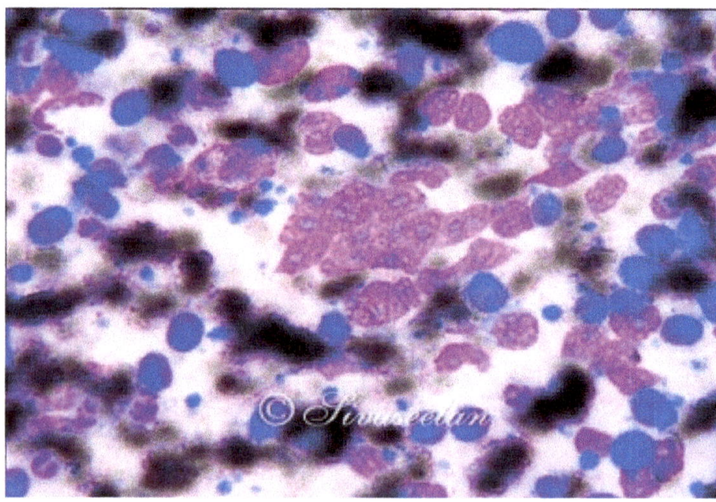

Fig. 51. Anaplastic lymphoma of multicentric origin of a dog revealing more number of anaplastic cells with multiple angular nucleoli adhering with each other. (A special stain was developed and used to differentiate neoplastic cells from normal cells).

Lymphocytic leukemia v_s leukemic lymphoma and lymphocytosis

★ Lymphocytic leukemia is a true leukemia in which the lymphocytic series cells of bone marrow are transformed into neoplastic cells from which neoplastic lymphocytes (with anisocytosis and anisokaryosis) are finding way to the blood (leukemia)
★ This tumour may co-exist with multicentric lymphoma also
★ Leukemic lymphoma is the leukemic phase of lymphoma of lymphnodes and other lymphoid organs. In the terminal phase, in about one third of these type of tumours, neoplastic lymphocytes are moving to the blood to produce leukemia. This phase is called as leukemic leukemia. If tumour is restricted only to lymphoid organs without presence of neoplastic

lymphocyte in the blood, then this condition is known as aleukemic leukemia. It is difficult to distinguish true leukemia from leukemic lymphoma, if the investigation is done at the terminal stage of the disease

★ Lymphocytosis is a condition in which more numbers of lymphocytes are present in the blood, which rarely show atypia (atypical morphology)

Plasma Cell Tumour (Plasma cell myeloma, Multiple myeloma, Plasmacytoma, Ewing's tumour)

★ Plasma cells are modified B lymphocytes meant for production of immunoglobulin that are normally seen in lymphoid organs. They are ovoid cells with bluish cytoplasm and eccentric nucleus where chromatin granules are arranged as clock-dial or cart wheel appearance. Laden immunoglobulin may be seen in the cytoplasm

★ Tumour may arise from these cells

★ This rare tumour occurs in older animals

★ Usually occur in bone marrow with the clinical sign of pain in the affected bones

★ Affected bones may be fractured easily

★ Since the bone marrow is completely replaced by tumour cells in advanced cases, anaemia and weight loss can be observed

★ Multiple radiolucent areas within the bone marrow with or without encroachment to the peripheral compact bone are seen in x-ray (punched out areas)

★ It may also occur in other lymphoid organs also

★ Abnormal protein (immunoglobulin- Bence Jones protein) called as para protein is excreted through urine of human, which is seldom observed in animals

★ Tumours in other visceral organs like liver, spleen and intestine may also occur with or without involving the bone marrow

Gross appearance

★ Focal or diffuse masses within the bone marrow, which sometimes rupture the bone to invade adjacent areas can be seen

★ This tumour grows as a nodular or diffuse reddish grey mass in different visceral organs

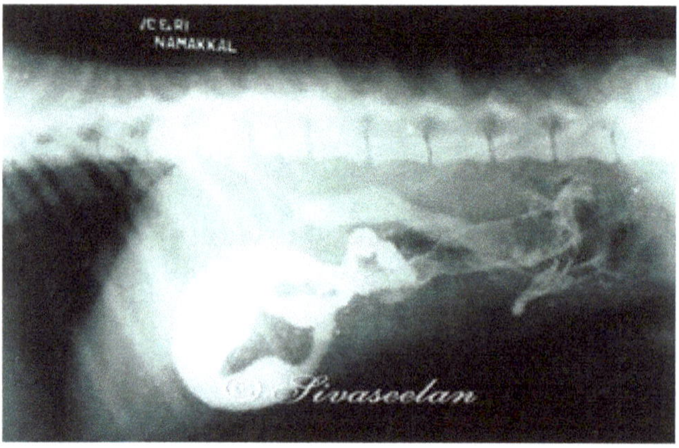

Fig. 52. An abdominal radiograph of a dog showing abnormal thickness of the intestine wall, which was confirmed as plasma cell tumour histopathologically.

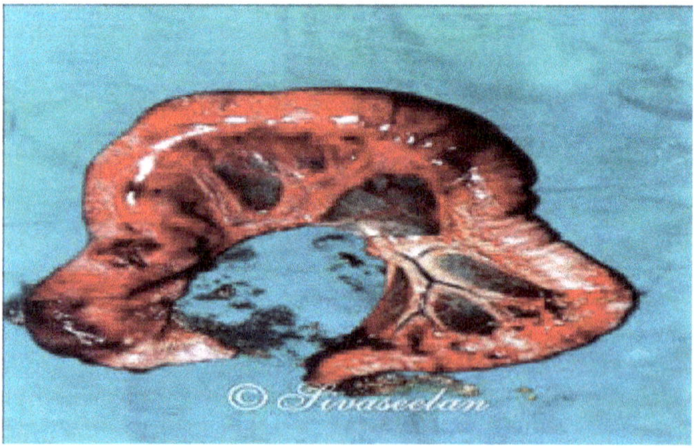

Fig. 53. An excised portion of the affected intestine shown in fig. 52.

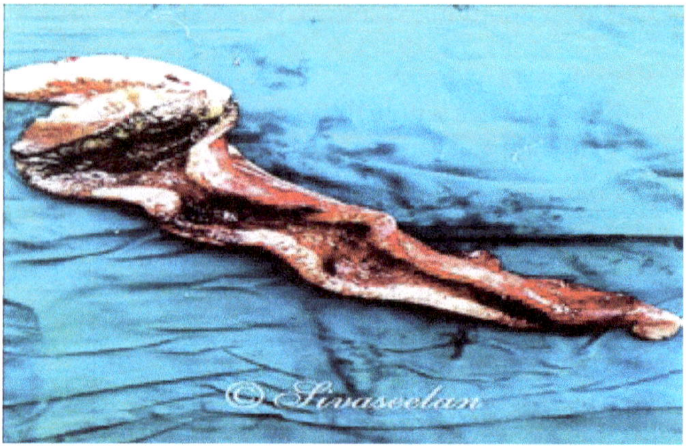

Fig. 54. Cut opened intestine shown in fig. 52 revealing markedly thickened wall.

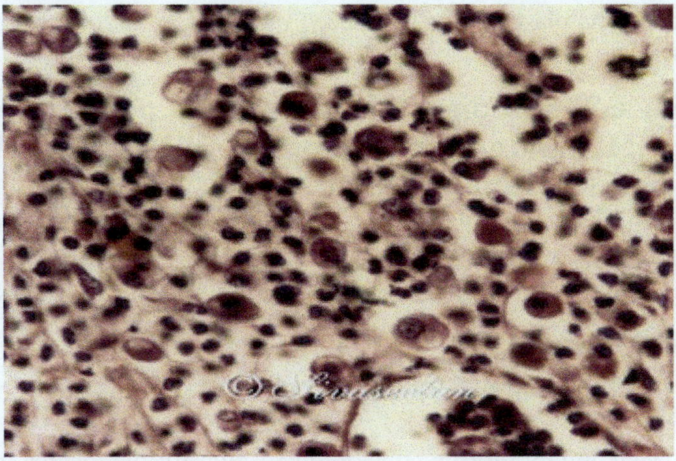

Fig. 55. Plasma cell tumour shown in fig. 53 revealing loosely arranged pleomorphic plasma cells.

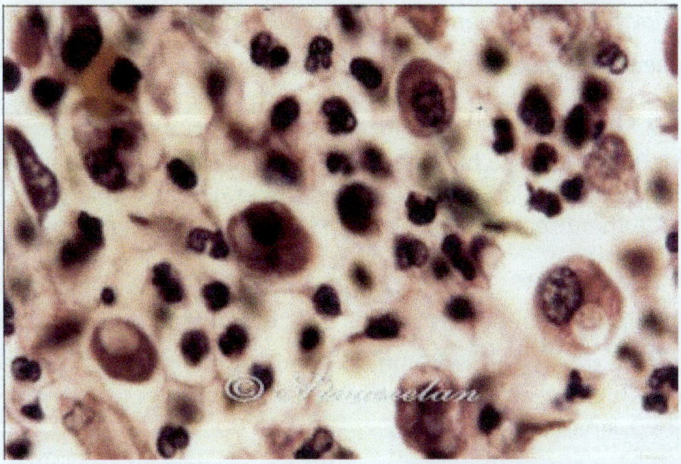

Fig. 56. Plasma cell tumour shown in fig. 54 revealing pleomorphic plasma cells with eccentrically placed nucleus and cytoplasmic immunoglobulin vacuole.

Histological feature

- ★ Tumour reveals pleomorphic plasma cell with eccentric or centrally placed nuclei
- ★ The nuclear chromatin is more homogenous in contrast to the peripherally clumped cartwheel shaped appearance of normal plasma cells
- ★ Basophilic cytoplasm may contain vacuoles
- ★ Eosinophilic secretion (immunoglobins) containing cells can be observed commonly
- ★ Giant cells are rarely seen

- ★ Neoplastic plasma cells have been recorded in peripheral circulation in few cases.

Reticulum cell sarcoma / Mononuclear phagocytic system tumour / Malignant histiocytosis / Histiocytic Medullary Reticulosis / Histiocytic tumour

Supporting cells (histiocytes/macrophages/sinus cells/reticulum cells) of lymphoid organs may involve in neoplasia. In this rare tumour, progressive enlargement of lymphoid organs like lymph nodes, spleen and liver can be seen.

Histological features

- ★ Pleomorphic histiocytic cells with vesicular nucleus dominate the functional lymphocytes
- ★ Nuclear indentation is considered to identify histiocytes even among atypical morphology of these cells
- ★ Phagocytosis of erythrocytes (erythrophagocytosis by neoplastic histiocytes), rarely leucocytes and thrombocytes can be observed
- ★ Anaemia, leucocytopenia and thrombocytopenia may be noticed.

Hodgkin's disease

Hodgkin's like disease has been reported in dog, horse and pigs. Similar to multicentric lymphoma, all peripheral and visceral nodes, spleen and liver show enlargement. Other organs like lung and skin may also reveal multiple growths.

Histological features

- ★ Mixture of lymphocytes, plasma cells, eosinophils and neutrophils are seen
- ★ Reed-Sternberg cells with nuclei of mirror image of each other can be seen. Actually deeply indented nuclei in fastly multiplying cells give impression of two separate nuclei
- ★ Some cells may also depict multiple nuclei and basophilic nucleoli are appreciated within the nucleus
- ★ Local or diffuse presence of fibrous tissue and proliferating fibroblasts are also seen
- ★ Neoplastic cells proliferate fastly to invade almost all organs of the body replacing the original cells, thus causing organ failure
- ★ Apart from lymph nodes, neoplastic cells infiltrate into liver, spleen, heart, stomach, intestine, nerve and brain

Myeloid tumours

These tumours are arising in the bone-marrow from precursors of the granulocytes (myeloblasts/myelocytes of neutrophils/eosinophils/basophils). In later stages, these cells may be found infiltrating into other organs like lymph nodes, spleen, liver, intestine, kidney and other organs. This type of tumour has been reported in the dog, cat, pig, cattle and small ruminants. Eosinophilic enteritis and diarrhoea is commonly seen in eosinophilic leukemia of cat.

Gross appearance

Since the tumour is composed of blast cells of granulocytes, the colour may appear as greenish (**chloroma**), which disappear on exposure to air and reappear on applying hydrogen peroxide. Lymphoid organs show nodular whitish/grayish spots in localised type and the organs enlarge with friable consistency in diffused type.

Histological features

- ★ Myeloid neoplasia may be acute or chronicAcute granulocytic leukemia is characterised by the presence of large numbers of myeloblasts and progranulocytes in the circulation and bone-marrow. This type is known as **progranulocytic or promyelocytic leukemia**
- ★ In chronic type, different stages of development of cells from myeloblasts to well differentiated myelocytes can be observed
- ★ The name **Myelocytic myeloma** can be applied to the well differentiated type of particular series *i.e.* neutrophilic, eosinophilic and basophilic, and they are diagnosed based on their morphology in the blood/bone-marrow smear accounting their enormous numbers and atypia
- ★ If only myeloblasts alone are observed in enormous numbers, the name **Myeoblastic myeloma** can be applied
- ★ Myeloblasts can be identified based on the criteria of large, round or polyhedral cells with prominent round/oval eccentrically placed vesicular nuclei.

Monocytic tumours

Involvement of Monocytic series of cells in the bone-marrow leads to Monocytic leukemia alone or it may also appear along with granulocytic series often. Enormous numbers and atypia, but with nuclear indentation are the criteria for the diagnosis.

Erythroleukemia / Erythremic Myelosis

Neoplastic involvement of erythrocytes has been detected in cats and dogs. In most of the cases granulocytes also show neoplastic changes. Blood and bone-marrow smears reveal more bizarre nucleated cells. Enormous packed cell volume of RBCs is usually seen in all cases.

Avian Leucosis (AL), Marek's Disease (MD) and Reticulo-Endothelial Viral Disease (REVD)

All these three viral diseases exist in birds. Single entity or in combinations have been reported not only in fowl, but also in other birds like quail and turkey. Though Avian leucosis was previously described under four headings of Visceral lymphomatosis, Osteopetrosis, Erythroblastosis and Myelocytosis, now only lymphomatosis alone are observed among birds. Lot of differences between AL and MD were previously listed including age of occurrence and organ of preference, but now even these differences could not be taken into account, owing to the fact that both AL and MD show almost same sort of lesions. Nerve enlargement and ocular defects, if present may be helpful to consider MD, but these lesions are very rarely noticed in the recent year outbreaks. Reticulo-Endothelial Viral Disease almost always occurs with either AL or MD or both.

Histological features

Histological appreciation of cells pertaining to these diseases is also confusing even with the use of special stains. So, grossly and microscopically these diseases altogether should be classified as lymphoproliferative disorder. Molecular techniques like PCR can only confirm these diseases based on the identification of the viral etiological agent(s).

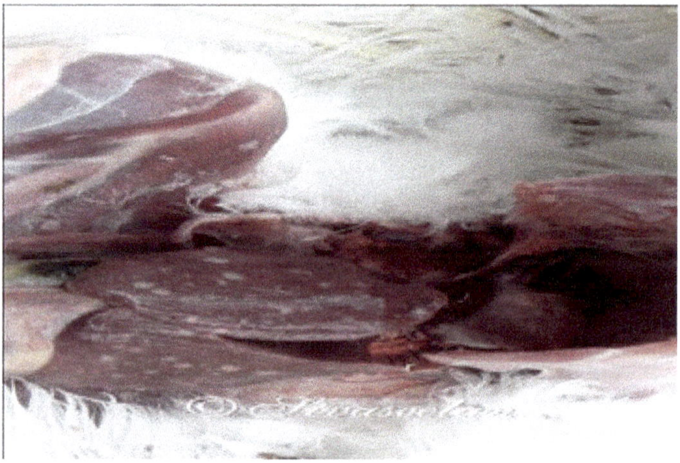

Fig. 57. Avian Leucosis affected liver of a chicken revealing multiple foci of studded tumours without elevating from the surface of the organ.

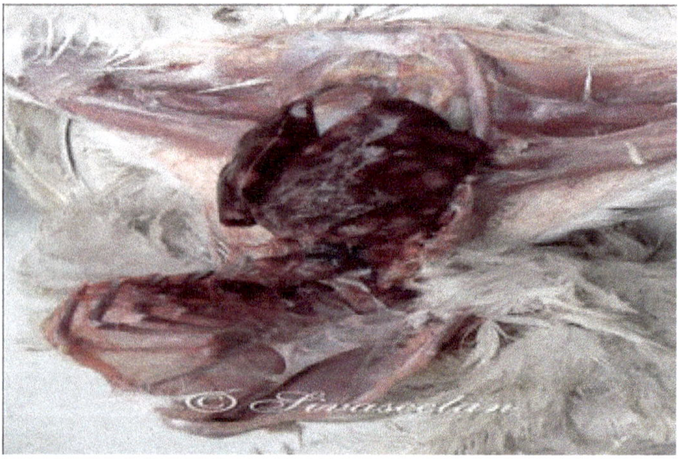

Fig. 58. Avian Leucosis affected liver of a turkey revealing multiple foci of tumours elevating from the surface of the organ.

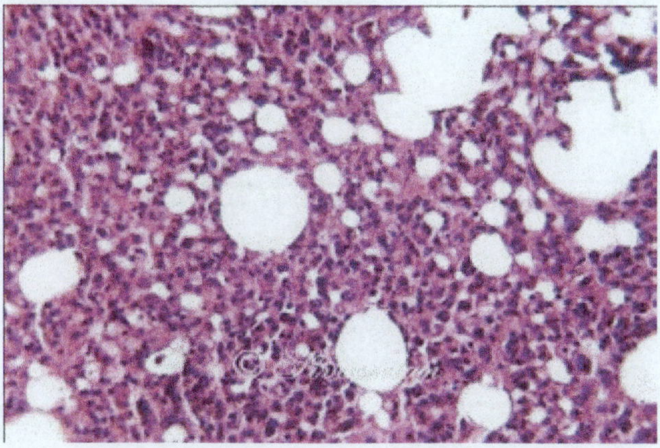

Fig. 59. Avian Leucosis affected lung of a chicken revealing infiltration of neoplastic lymphocytes in the interstitial areas.

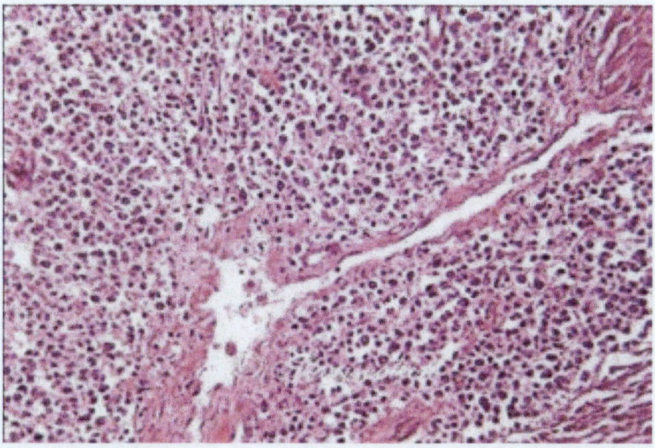

Fig. 60. Avian Leucosis affected uterus of a chicken revealing infiltration of neoplastic lymphocytes in the myometrium replacing the normal sturctures.

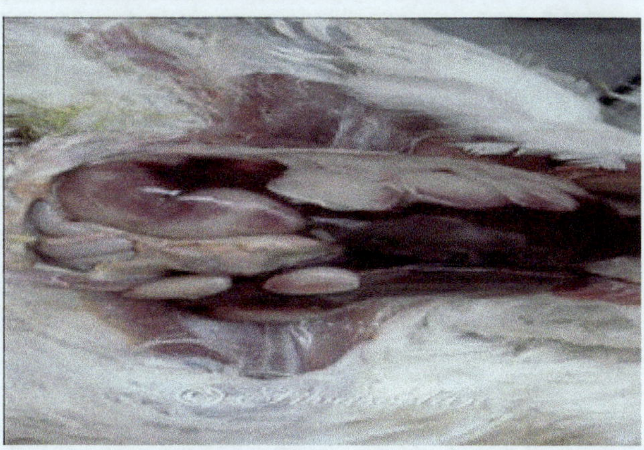

Fig. 61. Marek's Disease affected liver of a chicken revealing multiple elevated nodular growths resembling fat deposits.

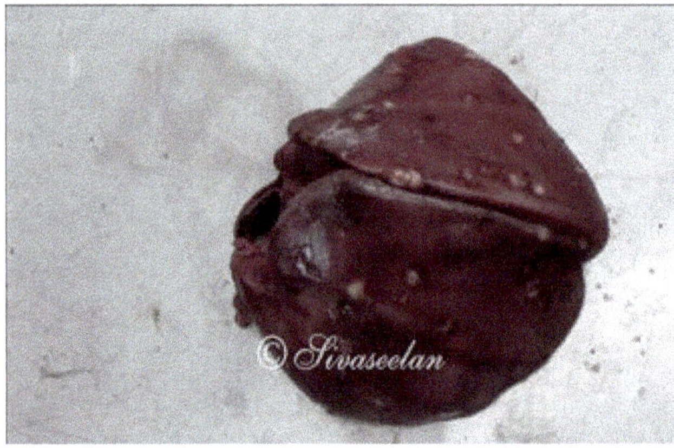

Fig. 62. Marek's Disease affected liver of a chicken revealing multiple studded growths without elevating from the surface.

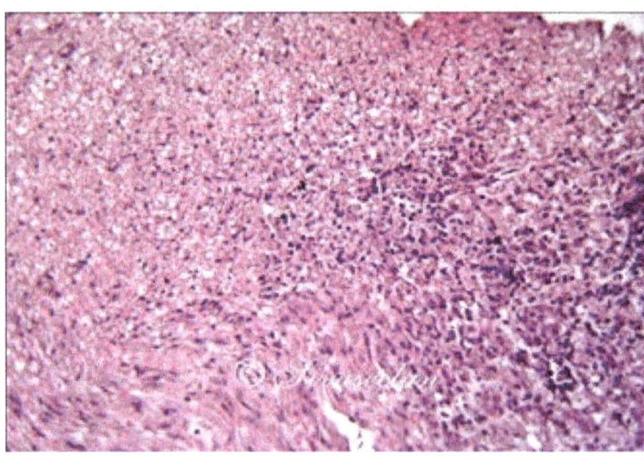

Fig. 63. Marek's Disease affected peripheral nerve of a chicken revealing Infiltration of lymphocytes.

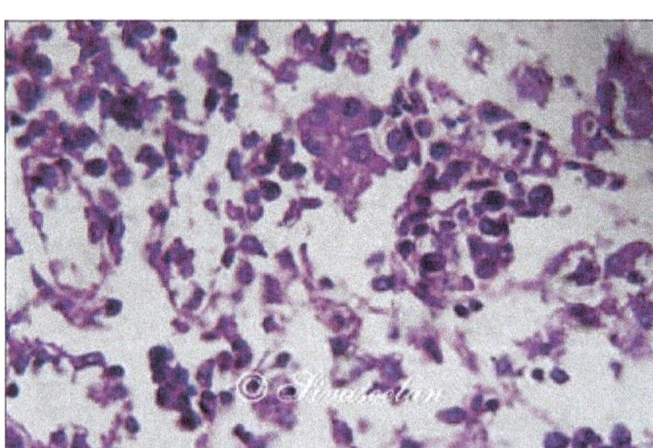

Fig. 64. Marek's Disease affected liver of a chicken revealing infiltration of lymphocytes and MD cell.

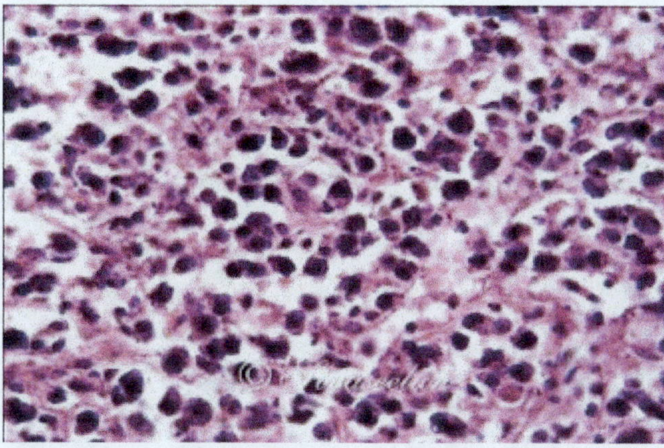

Fig. 65. Marek's Disease affected Bursa of a chicken revealing infiltration of pleomorphic lymphocytes.

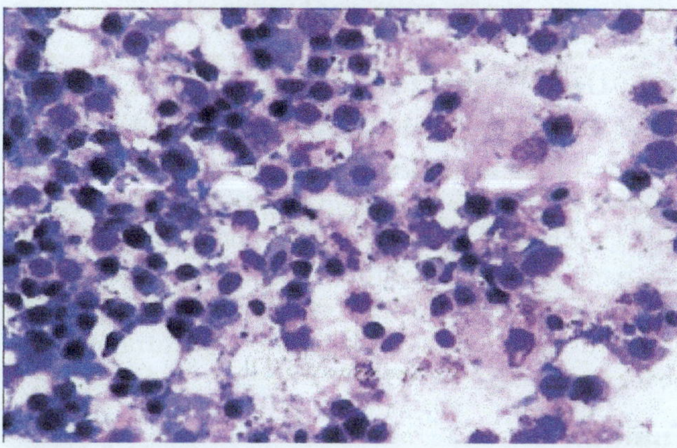

Fig. 66. Cytology of Marek's Disease affected liver of a chicken revealing pleomorphic lymphocytes.

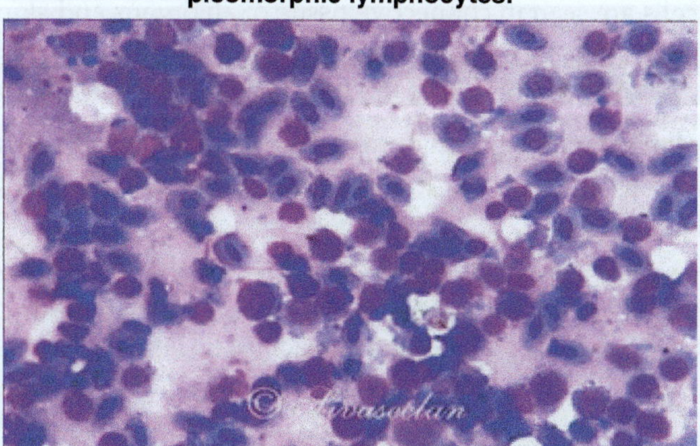

Fig. 67. Cytology of Marek's Disease affected kidney of a chicken revealing pleomorphic lymphocytes.

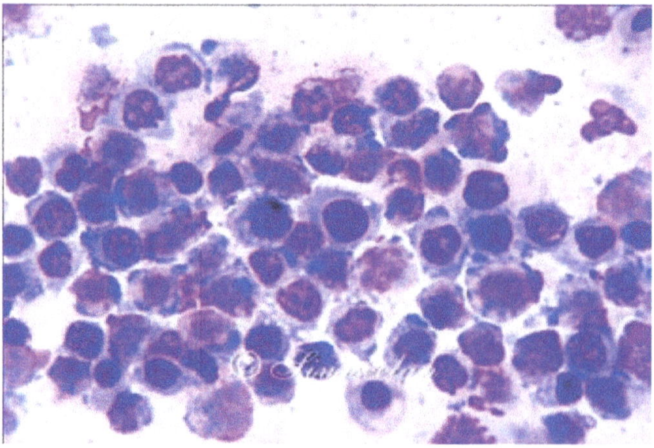

Fig. 68. Cytology of Marek's Disease affected hair follicle of a fowl revealing almost same size lymphocytes.

Megakaryocytic Myelosis / Megakaryocytic Leukemia / Malignant Megakaryocytosis / Thrombocytic leukemia

Megakaryocytic / Thrombocytic cell abnormal proliferation in the bone-marrow and other haemopoietic system results in this type of leukemia. Bizarre type of megakaryocytes including small/blast (dwarf) cells with round nucleus (no nuclear lobulations) and giant platelets with multiple lobulations are seen in the circulation. High platelet count of more than a million / µl can be observed. Since neoplastic platelets cannot participate in blood coagulation, post-traumatic haemorrhage is common in the affected dogs.

Mast Cell Tumour

- ★ Mast cells are analogue of basophils of blood
- ★ The cells are seen in connective tissue of all organs and skin
- ★ They are spherical or fusiform cells with round or ovoid non-lobulated nucleus when compared to lobulated basophils
- ★ They have intracytoplasmic granules, which contain heparin and histamine
- ★ Heparin is acidic and responsible for metachromasia with toluidine blue or Giemsa stain
- ★ Immature cells have many tiny granules with lesser heparin, which stain bluish whereas fully matured cells have larger few granules with more heparin to exhibit pink colour (metachromasia)

Incidence

- ★ Older dogs are commonly affected
- ★ Other animals show lesser incidences
- ★ Skin is the commonest site, but can be seen in other organs also

Clinical characteristics

Since proliferating neoplastic cells produce more heparin, which circulate in blood leads to defective blood coagulation (prolonged blood coagulation time). So, blood mixed excretions and secretions are commonly noticed in the affected individual.

Gross appearance

★ Occur as a cutaneous nodules ranging from 1-10 cm in diameter

★ Very rarely, this tumour appears as poorly demarcated skin swelling

★ Fastly growing tumour may invade into the below lying musculature

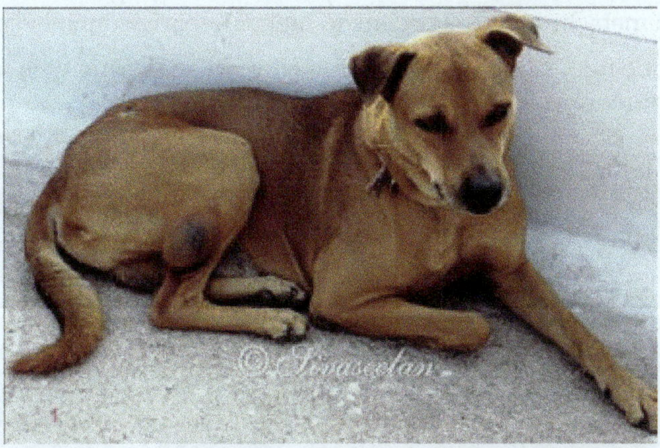

Fig. 69. A Mast cell tumour on the thigh region of leg of a dog.

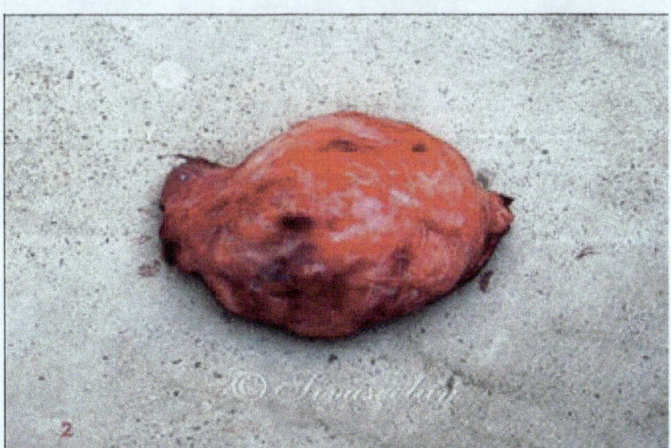

Fig. 70. Removed mast cell tumour shown in fig. 69 revealing non-encapsulation and invasion into the muscle.

Histological feature

★ Histologically, mast cell tumour is classified as grade I (well differentiated type), grade II (intermediate type) and grade III (poorly differentiated type/anaplastic type)

- ★ Clinically, severity increases with grade
- ★ Grade I shows uniform cells with distinct cytoplasmic borders and grade II reveals moderate pleomorphism of cells and indistinct cytoplasmic borders
- ★ Both grade I and II reveal enormous number of tiny/dust like cytoplasmic granules that stain blue with metachromatic stain due to lesser heparin content
- ★ In grade I, loosely arranged cells are divided by collagen bundles. Cells may also be arranged as cords or nests
- ★ Grade III reveals highly pleomorphic cells with indistinct cytoplasmic borders and the cells show only a few matured granules that stain pink with metachromatic stain due to higher heparin content
- ★ Mitotic figures are rarely observed, but in anaplastic type mitotic figures are numerous

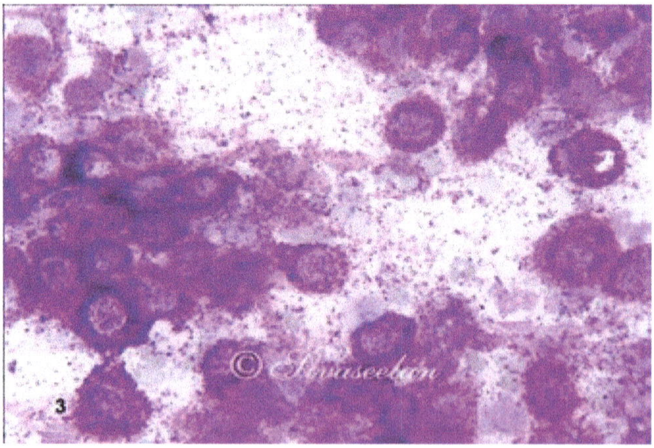

Fig. 71. Cytology of the mast cell tumour shown in fig. 69 revealing enormous number of granules in the cytoplasm of the cells under Giemsa staining.

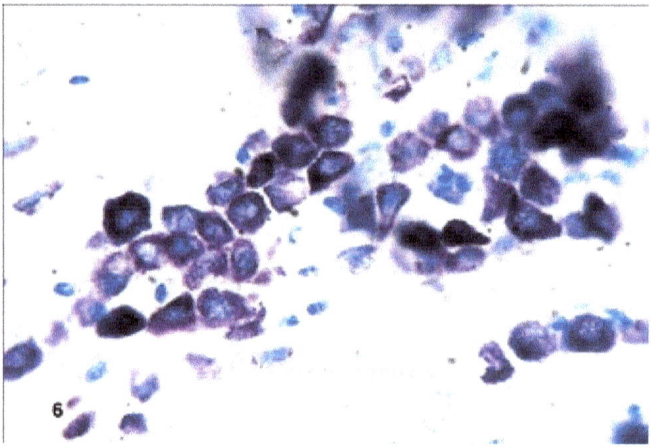

Fig. 72. Cytology of the mast cell tumour shown in fig. 69 revealing enormousnumber of metachromatically stained granules in the cytoplasm of the cells under Toluidine blue staining.

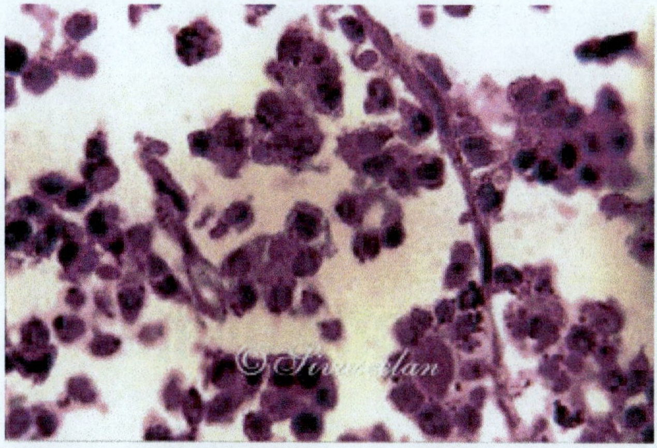

Fig. 73. Poorly differentiated type (grade III) mast cell tumour of the skin of a dog revealing pleomorphic cells with indistinct cytoplasmic borders and the cytoplasm contains only a few large granules .

11

Mesothelioma

Mesothelioma arises from mesothelial layers of visceral organs like liver, spleen, outer layer of intestine and the serosal layer that lines the three main coelomic cavities (pleura, peritoneum, pericardium). Mesothelial cells resemble squamous epithelium or endothelium and rest on a thin basement membrane supported by a thin strand of connective tissue to form membrane like supporting structure from which Mesothelioma may arise. Normal mesothelial cells cannot be seen microscopically, if cut crossly. Since they are occurring on the serosal, transcoelomic spread is common.

Gross appearance

- ⋆ They are small, discrete and nodular structures measuring about 1-5 cm in diameter
- ⋆ Multiple Mesothelioma of peritoneum often resemble pearly disease (peritoneal tuberculosis)
- ⋆ Cauliflower like fissures can also seen on some tumours
- ⋆ The colour varies from grey to red
- ⋆ Growth of tumour is restricted to serosal layer most of the times.
- ⋆ Cut surface often show no evidence of infiltration into the underlying tissue

Histological feature

- ⋆ The tumour mimics papilloma
- ⋆ Neoplastic mesothelial cells, which resemble cuboidal epithelial cells cover the papillary projection of fibrous tissue with collagen and fibroblast
- ⋆ Thin walled blood vessels, metaplastic cartilages, osteoid may be seen in the fibrous core
- ⋆ Tree like branching type can also be observed, in which fibrous core branches are covered by cuboidal epithelium

12

Epithelial Tumours

Tumours may arise from both glandular and non glandular epithelium. These are classified as:

Benign

1. Squamous papilloma arising from stratified squamous epithelium
2. Fibrous papilloma arising from epithelium and connective tissue
3. Adenoma arising from secretary epithelium
4. Polyp is a nodular outgrowth arising from non glandular lining or surface epithelium

Malignant

1. Squamous cell carcinoma arising from squamous epithelium
2. Adenocarcinoma arising from secretary or glandular epithelium

Papilloma

It may arise from epithelial surface of non secretary epithelium (squamous or transitional or columnar epithelial cells). Young animals of all species are most affected. Breed or sex predisposition are not noticed.

Etiology

★ Papilloma virus is causing this tumour in many of the animal species. This virus is a member of PaPoVa DNA virus, which is host specific except Bovine papilloma virus, which can cross infect other species also

★ Bovine papilloma virus is also having the ability to cause fibropapilloma, but other papilloma viruses can induce only squamous papilloma

★ Bovine papilloma virus, in addition to cutaneous papilloma, it can induce intestinal, bladder and meningeal tumours. It can cause meningioma and chondroma in laboratory animals

★ Cutaneous papilloma may regress spontaneously after certain period due to development of immunity

- ★ In papilloma, the virus can be demonstrated by Electron microscopy, Immunoperoxidase test and PCR techniques

Gross appearance

- ★ Common sites of occurrence are skin, oral mucosa, gastro-intestinal and genital tract, and mammary duct
- ★ In ruminants and horses, papilloma are usually multiple, whereas in dogs, it is usually solitary
- ★ Shape varies from nodular to cauliflower like and the attachment may be pedunculated or broad based
- ★ Large size tumours may ulcerate

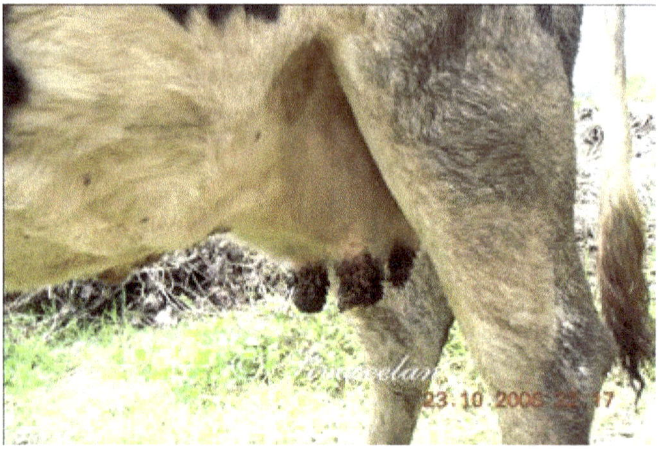

Fig. 74: Bovine Cutaneous Papilloma – Teat. Multiple papillomatous warts on the teat of a milch cow.

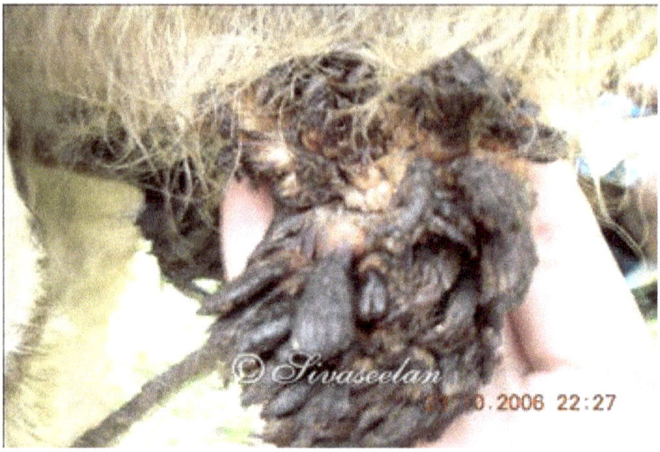

Fig. 75: Bovine Cutaneous Papilloma – Teat. Mutilated teat due to multiple warts.

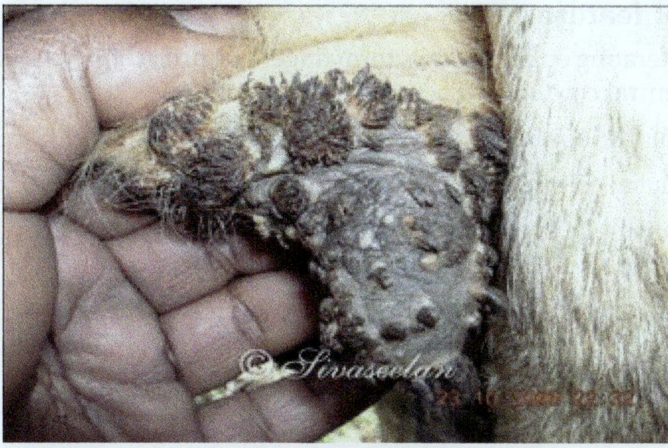

Fig. 76: Bovine Cutaneous Papilloma – Teat. Spontaneous regression of tumour shown in fig. 75.

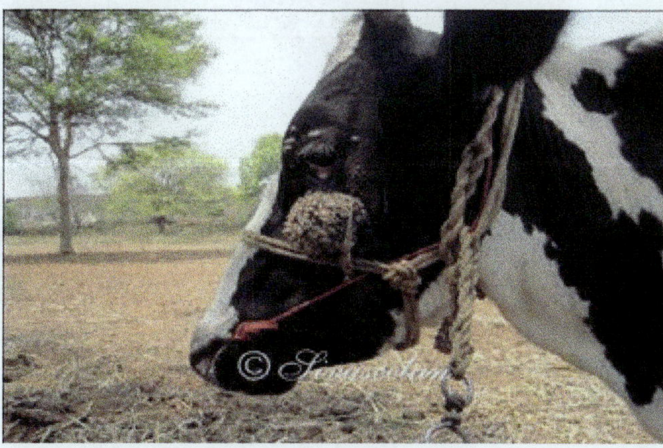

Fig. 77: Bovine Cutaneous Papilloma. Multiple tumours collectively forming a cauliflower like appearance.

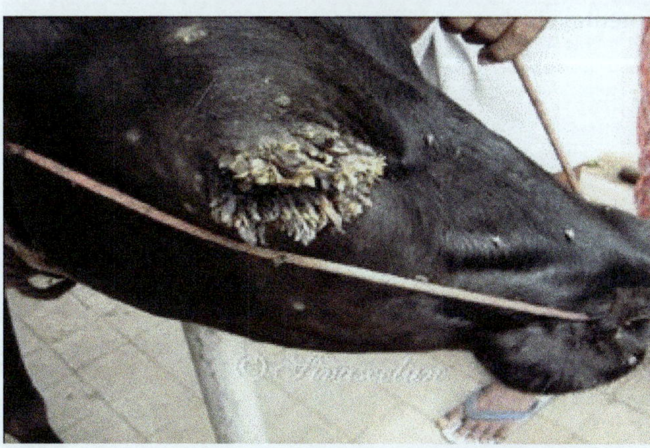

Fig. 78: Bovine Cutaneous Papilloma. Multiple warts arising from both eyelids of a cow masking the vision.

Histological feature

- ★ Proliferating epithelial cells form finger like projection (papillae) supported by central core of connective tissue with blood vessels
- ★ Neoplastic epithelial cells are covered by hyperkeratotic epidermis
- ★ Epithelial cells near the tip of projection will show more proliferation
- ★ Stratum spinosum and granulosum layers show cytoplasmic vacuolation indicating degenerative changes
- ★ Proliferating cells will not enter into dermis, which differentiate it from malignant type (squamous cell carcinoma)

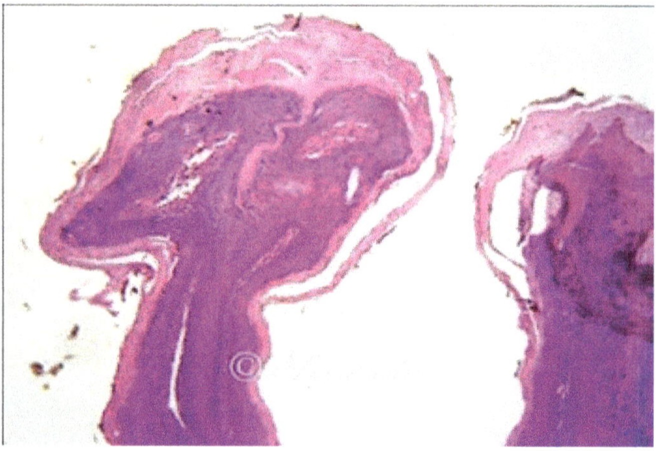

Fig. 79: Papilloma showing proliferating cutaneous epithelial cells forming finger like growth covered by hyperkeratotic layer.

Note

Bovine papilloma virus induced papilloma tissue can be stored in 50 % glycerol-saline at 4°C for several months without loss of infectivity and can be used for further experimental study.

13

Squamous Cell Carcinoma

It is a malignant tumour of squamous and stratified squamous epithelium. This is a common neoplasm, which affects aged animals regardless of species and sex.

Etiology

Action of Papilloma virus, which is activated by UV rays in non pigmented areas of the skin and mucosa is suspected.

Sites

- ★ The mucocutaneous junction is the commonest site in horse and cattle apart from other regions of non-pigmented skin (nasal mucosa, pinna, lips, eyelids, conjunctiva and horn core)
- ★ Tumours can also be seen in pigmented skin

Gross appearance

- ★ Varying shapes of nodular to cauliflower like growth are seen
- ★ The surface ulcerate and bleeds easily
- ★ Slowly growing tumours are horny in consistency

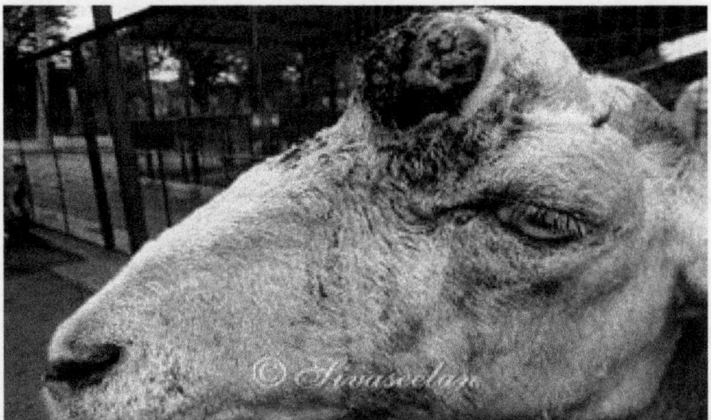

Fig. 80: Squamous cell carcinoma on the head of a sheep revealing ulceration and bleeding.

Ocular squamous cell carcinoma

This occurs in older animals, especially in cattle. Hereford breed in U.S. is the most susceptible breed due to poor pigmentation around eyes.

Etiology

A virus, which is activated by UV rays of sun light is suspected.

Site

About 75 % of the incidences are found on the bulbar conjunctiva and cornea, and about 25 % on the eyelid conjunctiva, membrane nictitans and outer skin of eyelids.

Gross appearance and histological feature

The four different forms of this tumour are

1. Plaque
2. Papilloma
3. Non-invasive carcinoma
4. Invasive carcinoma

1. Plaque

This is often seen in limbus area (junction of cornea and sclera) as a round or oval shaped nodular growth with white smooth surface. Microscopically, the picture varies from hyperplastic changes of epithelium to papilloma.

2. Papilloma

Hard spine like multiple projections of variable sizes resembling the shape of cauliflower or mushroom with narrow stalk are often found on corneum. Microscopically it is a squamous papilloma.

3. Non-invasive Carcinoma

This type may develop from the previous varieties (plaque and papilloma type). These tumours resemble papilloma. Microscopically, the picture is non invasive malignant neoplasm characterised by anisocytosis and anisokaryosis with mitotic figures and loss of polarity.

4. Invasive Carcinoma

This is a large growth, which may replace the entire eyeball. It may arise from conjunctiva, membrane nictitans or cornea. Ulceration and haemorrhages are commonly seen. Microscopically, It is a typical squamous cell carcinoma.

Metastasis

and papilloma types are benign. So these can be removed without recurrence. Carcinoma type may metastasize to regional lymph nodes and lungs.

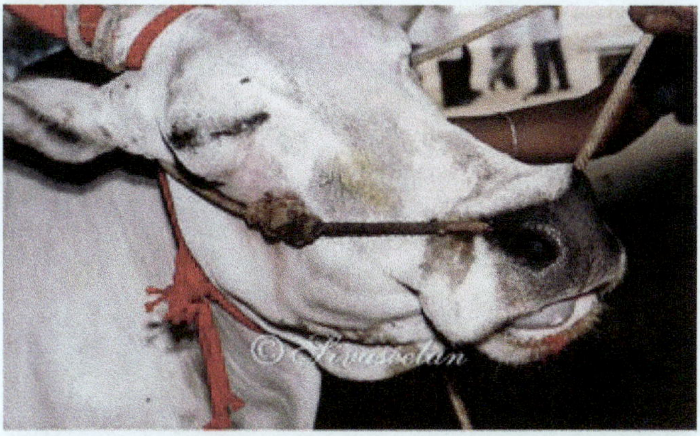

Fig. 81: Squamous cell carcinoma of the eye of a bullock causing fusion of eyelids.

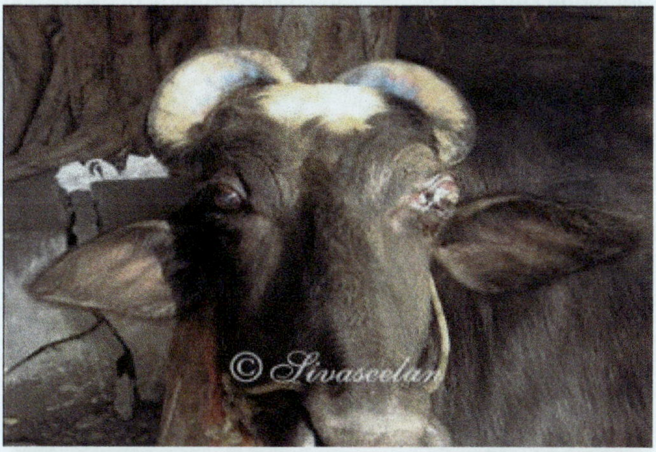

Fig. 82: Squamous cell carcinoma of the cornea portion of eye of a buffalo.

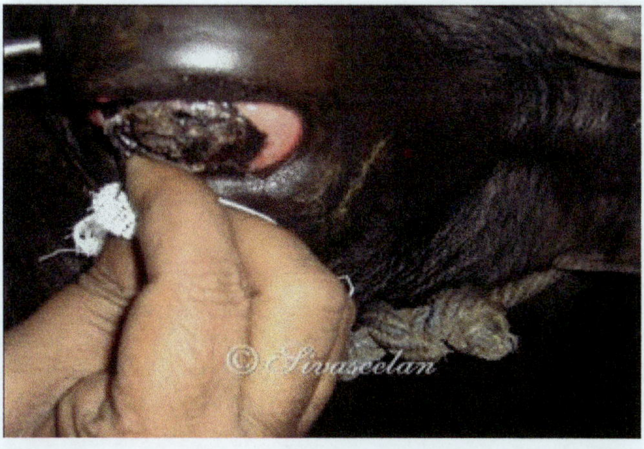

Fig. 83: Closure view of the tumour shown in fig. 81depicting total destruction of cornea.

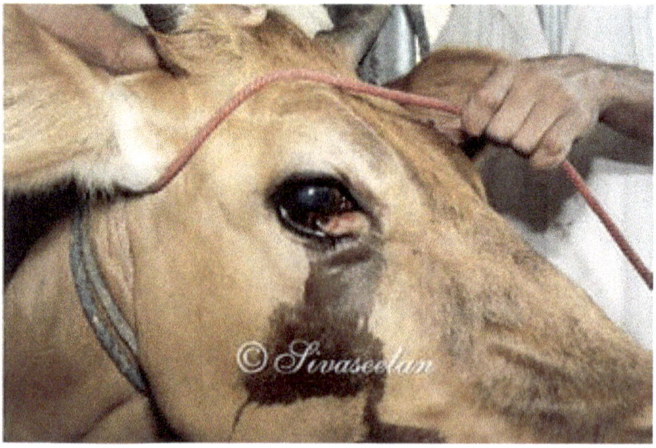

Fig. 84: Squamous cell carcinoma of the inner-canthus of eye of a Jersey cow.

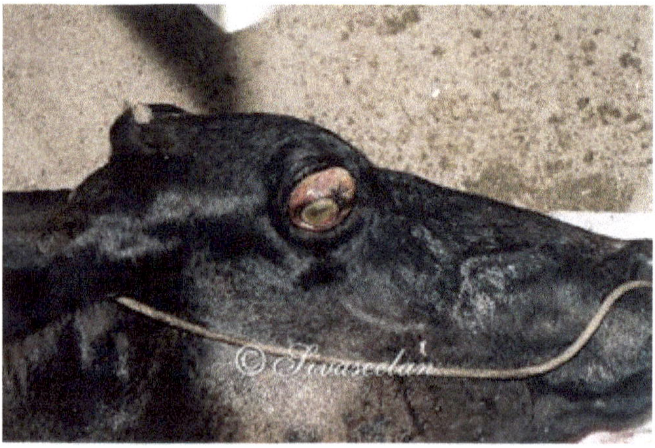

Fig. 85: Squamous cell carcinoma of the sclera portion of eye of a cow.

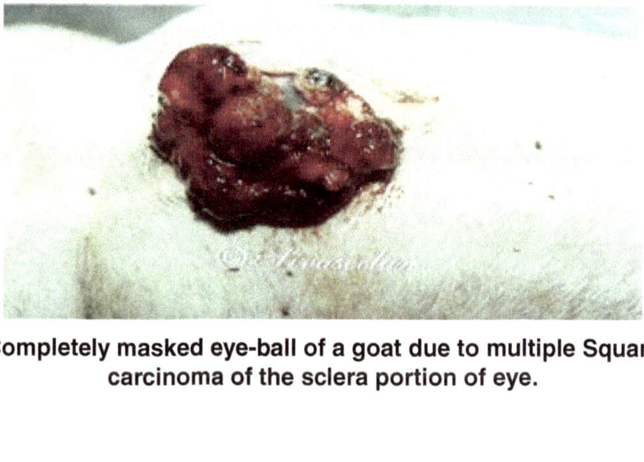

Fig. 86: Completely masked eye-ball of a goat due to multiple Squamous cell carcinoma of the sclera portion of eye.

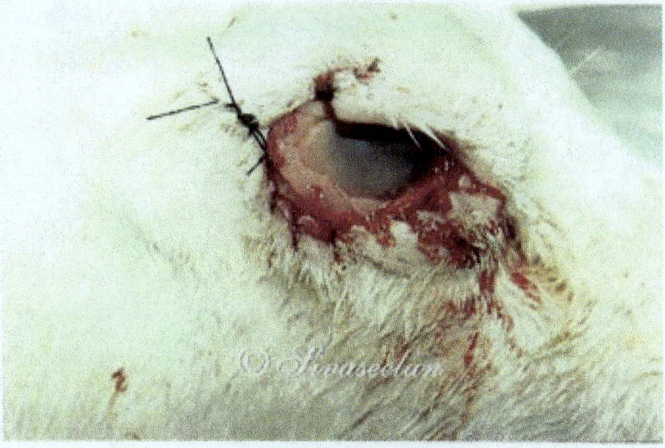

Fig. 87: Squamous cell carcinoma affected eye shown in fig. 86 after surgical removal of tumours.

Histological features

- ★ Proliferating squamous epithelial cells form cell nests (irregular cords of epidermal cells) with centrally placed keratin pearls
- ★ Stratum spinosum (prickle cell layer with intercellular bridges) is the major cell involving in neoplastic changes, which acts as a seed for cell nests
- ★ Proliferating prickle cells give rise to strata of stratum granulosum, stratum lucidum and stratum corneum (keratin producing layer), which are concentrically arranged to make cell nests with prickle cells at the periphery and keratinocytes as inner most layer that produces keratin pearls
- ★ In highly proliferating type (poorly differentiated type) keratin pearls cannot be seen within the cell nests due to non formation of stratum corneum from other layers
- ★ Proliferating cells enter into the dermis and subcutis
- ★ In anaplastic type, epidermal cells are elongated, which mimic fibrosarcoma, but the presence of inter-cellular bridges of prickle cells will help to differentiate
- ★ Fine Needle Aspiration Cytology will help to distinguish squamous cell carcinoma from inflammatory swelling. In inflammatory swelling, in addition to inflammatory cells, normal flat squamous cells with tiny nucleus can be observed, whereas in squamous cell carcinoma, anisocytosis, anisokaryosis and poikilokaryosis are appreciated

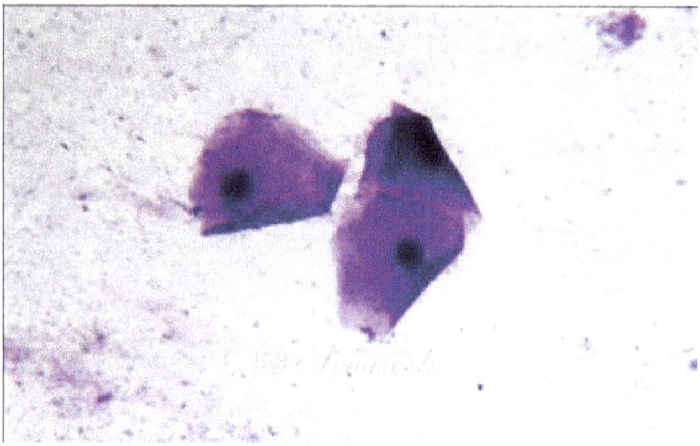

Fig. 88: FNAC smear of non-tumour mass showing normal squamous epithelial cells with uniformly tiny nucleus.

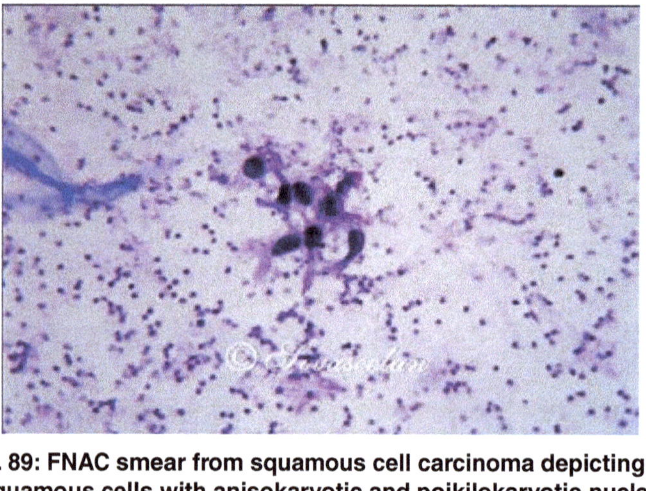

Fig. 89: FNAC smear from squamous cell carcinoma depicting neoplastic squamous cells with anisokaryotic and poikilokaryotic nuclei.

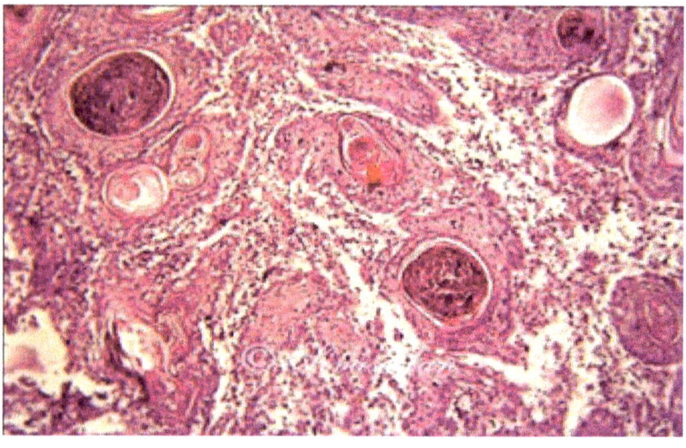

Fig. 90: Squamous cell carcinoma of the eye revealing cell nests with keratin pearls. Almost equal proportion of cell nest and pearl indicates moderately proliferating tumour.

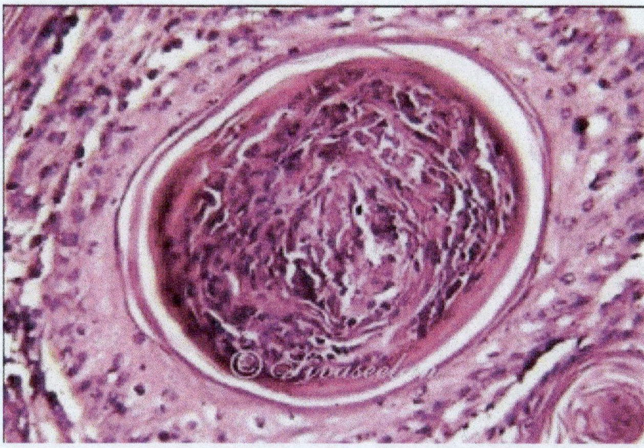

Fig. 91: Magnified view of single cell nest with keratin pearl.

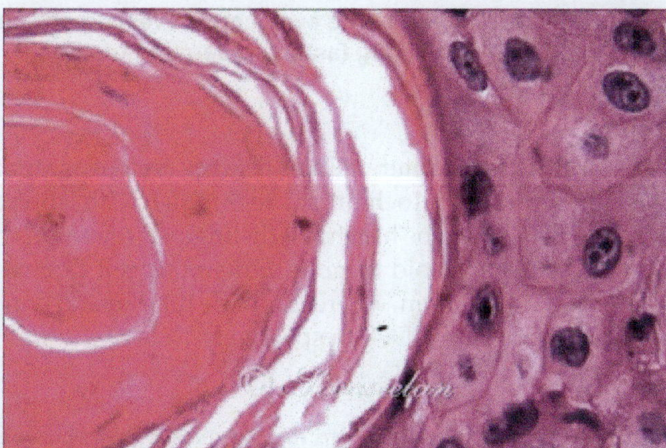

Fig. 92: Highly magnified cell nest and pearl revealing the neoplastic squamous cells with enlarged nucleus. Multiple angular nucleoli are also seen within nucleus.

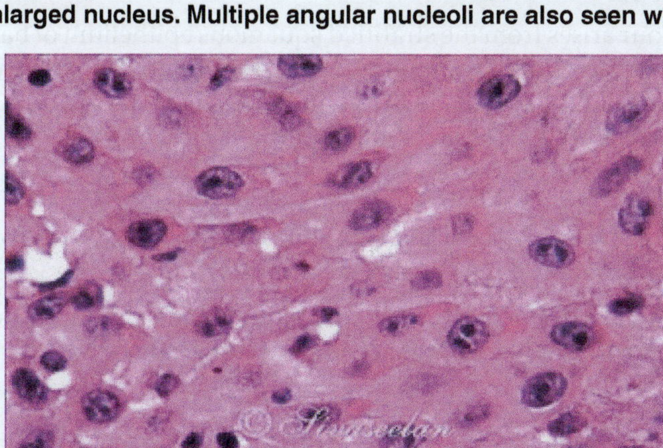

Fig. 93: Neoplastic squamous cells (prickle cells) of a cell nest revealing typical intercellular bridges and anisokaryosis with multiple angular nucleoli.

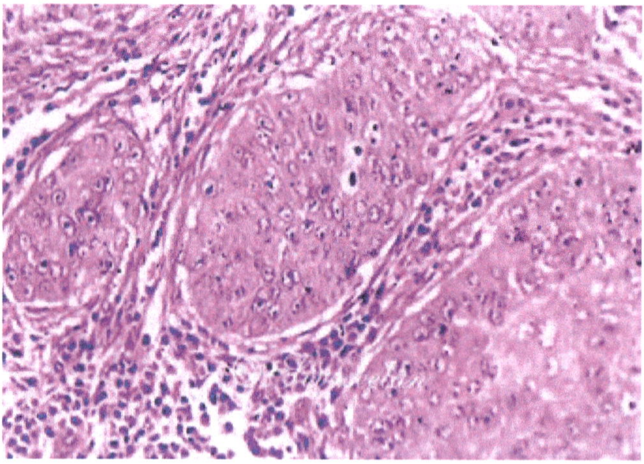

Fig. 94: Squamous cell carcinoma of the eye of cow revealing cell nests without keratin pearl indicating fastly proliferating tumour.

Note:

In highly anaplastic type, if inter-cellular bridges are not ascertained between prickle cells, use of immunohistochemical technique with antibodies against cytokeratin, actin and CD-45 will be helpful to distinguish squamous cell carcinoma from muscle tumour and lymphoid tumour. Squamous cell carcinoma will yield positive response only to cytokeratin, whereas muscle tumour and lymphoid tumour will yield positivity to actin and CD-45 respectively.

Metastasis

It is locally invasive and metastasis to regional lymph nodes is seldom seen.

Horn Cancer

This tumour arises from the stratified squamous epithelium of base of the horn or mucus membrane lining the frontal sinus. This tumour occurs in about 1% of cattle population in India. This is the commonest tumour found in Indian cattle. Bilateral occurrence has also been reported.

Etiology

- ★ Paring of horns for beautification, chronic yoke friction of working bullock are considered as the predisposing causes
- ★ UV radiation acting especially in castrated bulls (bullocks) is suspected to induce virus, which might act as an exciting cause

Symptoms

Affected animal often shakes its head due to irritation and pain, the horn tilt to a side and horn avulsion occurs exposing the tumour.

Gross appearance

- ★ Growth of varying sizes and shapes (nodular to cauliflower like) is seen
- ★ It is pinkish in colour, friable and bleeds easily
- ★ Growing mass may invade the frontal sinus and may even ramify the cranial bone

Histological feature

Microscopically, typical squamous cell carcinoma can be appreciated.

Metastasis

Recurrence is common with rare metastasis.

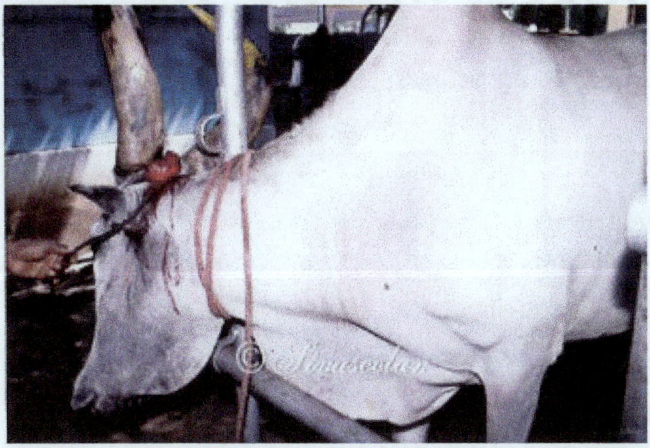

Fig. 95: Squamous cell carcinoma arising from the horn of a bullock (horn cancer) showing tendency to bleed easily.

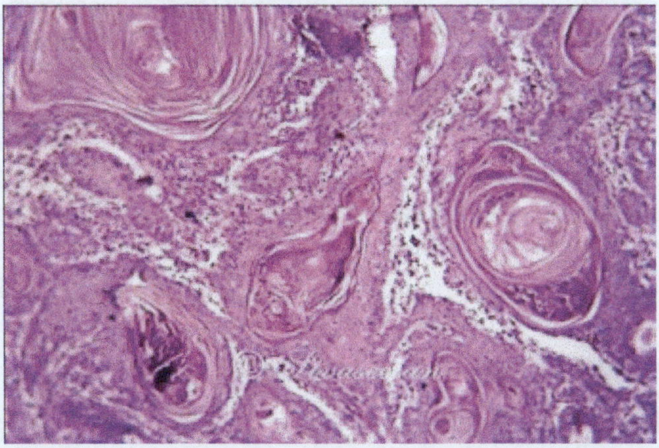

Fig. 96: Squamous cell carcinoma of the horn shown in fig. 95 depicting lesser cellular component than pearl indication slowly proliferating tumour.

14

Basal Cell Tumour (Basal Cell Carcinoma)

Synonyms

- ★ Rodent ulcer
- ★ Jacob's ulcer
- ★ Hair matrix carcinoma
- ★ Basaloid tumour

Gross appearance

- ★ Common in aged dogs and cats
- ★ Usually solitary, but multiple cases also occur
- ★ Commonly found on dermis, sub cutis and ranges from 0.5-10 cm in diameter
- ★ Surface skin is often ulcerated (rodent ulcer)

Histological feature

- ★ Basal cells originate from undifferentiated generative cells or small uniform cells with prominent oval nuclei and relatively little cytoplasm, which differentiate into the cells of hair follicles, sebaceous gland and sweat glands
- ★ When these basal cells involve in neoplastic changes, they lack cytoplasmic borders, which are normally seen

Based on the histological feature, four types are observed.

1. Solid Basal Cell Tumour

- ★ Proliferating basal cells are forming islands of cellular masses of variable sizes
- ★ In the outer layers of island, the basal cell nuclei are pallisading, but in the inner layers, nuclei are haphazardly arranged

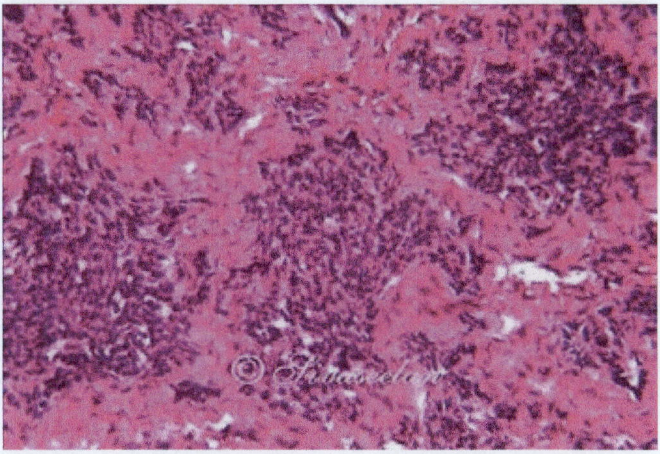

Fig. 97: Solid type of basal cell tumour revealing islands of cellular masses of variable sizes. The cells are indistinguishable from each other due to prominent nuclei and scanty cytoplasm.

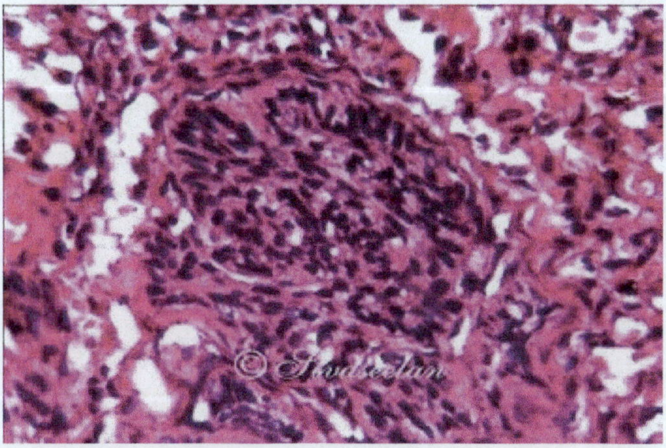

Fig. 98: In the outer layers of an island, the basal cell nuclei are pallisading, but in the inner layers, nuclei are haphazardly arranged.

2. Cystic Basal Cell Tumour

★ This type resemble the solid basal cell tumour, but the neoplastic basal cells encompass the cystic spaces

★ These cystic spaces indicate the differentiation of epidermal basal cells into sebaceous glands

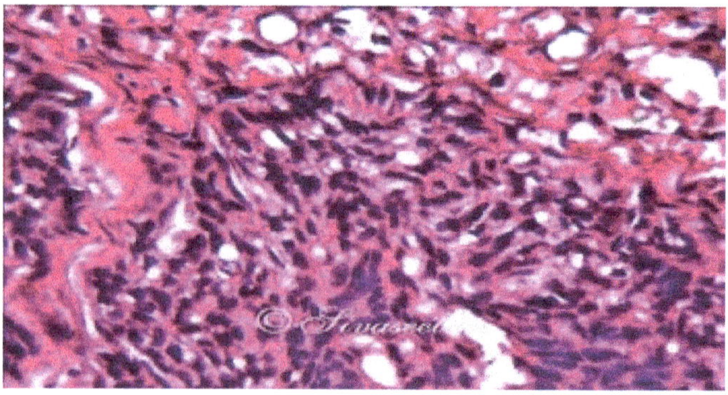

Fig. 99: Cystic type of basal cell tumour showing the neoplastic basal cells encompassing the cystic spaces.

3. Ribbon type

- ★ This type shows strands consist of one, two or three rows of basal cells resembling ribbon intervening to exert snake like appearance
- ★ The stroma between the cells often show mucinous degeneration
- ★ Mucin dominated type is called as **"adenoid basal cell tumour"**
- ★ Mucin formation indicates early sweat gland differentiation

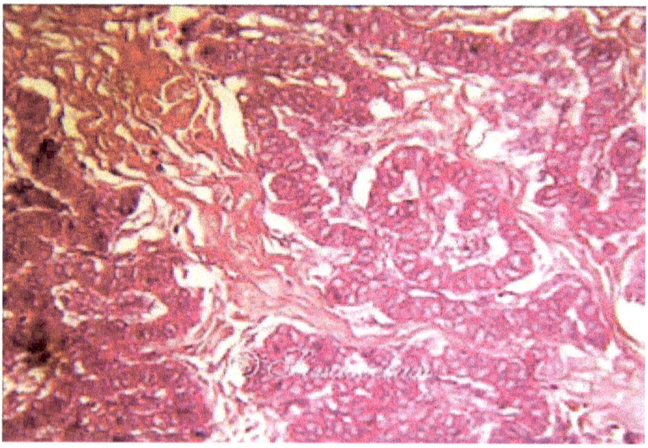

Fig. 100: Ribbon type of basal cell tumour showing strands consisting of one or two rows of basal cells resembling ribbon intervening to exert snake like appearance.

4. Medusoid Basal Cell Tumour

- ★ This type shows radiating strands of basal cells from a central mass of parallel arrangement of group of basal cells
- ★ This arrangement mimic Medusa's head (A Greek Goddess) or an octopus with tentacles
- ★ Mixed types of tumours with mixture of more than one type have also been reported

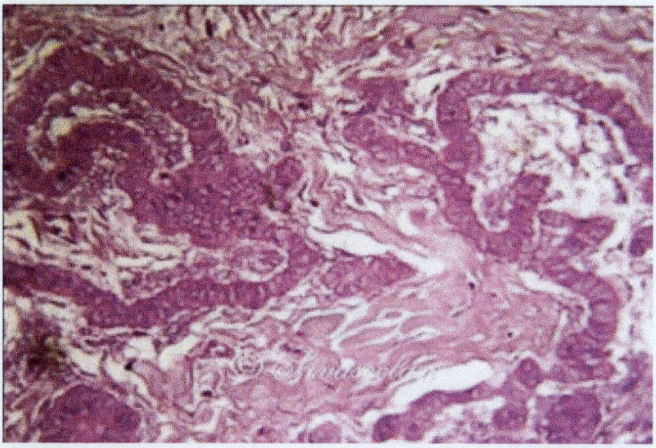

Fig. 101: A mixed type of basal cell tumour showing both Medusoid appearance of radiating strands of basal cells from a central mass of parallel arrangement of group of basal cells (left) and ribbon like arrangement (right).

Metastasis

This tumour is benign and rarely metastasizes, except solid type, which is considered as the most aggressive type.

15

Hair Follicle Tumour

The normal hair follicle of skin has two distinct portions

- Follicular sheath
- Hair bulb

Follicular sheath is an invagination of epidermis consisting all the layers of epidermis with outer basal cell layer and innermost keratin producing corneum cell layer. Hair bulb is composed of basophilic cells (hair matrix cells) from which hair forms. These cells resemble basal cell layer of skin with prominent nuclei, but without distinct cell border.

Trichoepithelioma and Pilomatricoma

Gross appearance

- ★ Trichoepithelioma arises from follicular sheath and Pilomatricoma arises from hair bulb
- ★ Co-existence of these two types has also been reported
- ★ Trichoepithelioma is common in dog and limited to skin and subcutis

Gross appearance

- ★ Grossly, it resembles basal cell tumour and solitary in most of the incidences
- ★ The surface is often ulcerated similar to basal cell carcinoma

Histological feature

- ★ Basal cells proliferate into many layered mass, which resemble basal cell tumour, but inside which all other layers of epidermis present encompassing keratinised centre
- ★ The inner most layer produces the keratin
- ★ This structure is called as "horn cyst"
- ★ Abrupt transition is seen from basal cell layer to the central keratinocytes with indistinct central layers

- ★ Poorly differentiated type shows numerous solid islands of basal cells with only few horn cysts
- ★ In well differentiated type, rudimentary hair can be seen, which is surrounded by many layered neoplastic basal cells
- ★ Superficial tricoepithelioma in which squamous cell proliferation is observed is called as **"baso squamous epithelioma"**
- ★ Extensive melanin pigmentation can also be seen in tricoepithelioma
- ★ Recurrence and metastases are rare

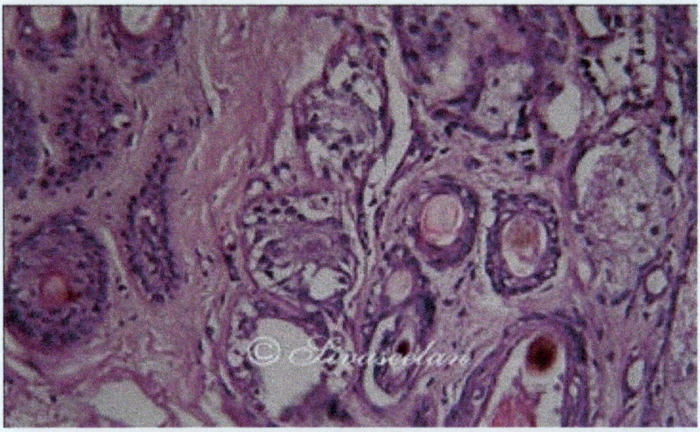

Fig. 102: Trichoepithelioma of a dog showing many layered hair follicle basal cells encompassing the keratin material.

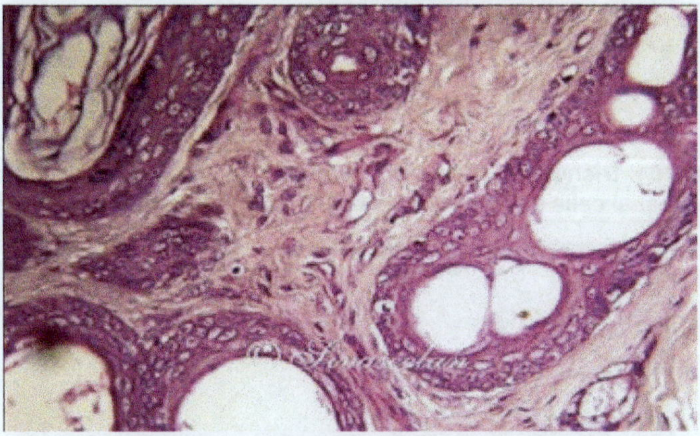

Fig. 103: Magnified view of Trichoepithelioma of a dog showing proliferation of hair follicle basal cells.

Pilomatricoma (Calcifying Epithelioma)

It is found in aged dogs and almost always occurs as a solitary growth. Grossly, it resembles basal cell tumour.

Histological feature

- ★ Basophilic cells proliferate to produce many layered cells
- ★ These cells are small and deeply staining with only scant amount of cytoplasm
- ★ The cellular borders are indistinct and seen as a chain of nuclei
- ★ These proliferating basophilic cells give rise to layers of fully keratinised "**shadow**" cells which stain faintly eosinophilic with H&E
- ★ Shadow cells have distinct border with a central unstained area at the sites of nuclei (shadow cells)
- ★ Tumour of recent origin shows the basophilic cells predominantly while in older lesions the shadow cells dominate
- ★ Frequently calcified areas are seen on shadow cells area, which gives the name calcifying epithelioma
- ★ Pilomatrichoma is benign tumour which, rarely recurs or metastasizes

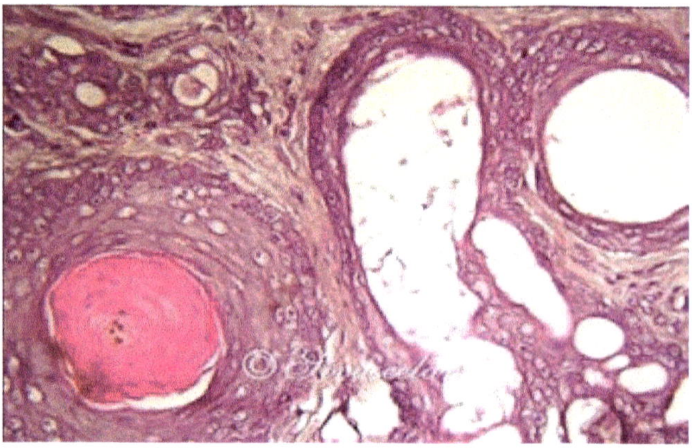

Fig. 104: Trichoepithelioma of a dog showing many layered neoplastic hair follicle basal cells encompassing the keratin centre making a horn cyst.

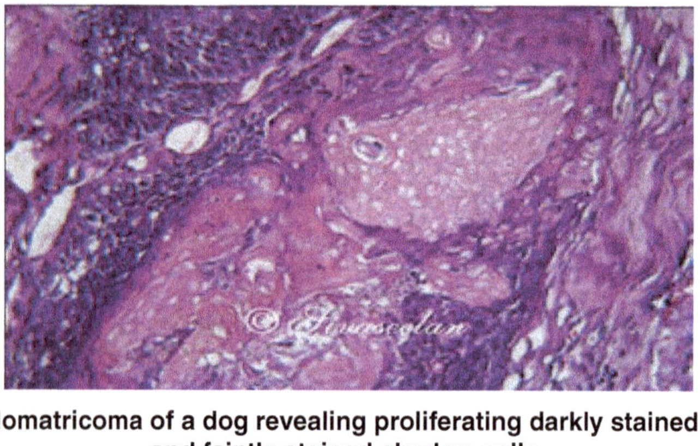

Fig. 105: Pilomatricoma of a dog revealing proliferating darkly stained basal cells and faintly stained shadow cells.

16

Sebaceous Gland Tumours

This is a common skin epithelial tumour of aged dog. Occasional incidence in cats is reported, but not in other animals. Frequent site of occurrence is Meibomian gland modified sebaceous gland found in eyelids. Sebaceous gland neoplastic growth occurs in different forms as mentioned below.

Nodular type (Hyperplastic type)

This is a small growth that varies from 2-5 cm in diameter, which occurs as yellowish single or multiple mass.

Histological feature

This type shows lobules containing fully matured sebaceous cells arranged around sebaceous duct, which is composed of stratified squamous epithelium.

Sebaceous Adenoma

This is comparatively larger than hyperplastic type (2cm in diameter).

Histological feature

- ★ Irregularly sized and shaped lobules containing fully matured sebaceous cells
- ★ Undifferentiated generative cells (smaller cells) from which sebaceous cells are differentiating are also found in between lobules of sebaceous cells

Sebaceous Epithelioma

- ★ This type resembles solid basal cell tumour and Trichoepithelioma
- ★ This tumour is composed of undifferentiated basal cells with prominent nuclei admixed with transititional cells (transititional cells are intermediate transforming cells from basal cells to matures sebaceous cells, which show vacuolation in the cytoplasm)

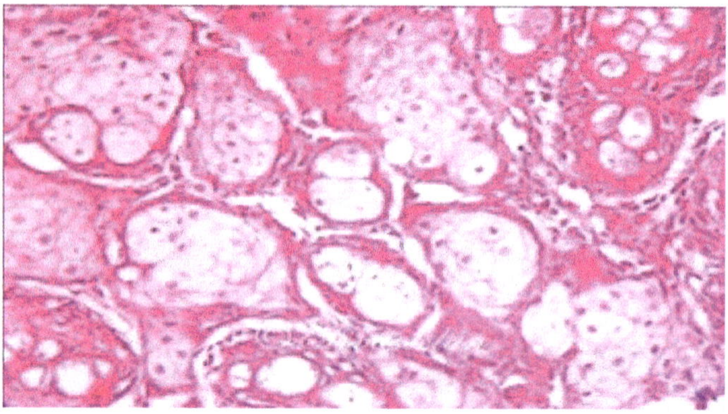

Fig. 106: Sebaceous Gland Adenoma of a dog showing irregularly shaped and sized lobules containing matured sebaceous cells.

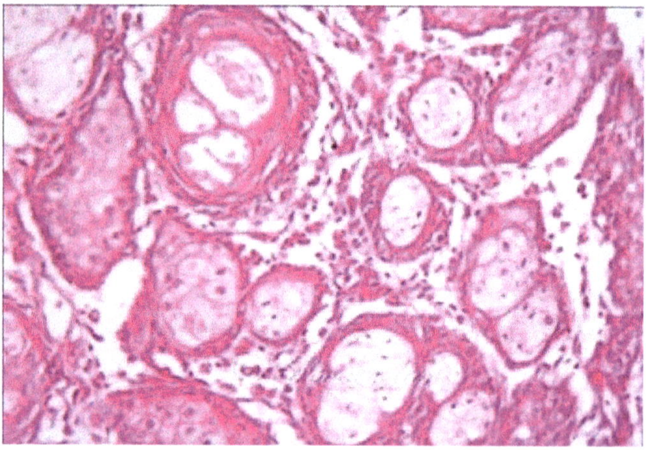

Fig. 107: Sebaceous Gland Adenoma of a dog showing degenerating sebaceous cells indicating regressive type. Undifferentiated generative cells are seen in-between the lobules.

Sebaceous Adenocarcinoma

- ★ This is a rare malignant type of tumour and occur with ill defined borders and ulcerations
- ★ Histologically, this tumour resembles the sebaceous epithelioma, but with more anisocytosis and anisokaryosis

In all these types, melanocytes and plasma cells may also be seen with proliferating squamous epithelium attempting to from ducts.

Metastasis

Sebaceous hyperplasia and adenoma are benign. Epithelioma behaves like basal cell tumour and sebaceous adenocarcinoma is a true malignant type, which will often metastasize to regional lymph nodes and lung.

17

Sweat Gland Tumour

★ Sweat glands are coiled tubular or saccular glands found in association with hair follicles

★ The secretory parts are located in dermis and subcutis and excretory ducts pass up through the dermis and empty into the hair follicles above the ducts of the sebaceous gland

★ Sweat gland bears the histological feature of any acini, but a myo-epithelial cell layer is interposed between secretory epithelium and basement membrane (bilayered cells)

★ Sweat gland tumour is the least common tumour of skin and found in aged dog and cats

Different types of sweat gland tumour are narrated below

Cystic Hyperplasia

This type is the most frequently observed sweat gland tumour found on the head and neck of dogs, which usually measures about 1- 4 cm in diameter. Cut surface show cysts of varying size and number. Cysts are filled with clear yellow or brown serous gelatinous material.

Histological feature

★ Cystic spaces are lined by bilayered cells (inner cuboidal and outer elongated myo-epithelium)

Sweat Gland Adenoma and Adenocarcinoma

★ Sweat gland adenoma in the early stage resembles mammary gland tumour all the way, except bilayered acini

★ Adenoma often reveals papillary cystic adenomatous changes

★ Some benign tumours show irregular glands lined only by cuboidal cells

★ Due to malignant changes, bilayered cells cannot be appreciated in adenocarcinoma and pleomorphic cells evade the basement membrane of acini

18

Adenoma of Gland

This is a benign tumour of secretory epithelial cells of acini in any gland.

Gross appearance

- ★ They are nodular and encapsulated, solitary or multiple in occurrence and firm or soft in consistency
- ★ Adenoma of hollow organs shows reddish polypoid growth

Histological feature

- ★ Acini show multiple layered neoplastic epithelial cells, but they do not pierce the basement membrane
- ★ Adenoma is supplied with plenty of thin walled blood vessels
- ★ Since, these acini lack duct, secretory product accumulate within the lumen of acini to make it as cyst, which is called as "cystadenoma"
- ★ If proliferating epithelial cells projects towards the lumen as a secondary and tertiary structure, then the name "papillary cystadenoma" is given
- ★ Neoplastic involvement of fibrous stroma in addition to epithelial changes gives the name as "fibroadenoma"
- ★ This tumour can safely be removed and will not recur in most of the cases

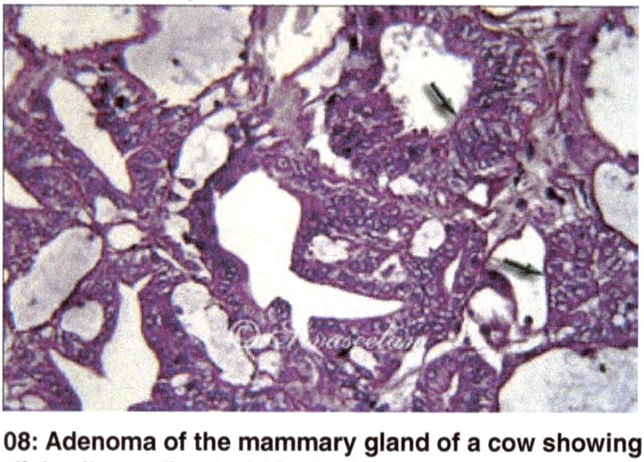

Fig. 108: Adenoma of the mammary gland of a cow showing proliferating epithelial cells confined within the basement membrane of acini.

19

Adenocarcinoma

- ★ Malignant type of glandular epithelium depicts multi layered neoplastic epithelial cells within the acini, which usually lack polarity, pierce the basement membrane and evade to the inter-acinar spaces
- ★ More mitotic figures are usually observed
- ★ Frequent metastases are the other features
- ★ Removal is not advisable, as this often recur. So radiation and other advanced therapy are advocated

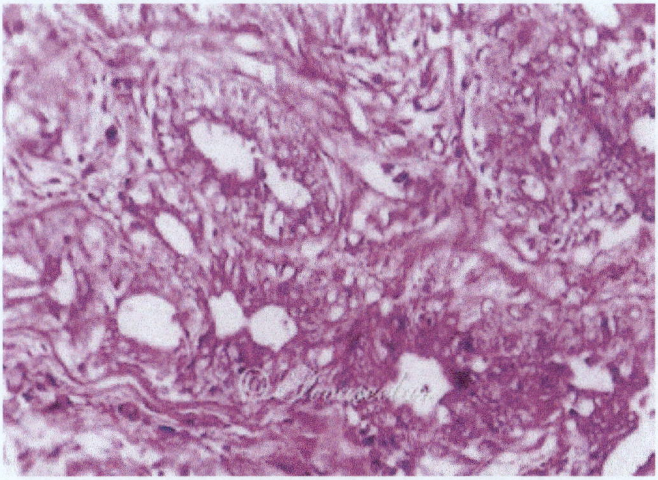

Fig. 109: Adenocarcinoma of the mammary gland of a cow showing proliferating acinar cells breaking and evading the basement membrane.

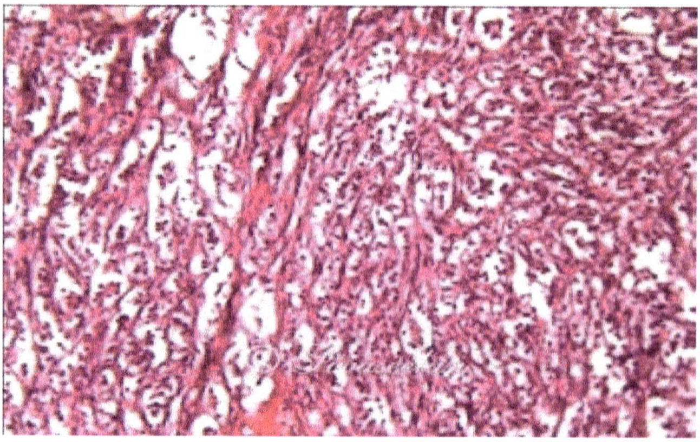

Fig. 110: Adenocarcinoma of the intestine of a fowl showing proliferating epithelial cells forming irregular acini.

20

Salivary Gland Tumour

Incidence

Unilateral occurrence is more when compared to bilateral incidence. Benign form is seen as a single mass surrounded by normal gland and malignant type may replace the entire gland. Incidence is common in dogs.

Pleomorphic adenoma

This type of tumour is composed of mixed tissues of epithelium, myoepithelium, cartilage and bone.

Monomorphic adenoma

This tumour arises from the duct lining epithelium and myoepithelium or from mucous acini. Involvement of mucous acini can be ascertained by demonstrating mucous with alcian blue or PAS stains.

Acini cell tumour

It is a common tumour of parotid glands of dog arising from serous glandular epithelium, mucus cannot be demonstrated with PAS or alcian blue. Neoplastic cells are polyhedral cells with tiny nuclei arranged in several layers within acini, some may show papillary projections.

A bilateral sub-mandibular salivary gland tumour in a goat was reported by **Sivaseelan** *et al*. (IVJ, 88-4: 68-69). Since the cytoplasm of neoplastic cells could not be stained with alcian blue, involvement of mucous acinar cells was ruled out and the tumour was confirmed as serous acinar type.

Adenocarcinoma

It may arise from either mucous or serous glands, which shows the histological feature of typical adenocarcinoma with follicular arrangement of neoplastic epithelial cells divided by fibrous stroma.

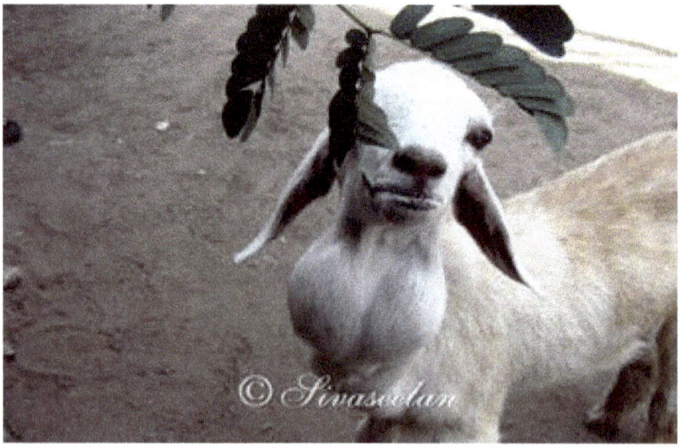

Fig. 111: Bilateral Adenocarcinoma of the salivary gland of a kid showing highly prominent enlargement of the gland.

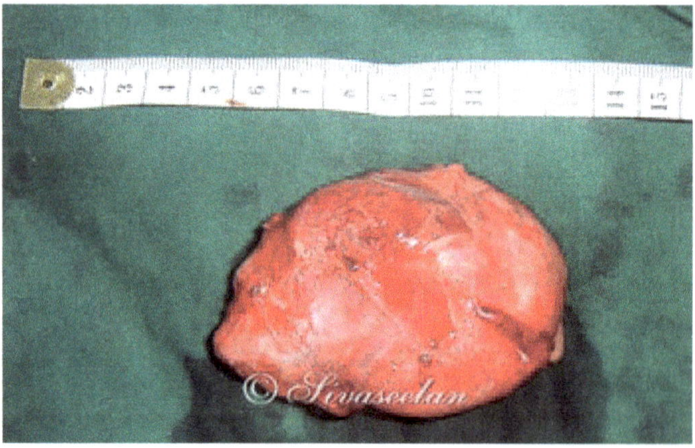

Fig. 112: Removed tumour shown in fig. 111.

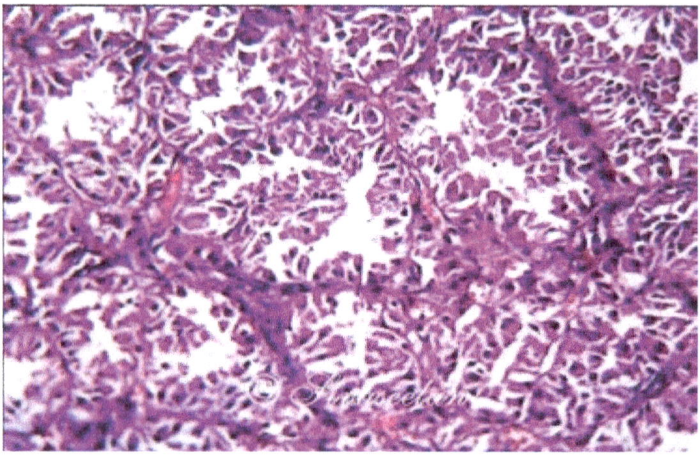

Fig. 113: Histological photomicrograph of the tumour shown in fig. 112 revealing irregular acini formed due to proliferating secretory epithelial cells.

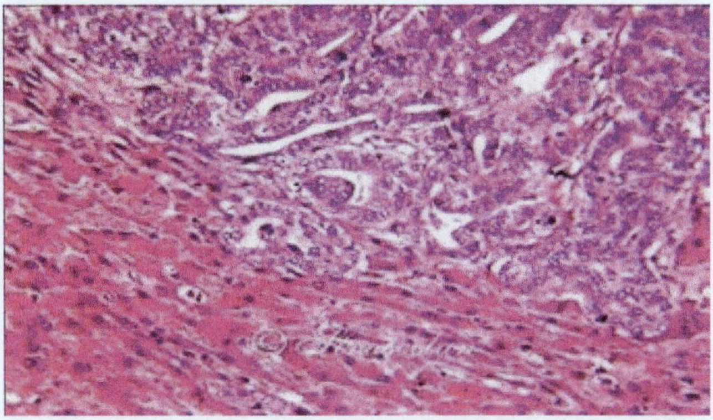

Fig. 114: Metastasis of the salivary gland shown in fig 111 to liver (Irregular acini formed due to proliferating neoplastic salivary gland cells growing into the hepatic cells by infiltration).

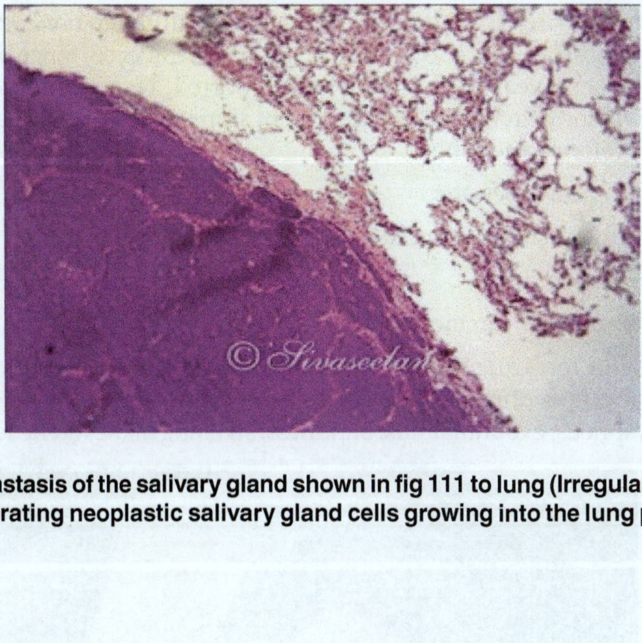

Fig. 115: Metastasis of the salivary gland shown in fig 111 to lung (Irregular acini formed due to proliferating neoplastic salivary gland cells growing into the lung parenchyma).

21

Nasal Tumours

Ethmoturbinate tumour

This tumour arises from mucosa of the ethmoturbinate bone, often occur as endemic form in ruminants and horses. In India, several occurrence of this tumour in aged cattle over 6 years of age have been reported. The tumour develops from ethmoid region and often invades the adjacent sinuses. Metastasis occurs to many organs with preference to lungs.

The histological types are:

- ⋆ Undifferentiated carcinoma
- ⋆ Adenocarcinoma
- ⋆ Squamous cell carcinoma

The endemic form quickly spreads to all animals of the herd and viral etiology is suspected for the outbreaks. The affected animals manifest mucopurulent nasal discharge, dyspnoea, exophthalmus, blindness, swelling of the forehead and circling.

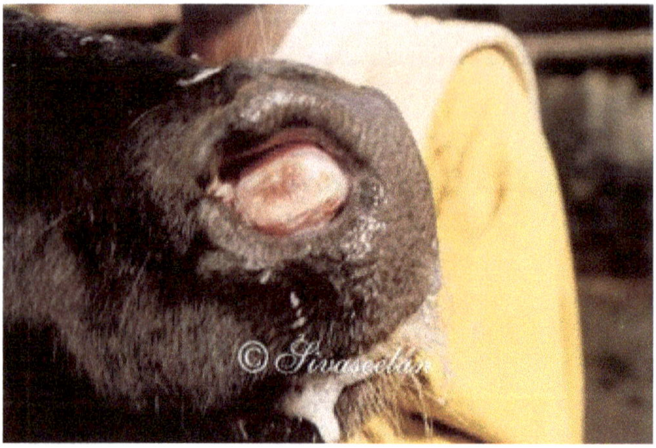

Fig. 116: Nasal septum of a cow revealing a carcinoma protruding from nasal cavity.

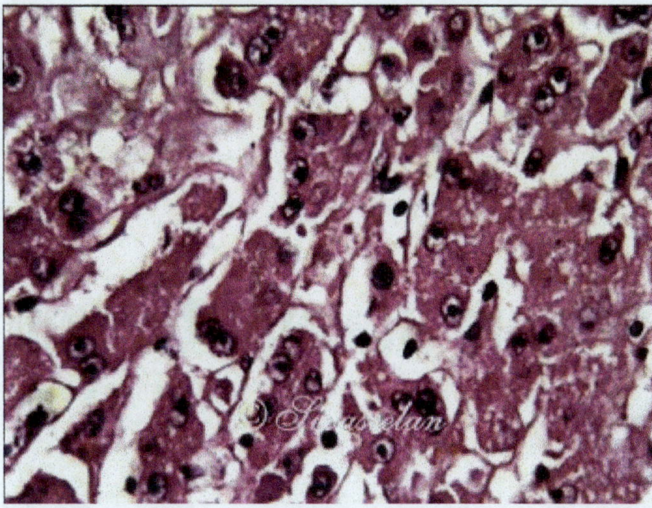

Fig. 117: Nasal septal tumour shown in fig. 116 depicting sheet arrangement of pleomorphic neoplastic epithelial cells with prominent nucleoli within vesicular nuclei.

22

Urinary Bladder Tumour

They occur as:

- ★ Transitional cell papilloma, that grows as projections of epithelium towards the lumen
- ★ Adenoma that occurs from pre existing glands in the mucosa or from the transitional epithelium through the metaplastic change
- ★ Carcinoma, that occurs as one of four types:
  - Transitional (urothelial) carcinoma
  - Squamous cell carcinoma
  - Adenocarcinoma
  - Undifferentiated carcinoma

Carcinoma

Incidence

It is endemic in certain areas (Ooty, Kodaikanal, Yercaud and other hilly regions) and is associated with a syndrome known as enzootic haematuria in cattle.

Gross appearance

Bladder carcinoma occurs as a papillary or non papillary growth or may have a cauliflower like appearance. Non papillary type occurs as a flat diffused growth increasing the thickness of mucosa of the urinary bladder.

Histological features

Transitional cell carcinoma appears as cords of cells with prominent stromal fibrosis. It may be infiltrative or non infiltrative. Squamous cell carcinoma reveals cell nests, adenocarcinoma appears with irregular glandular structure and undifferentiated carcinoma shows sheet of cells with anaplasia.

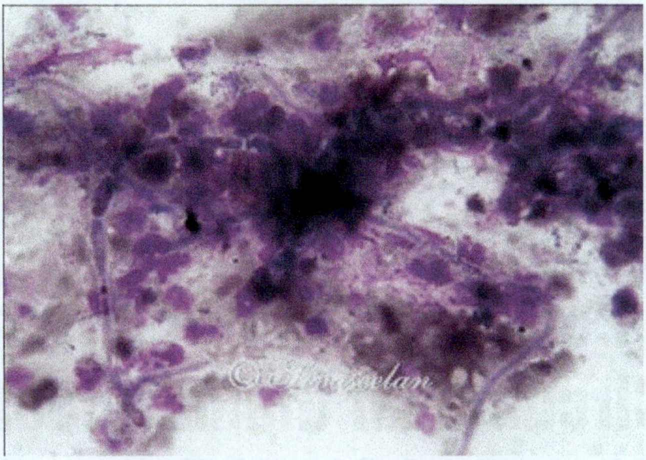

Fig. 118: Urine smear of a dog revealing pleomorphic carcinoma cells admixed with fungal filaments.

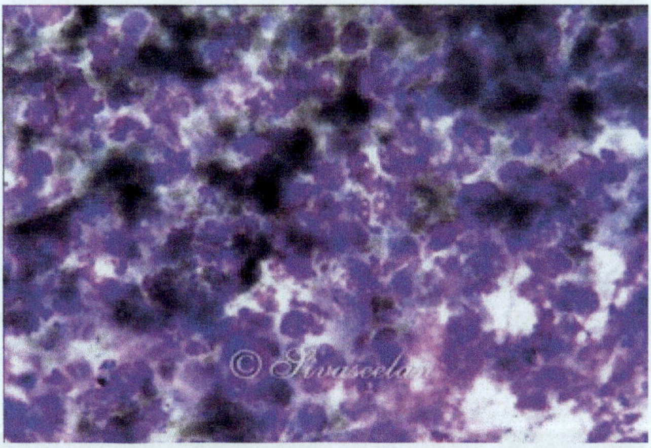

Fig. 119: Urine smear of a bitch showing pleomorphic carcinoma cells with multiple angular nucleoli.

23

Perianal Gland Tumour (Circumanal Gland Tumour, Hepatoid Gland Tumour)

- Perianal glands are modified sebaceous glands located in the subcutis encircling the anus and empty the secretion on to the skin through hair follicles and also to the neck of anal sac
- They are also found in the skin at lumbar region, tail, thigh and prepuce
- Perianal gland tumour is the most common tumour of aged male dogs and may occur as a solitary or multiple mass
- Ring like appearance around the anus indicates multiple occurrence
- Size varies from 1-10 cm in diameter
- They are well circumscribed and sometimes ulcerated

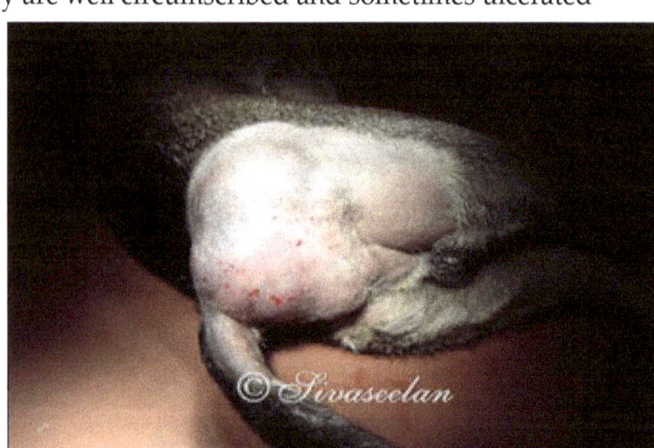

Fig. 120: Multiple Perianal gland tumours around the anus of a native breed dog.

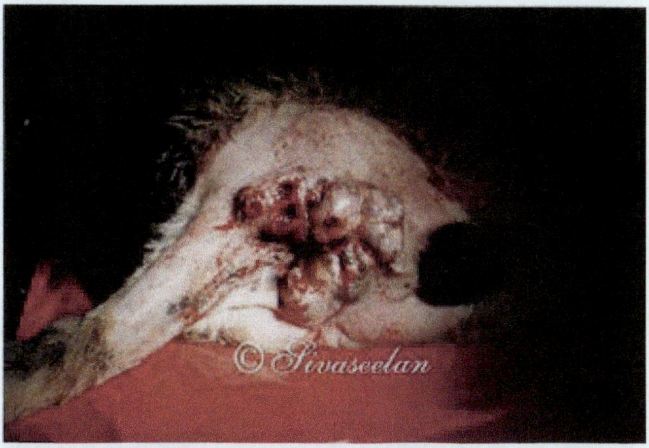

Fig. 121: Multiple Perianal gland tumours around the anus of a dog revealing haemorrhage.

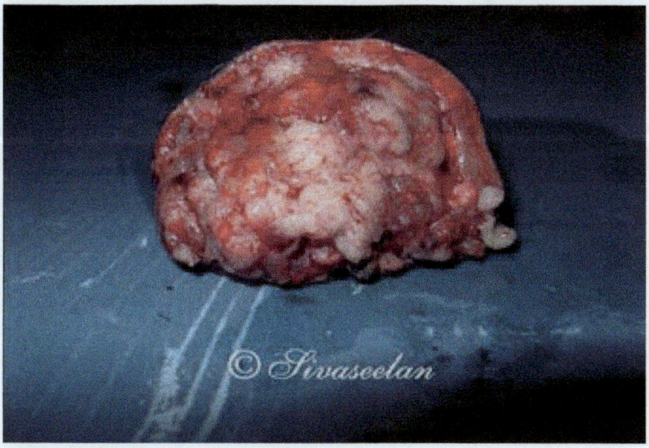

Fig. 122: An excised single tumour shown in fig. 121 depicting easily bleeding nature of Perianal gland tumour.

Histological feature

Nodular hyperplasia

- ★ Hyper active gland shows more layers of acinar epithelial cells with isometric architecture

Adenoma

- ★ Shows lobules of large discrete, round to polyhedral cells (liver like cells/ hepatoid cells) with vacuolated or granular cytoplasm
- ★ Basophilic small reserve cells are also seen in between the lobules
- ★ Inflammation and necrosis are commonly observed

Adenocarcinoma

* This type does not show lobulations
* Hepatoid cells and reserve cells are arranged as a mixed cell sheet

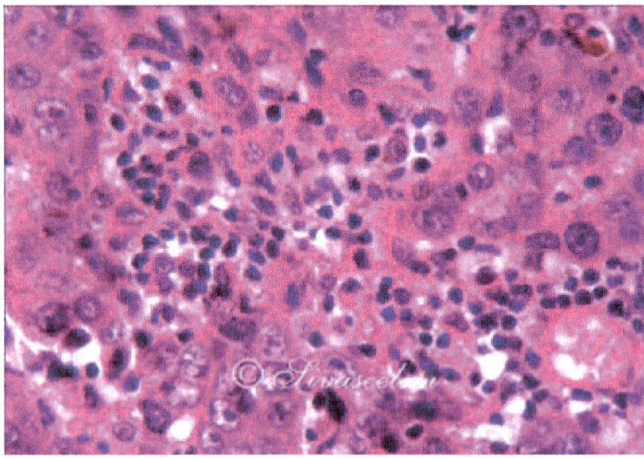

Fig. 123: An adenocarcinoma of Perianal gland of a dog showing Hepatoid cells and Reserve cells arranged as a mixed cell sheet.

Metastasis

* Recurrence and metastasis are very rare:

24

Melanocytoma and Malignant Melanoma

- ★ Melanocytes that contain a special organelle, melanosome are branching cells found at the junction of epidermis and dermis admixed with the basal cells
- ★ Melanin pigment is extruded along the dendritic processes to the surrounding basal cells to impart black colour to the skin
- ★ Melanocytic tumours are common among dogs and horses, but rare in ruminants
- ★ It can develop in the skin, mucous membrane, eye and oral cavity
- ★ The common sites are eyelids, extremities, gums and buccal mucosa
- ★ Most of the oral melanocytic tumours are malignant and those of skin are benign
- ★ The size varies from 1-10 cm in diameter
- ★ The tumours, which measure below 3 cm in diameter may be benign in growth
- ★ Colour varies from brown to black depending upon the melanin content
- ★ A rare case of cutaneous malignant melanoma in a Kangeyam bullock was reported by **Sivaseelan** *et al.* (IVJ, 2010, 8-11: 1144-1145). Ultraviolet-B rays with the wave length of 280 – 320 nm induced DNA damage was suggested for the induction of this tumour
- ★ In another study, **Sivaseelan** *et al.* (IJVP, 2010, 40-1: 74 – 76) observed primary melanoma on the skin and secondary metastasis to heart, lung, liver, kidney, bladder and intestine. Almost all viscera showed multiple tumour growths

Histological feature

- ⋆ Melanin pigment laden melanocytes show pleomorphism
- ⋆ Black or brown melanin pigments may obscure the nucleus of the cell
- ⋆ Masson's Fontana silver stain will give clear picture of melanin pigments within the cells when compared to H & E stains
- ⋆ Neoplastic melanocytes are arranged as diffuse single cells or as cell nests
- ⋆ In malignant melanomas, melanocytes are modified as pleomorphic epithelioid cells or spindle cells or mixture of both
- ⋆ More anaplasia and frequent metastasis are the other features

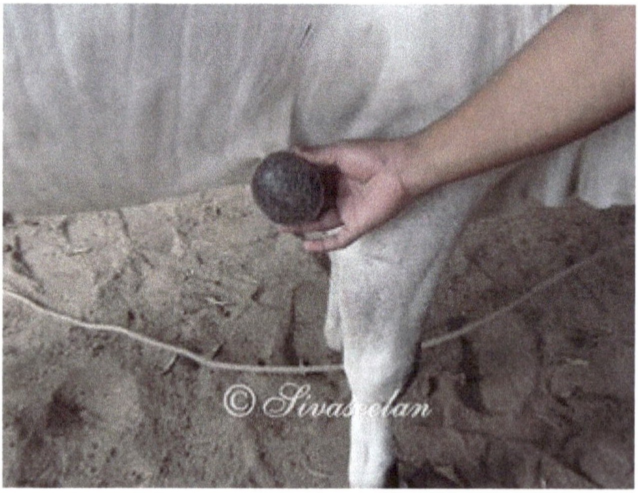

Fig. 124: A bullock showing a tennis ball size circumscribed and pedunculated melanoma on the skin.

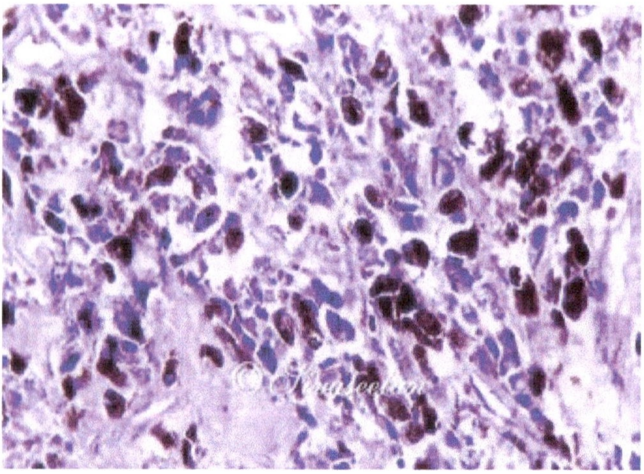

Fig. 125: Tissue section of the tumour shown in fig. 124 revealing pleomorphic darkbrown melanin pigment containing neoplastic melanoblasts.

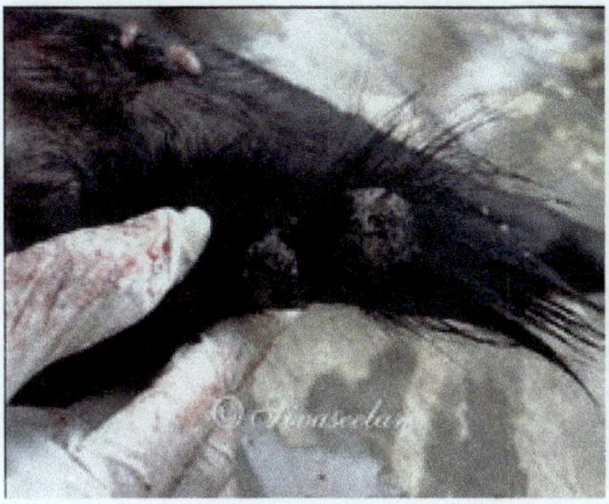

Fig. 126

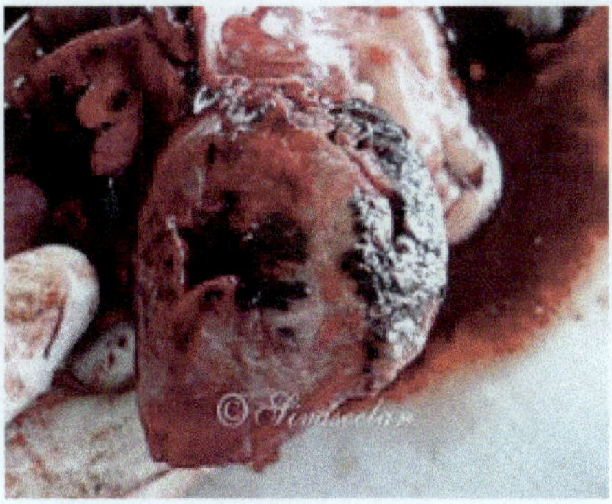

Fig. 127

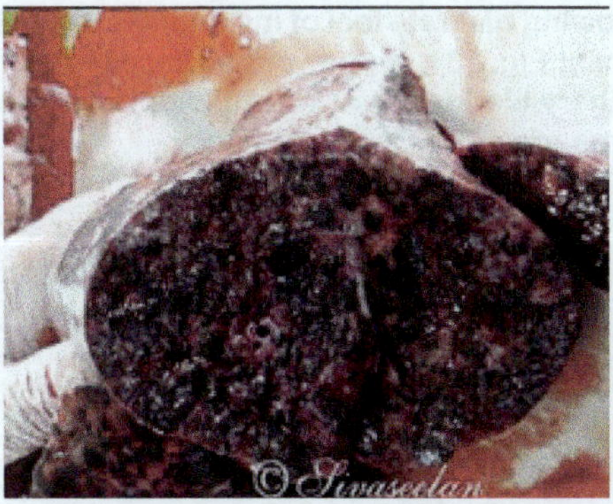

Fig. 128

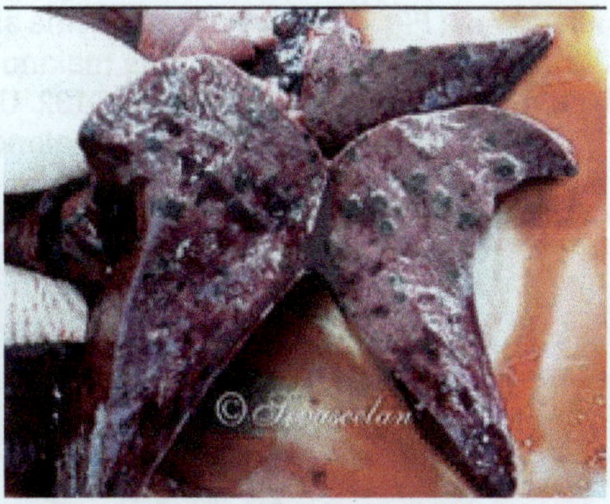

Fig. 129

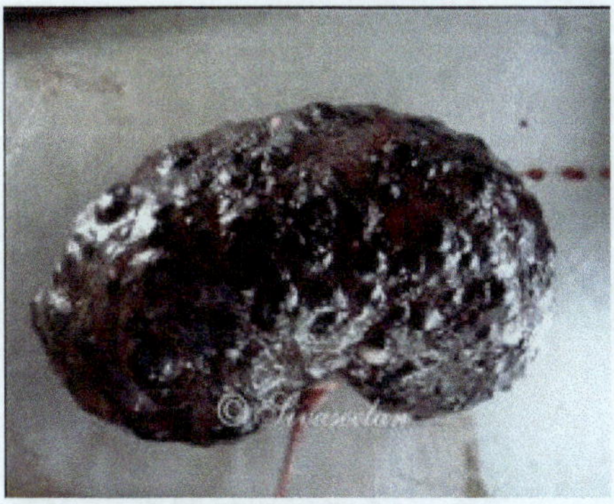

Fig. 130

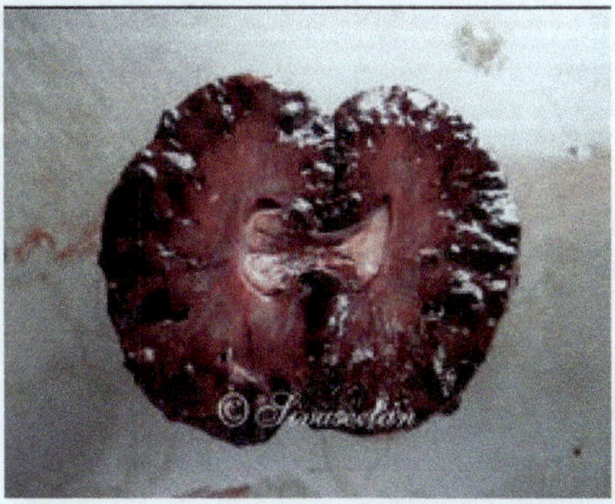

Fig. 131

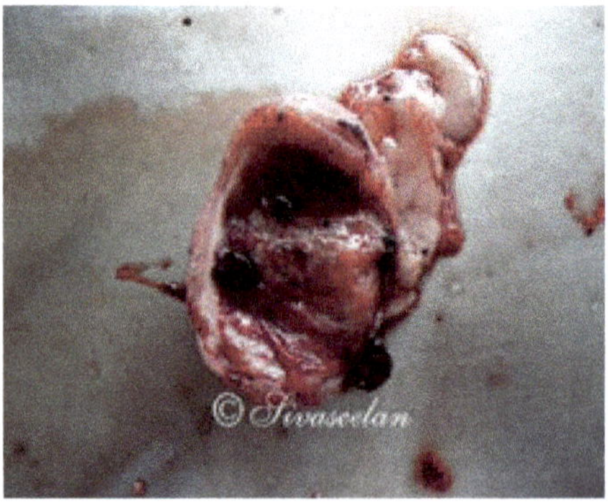

Fig. 132

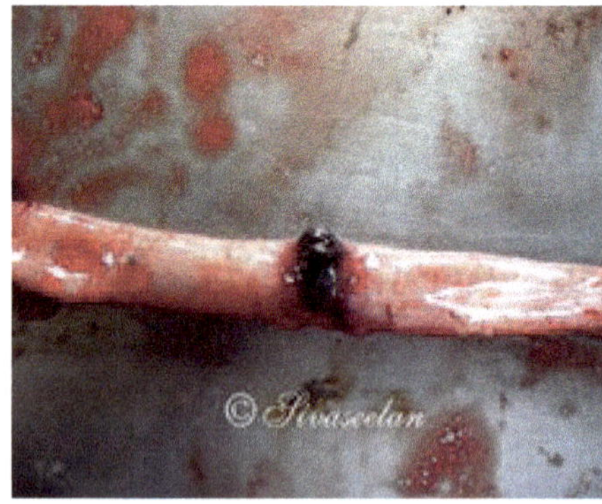

Fig. 133

Fig.126. Melanoma growths on the skin; Fig. 127. Heart revealing multiple foci of melanomas in the myocardium; Fig.128. Lung exhibiting multiple variable sized melanomas; Fig. 129. Liver parenchyma showing discrete foci of melanomas; Fig.130. Kidney surface showing multiple melanomas; Fig. 131. Kidney cut-surface revealing deeply embedded melanomas; Fig. 132. Urinary bladder showing melanoma nodules; Fig.133. Intestinal wall depicting a melanoma growth.

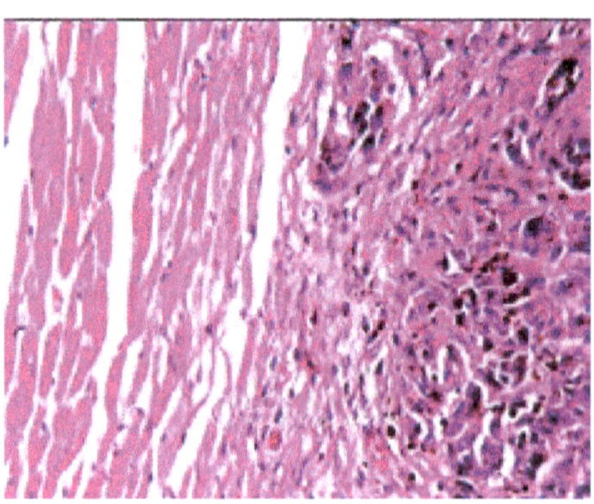

Fig. 134

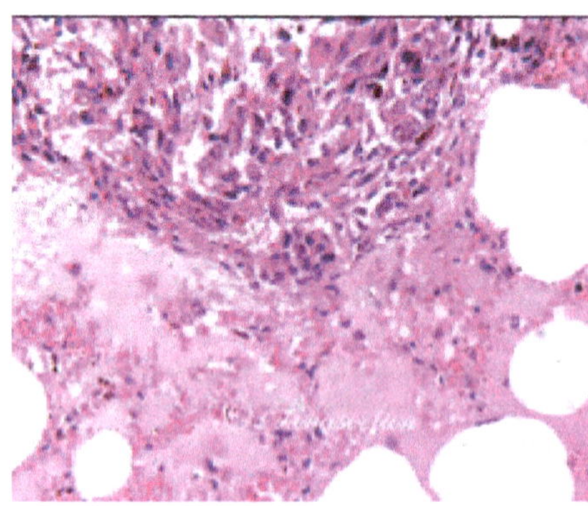

Fig. 135

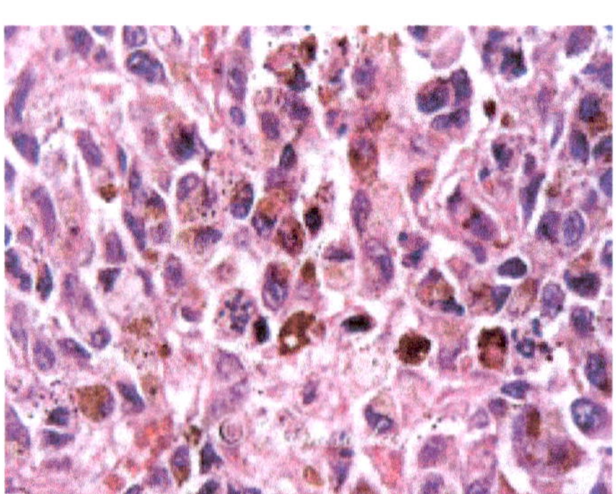

Fig. 136

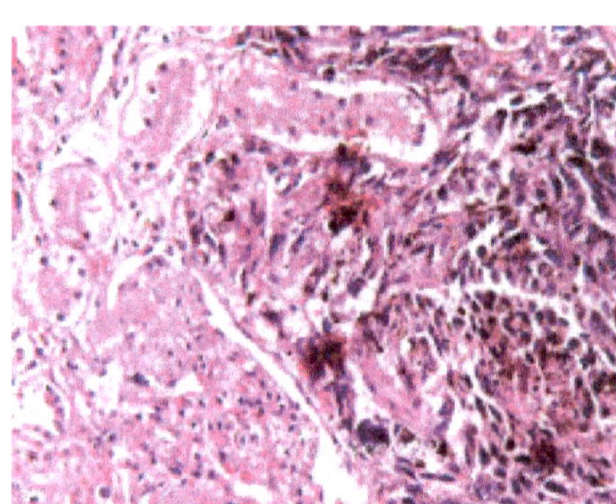

Fig. 137

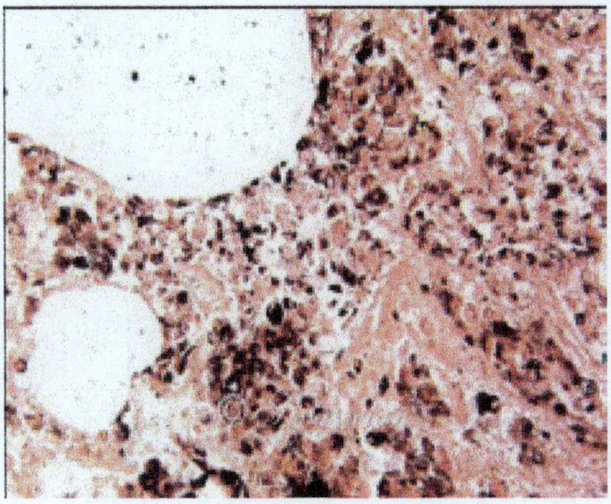

Fig. 138

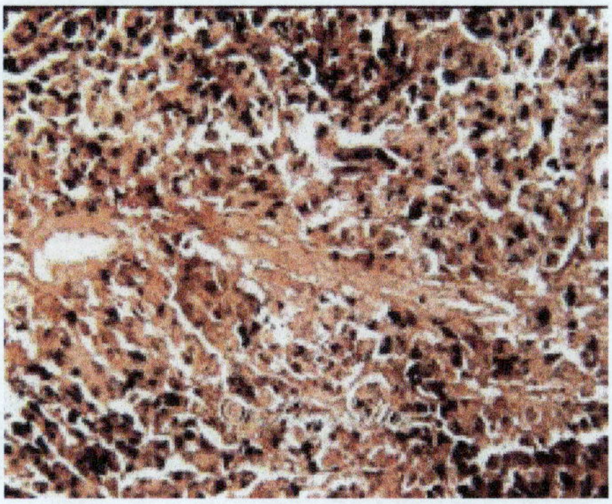

Fig. 139

Fig. 134. Heart showing pleomorphic neoplastic melanin laden melanocytes arranged in sheets, clusters or nests, H&E x400; Fig. 135. Lung showing pleomorphic neoplastic melanin laden melanocytes arranged in sheets or cords, H&E x400; Fig. 136. Liver section depicting melanin laden melanocytes with mitotic figures, H&E x1000; Fig. 137. Kidney section showing tubular necrosis and pleomorphic neoplastic melanin laden melanocytes arranged in sheets. H&E x400; Fig. 138. Lung revealing black melanin laden pleomorphic melanocytes, Masson-Fontana Silver stain x400. Fig. 139. Liver section exhibiting black melanin pigment laden neoplastic melanocytes, Masson-Fontana Silver stain x400.

25

Ceruminous Gland Tumours

- ★ These glands are coiled tubular modified sweat glands found in the external auditory meatus
- ★ The acini of this glands are bilayered similar to sweat gland
- ★ The ducts open onto the neck of hair follicles or onto the free surface of skin
- ★ Combined secretions of ceruminous gland and sebaceous gland are mixed with desquamated keratin to make up the waxy material called "**cerumen**" in the ear canal
- ★ Ceruminous gland tumours are found in aged cats and dogs
- ★ Grossly, small nodular or pedunculated masses are noticed in the ear canal

Histological feature

- ★ This tumour resembles sweat gland tumour
- ★ Orange or copper colour secretion with inflammatory cells may be found in the ear canal
- ★ Multilayered epithelial cells restricted to the bilayered basement membrane and secretions within the acini can be observed
- ★ Malignant type (adenocarcinoma) show solid sheet like arrangement without acinar pattern and may show anaplasia:

26

Mammary Tumour

- ★ Neoplastic changes may occur from any component of mammary gland (epithelium, myo-epithelium and fibrous tissue)
- ★ In mixed mammary tumour, chondromatous changes (cartilage formation) develop from myo-epithelium, but not from metaplasia of fibrous stroma and ossification (bone formation) may arise from fibrous stroma
- ★ Mammary tumour are common in aged dogs
- ★ Canine mammary tumours represent approximately 30-50 % of all types of tumours in bitches. Incidence of mammary tumour is reduced with the early spaying. Chances for development of mammary tumour before coming to first estrus, after one estrus and after two or more cycles are 0.5 %, 8 % and 26 % respectively. This infers that the hormone estrogen plays a vital role in causing mammary tumours
- ★ These tumours arise primarily in the females from secretary epithelial, myoepithelial or less frequently mesenchymal elements of mammary tissue. Involvement of only epithelium is called as "simple tumour"
- ★ Involvement of more than one cell type results in mixed mammary tumour, which may be benign or malignant.

Simple Mammary Tumour

Papilloma may arise from lining epithelium of teat canal and larger ducts. This benign type may extend to a malignant type of carcinoma.

Mixed Mammary Tumour

This type is more common than the simple tumour. Size of these tumours varies from 1-10 cm in diameter. Colour varies from brown to reddish and the consistency from soft to firm.

Benign Mixed Mammary Tumour

Combination of adenoma of acinar epithelium, spindle cell tumour of myo-epithelium, chondroma of myo-epithelial metaplastic cells and osteoma of fibrous metaplastic cells may arise from mammary gland.

Combination differs among the affected dogs. Depending upon the cell types, the name like fibrochondroadenoma is given, but the current terminology is simply benign mixed cell tumour.

Malignant Mixed Cell Mammary Tumour

- ★ Malignant changes may occur from all the cellular constituents, but adenocarcinoma of epithelial cells are common
- ★ Involvement of fibrous stroma should be differentiated from myo-epithelial cell neoplasia by Masson's Trichrome or Van Gieson stain
- ★ Giant cell formation from myo-epithelium and mitotic figures are common in malignant type
- ★ Early metastasis is often observed to regional lymph nodes and other viscera
- ★ A massive type of mixed mammary tumour weighing 5.2 Kg. occupying the posterior quarters of a bitch was reported by **Sivaseelan** *et al.* (IJVP, 2010, 34-2: 198-199). They also proved that in well matured mammary tumour, degree of malignancy increases from the outer area to the centre of the tumour.

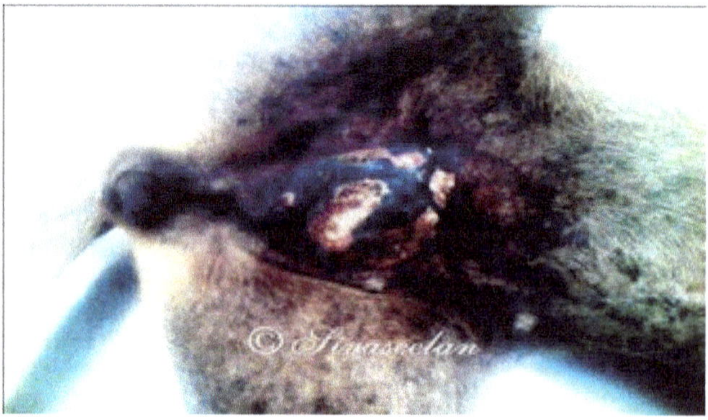

Fig. 140: Mammary tumour arising from the posterior pair of mammary gland of a bitch.

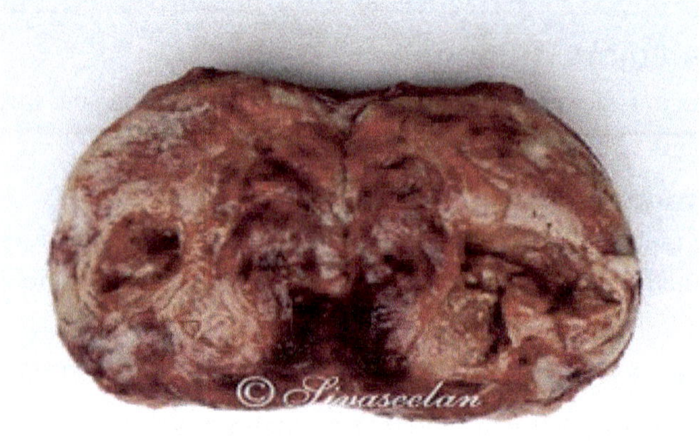

Fig. 141: Mammary tumour shown in fig. 140 revealing intermixed congested and necrotic areas.

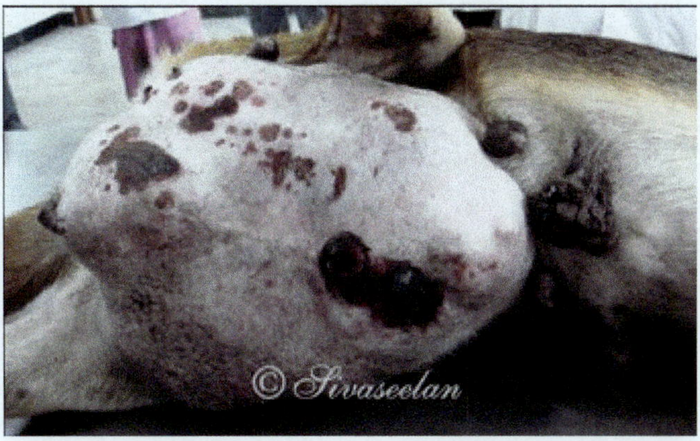

Fig. 142: A massive mammary tumour of a bitch involving posterior quarters.

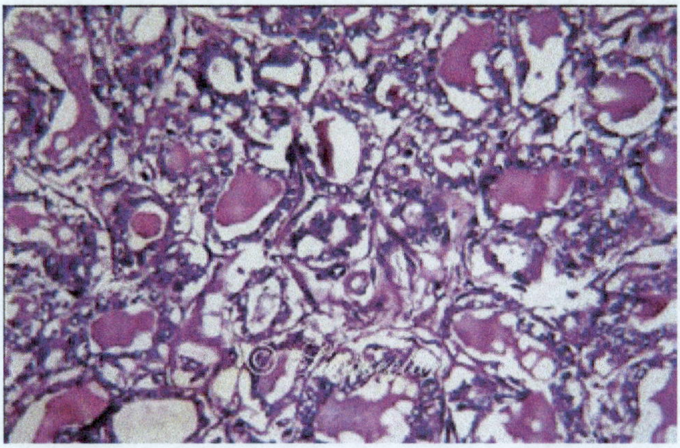

Fig. 143: Mammary tumour shown in fig. 142 depicting cystadenoma (note: variable size and shape of acini with retained secretion due to lack of outlets to release the secretion)

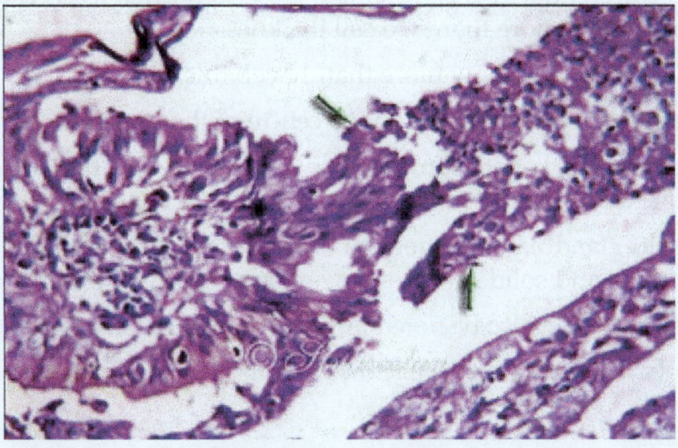

Fig. 144: Tissue from yet another location of Mammary tumour shown in fig. 142 depicting metaplastic transformation of myo-epithelium into chondrocytes (arrows) to form chondroma.

27

Liver Tumours

Hepatocellular Adenoma and Hepatocellular Carcinoma

This tumour is found in all species of animals, but aged dogs are more prone. Affected dogs show anorexia, vomiting, ascites, lethargy and weakness. Severely affected dogs show abdominal enlargement with palpable liver (liver is more palpable in hepatocellular carcinoma than cholangiocellular carcinoma and jaundice). Serum biochemical analysis will reveal liver abnormality.

Gross appearance

- ⋆ This tumour varies from small round discrete solitary lesion of one to several cm to multiple occurrence of variable sizes
- ⋆ The colour differs from tan to reddish
- ⋆ The soft and friable nature of hepatocellular carcinoma distinguishes it from cholangiocellular carcinoma, which is firm in consistency

Histological feature

- ⋆ Well differentiated type resemble close to normal liver, except the cords composed of more than two cell thickness
- ⋆ Some cords may show more than 10 cell thickness
- ⋆ Necrosis may be observed in the centre of the neoplastic cords
- ⋆ Since the thickened cords mimic the trabeculae, this type is called as "trabecular pattern"
- ⋆ Pseudo-glandular arrangement of irregular clusters of cells separated by sinusoids and solid sheets arrangements are other patterns observed
- ⋆ Some cysts can also be noted among the cluster of neoplastic hepatocytes
- ⋆ Poorly differentiated type shows anaplasia or pleomorphism

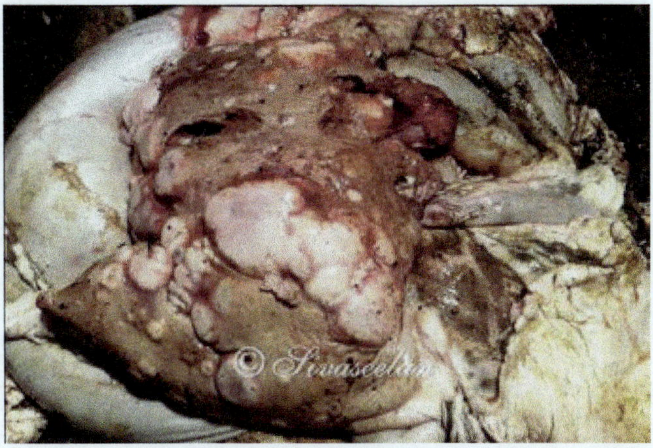

Fig. 145: Hepatocellular carcinoma of a rabbit revealing multiple tumours involving the whole liver.

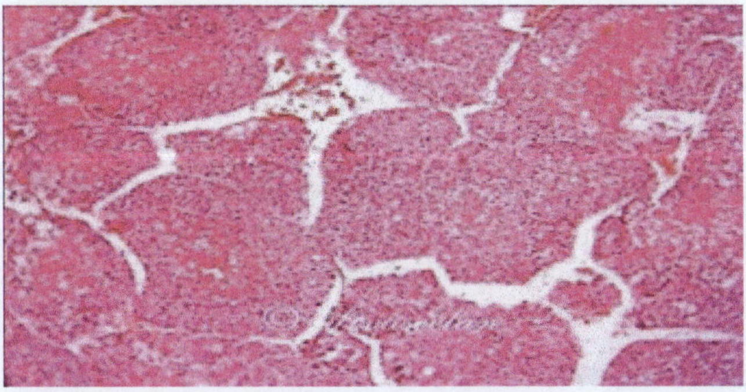

Fig. 146: Hepatocellular carcinoma revealing pseudo-glandular arrangement of neoplastic hepatocytes.

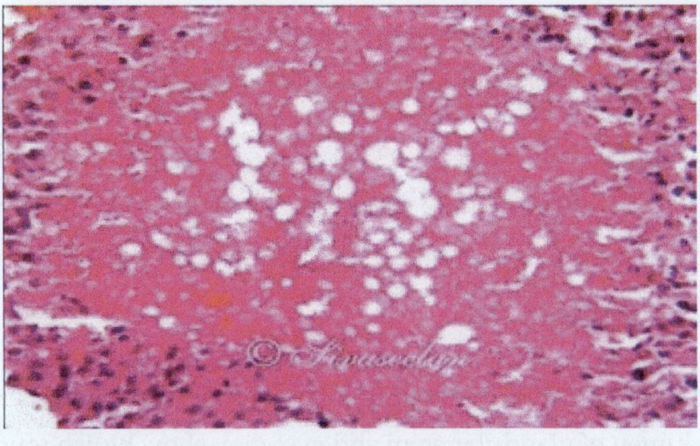

Fig. 147: A pseudo-gland depicting central necrosis with cystic changes

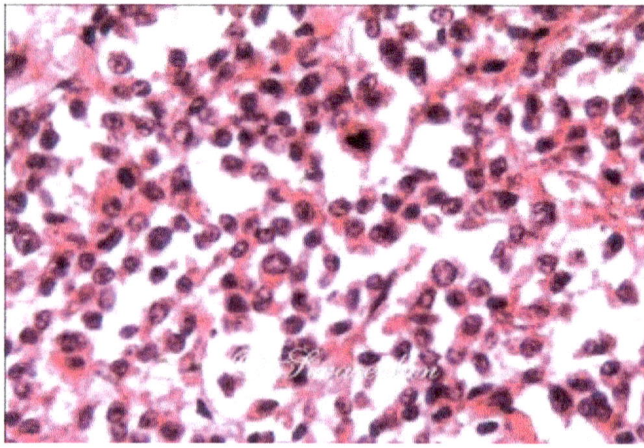

Fig. 148: Hepatocellular carcinoma revealing aniso and poikilo karyosis. Nucleoli are multiple in some cells depicting angularity.

Growth and Metastasis

Adhesion may form with surrounding structures. Metastasis occurs to regional lymph nodes and lung.

Cholangiocellular Carcinoma (Bile Duct Carcinoma)

It is rare, when compared to hepatocellular carcinoma. More incidences have been reported in the intra hepatic bile ducts of dogs, than in the extra hepatic bile duct, which leads to gall bladder.

Gross appearance

- ★ The size varies from few mm to several cm in diameter
- ★ Smaller tumours are invisible and embedded within the liver
- ★ Solitary or multiple occurrences is possible
- ★ The colour varies from grayish white to light brown
- ★ Light colour indicates more fibrous stroma, which accounts for firm consistency
- ★ Solid types are commonly seen, but cystic type may also occur
- ★ Necrotic central area may be filled with blood tinged fluid

Histological feature

- ★ This tumour shows either glandular or cystic pattern lined by pleomorphic neoplastic bile duct epithelium (cuboidal to columnar)
- ★ The lumen of glandular acini and cyst may show bluish mucus secretions with alcian blue stain
- ★ The surrounding liver may show hyperplastic bile duct or metastasis from primary foci

- ★ Pseudo glandular pattern of hepatocellular carcinoma should be differentiated from cholangiocellular carcinoma by observing polyhedral cells in the former and cuboidal to columnar cells in the later
- ★ More fibrous stroma can be seen in cholangiocellular carcinoma when compared to hepatocellular carcinoma

Metastasis

This tumour is more aggressive than hepatocellular carcinoma, and metastasizes to regional lymphnodes and other organs especially to lungs.

28

Lung Tumours

Lung tumours are rare in animals when compared to human. Smoking and environmental pollutions predispose human for lung cancers. Since, lung is the commonest organ for metastatic tumour growth from many of the other organ tumours, care must be taken to differentiate these.

Gross appearance

- ★ Both solitary and multiple tumours may occur
- ★ Diaphragmatic lobe of right lung is the commonest site of occurrence
- ★ Bronchi and bronchiolar epithelium is a source of most of the lung tumours
- ★ Involvement of alveolar epithelium may also occur rarely
- ★ They occur in different size, colour and consistency

Histological feature

- ★ Bronchi, bronchiolar columnar epithelium and cuboidal epithelium of bronchi acini are the source from which bronchiogenic carcinoma and adenocarcinoma may arise respectively
- ★ In adenocarcinoma, secretory cells with vesicular nucleus are arranged as a solid sheet to form acinar/tubular pattern
- ★ Mucin accumulation can be seen within the lumen
- ★ Papillary adenoma and papillary cyst adenoma may also arise from secretory epithelium of bronchi and bronchiole
- ★ Chronic irritants like cigarette and automobile smoke, industrial pollutants like cotton lint and coal particles, and unpaved road pollutants like mud/sand/silica can cause destruction of bronchi and bronchiolar columnar epithelium, in due course highly resistant type of epithelium (squamous epithelium) may form, from which squamous cell carcinoma with cell nest formation may occur

- ★ Metastasis of this squamous cell carcinoma may occur to the lung parenchyma and other organs through peribronchiolar lymphatics
- ★ Lung alveolar epithelium may involve in neoplasia in which neoplastic cells may proliferate from lung alveoli (cancer pneumonia)
- ★ In anaplastic type of alveolar epithelium, solid sheet is formed by large polyhedral to ovoid cells (**oat cells**) and some of the cells are tall columnar resembling fibrosarcoma

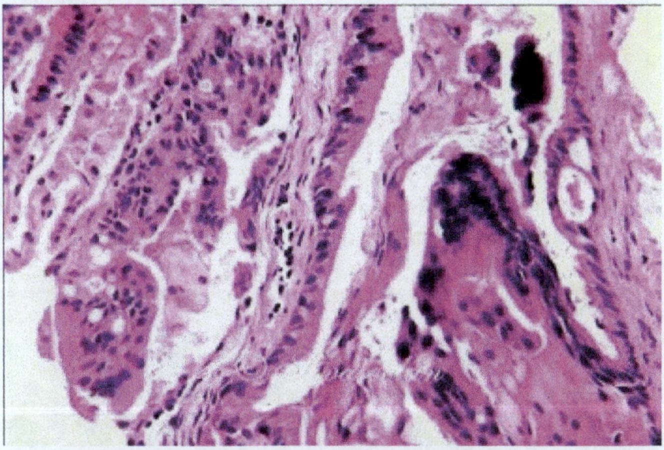

Fig. 149: Lung revealing loss of alveolar arrangements and depict solid sheet arrangement of epithelial cells.

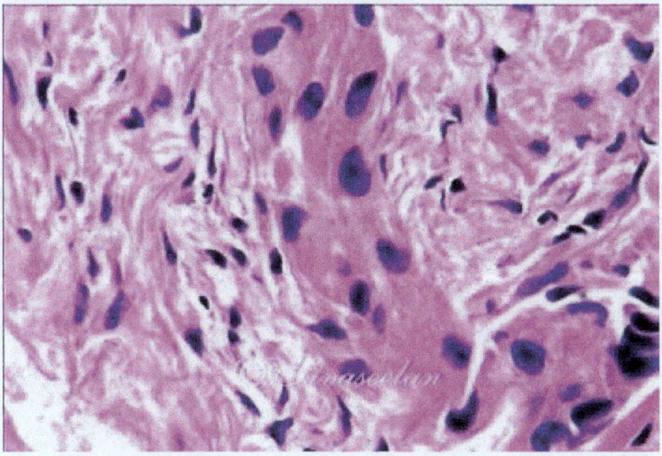

Fig. 150: Lung revealing solid sheet arrangement of epithelial cells (oat cells)

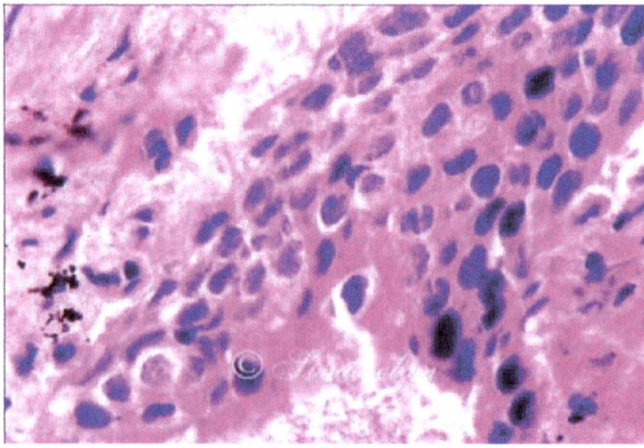

Fig. 151: Lung revealing solid sheet arrangement of epithelial cells with granular cytoplasm indicating accumulation of secretion.

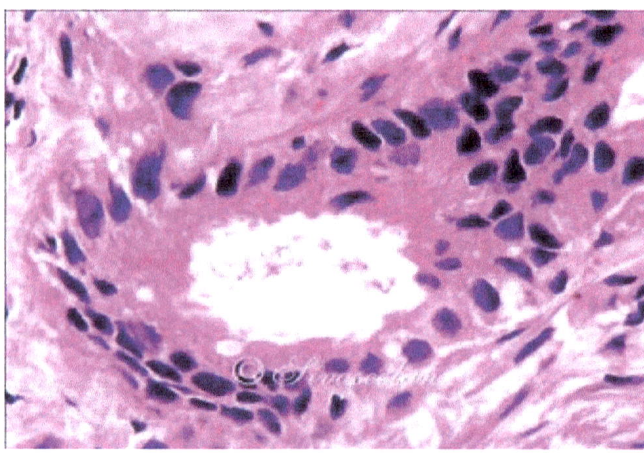

Fig. 152: Adenocarcinoma of lung showing formation of typical acini with multiple layers of epithelial cells.

29

Thyroid, Parathyroid and Pancreatic Tumours

Thyroid tumours are found in goiter belts among horses and aged dogs.

Adenoma

It is a small and well demarcated nodular growth.

Histological feature

Small irregular acini can be seen, which are demarcated from larger normal surrounding acini.

Adenocarcinoma

The size is larger than adenoma.

Histological feature

- ★ Typical adenocarcinoma with pleomorphic acinar cells, papillary projections and basement membrane breakages can be seen
- ★ Thyroid tumours that produce more thyroid hormone are called as thyrotoxic, which are more dangerous

Parathyroid Tumours

Primary tumours of parathyroid occur spontaneously and secondary tumours are due to overstimulation of acinar cells to maintain optimum calcium level of blood, which are encountered in millers' disease of horses, rubber jaw syndrome and interstitial nephritis of dogs, and Von Recklinghausen's disease of human (osteitis fibrosa cystica). Both adenoma and adenocarcinoma may occur as primary tumours.

Pancreas Tumours

Adenoma and adenocarcinoma may arise either from exocrine or endocrine acinar cells. Tumours of islet cells can cause hyper insulinism with hypoglycemia. To identify the particular cell type, specific antibody against the cell antigen must be used in Immunoperoxidase test.

30

Adrenal Gland Tumours

Cortical Tumours

Adenoma and adenocarcinoma of zona fasciculate, zona reticulosa, zona glomerulosa cells may occur in animals secreting more glucocorticoids, mineralocorticoides and androgen with consequent effects. In man, excretions of malformed 17 ketosteroids and estrogen have been reported.

Medullary Tumours

Pheochromocytoma (chromaffinoma) arises from medullary cells, which may secrete more adrenalin with consequent tachycardia, hypertension and hypertrophy of the heart, hyperglycaemia and glycosuria. Chromaffinoma indicates the tumour of dark staining cells, which are larger cells with central nuclei without distinct border (similar to basal cells). This feature distinguishes it from adrenal cortical tumours. Bilateral occurrence has also been reported and metastasis may occur to internal organs.

Sympathoblastoma

This tumour may arise from sympathetic nerve cells and fibres that normally found in the adrenal medulla, which can also occur in the spinal cord sympathetic ganglia (pelvic, thoracic and lumbar ganglia). It is firm in consistency due to more fibrous tissue.

Neuroblastoma (Tumours of immature Neuroblasts)

This tumour shows high cellularity and consists of immature undifferentiated small round cells (neuroblasts). Rosette of elongated cells around the central core of nerve fibre is a characteristic feature. The neoplastic neuroblasts proliferate fast to produce a malignant tumour.

Ganglioneuroma (Tumours of mature Nerve cells and Fibres)

This tumour shows mature well differentiated nerve cells with Nissl bodies and fibres arranged as a sheet. The cells proliferate slowly to produce benign tumour.

Aortic Body Tumour (Heart Base Tumour and Carotid Body Tumour)

- ★ These tumours arise from chemoreceptor cells that are normally found in the tunica adventitia of aorta and carotid arteries
- ★ These receptor cells regulate the respiration and blood circulation by detecting the co_2 and o_2 tension and pH of blood
- ★ These rare tumours have been reported from old dogs
- ★ Aortic body tumour is found in between aorta and pulmonary artery or encircling both at the base of the heart (heart base tumour)
- ★ Carotid body tumour is seen at the bifurcation of the carotid arteries
- ★ These tumours appear as firm, reddish and encapsulated masses

Histological feature

- ★ These tumours reveal lobules of packed polyhedral cells with granular or vacuolated cytoplasm and spherical nucleus
- ★ Connective tissue stroma divide the lobules
- ★ Metastasis may occur if tumour cells invade the tunica media and mix with the blood.

31 Ameloblastoma (Adamantinoma)

- ★ This tumour arises from alveolar border of maxilla and mandible (junction of teeth and gum)
- ★ It has been reported in all animals, but cattle are more commonly affected
- ★ Ameloblasts are odontogenic (adamantic) enamel producing epithelium from which this tumour may arise
- ★ The size varies from one to several cm in diameter and the consistency is soft (enamel is not found in this tumour)
- ★ Some bigger tumours may occupy the entire oral cavity
- ★ It can infiltrate into bone of maxilla or mandible
- ★ This tumour seldom metastasizes to other organs

Histological feature

Solid type

- ★ This type reveals island arrangement of neoplastic ameloblasts in mature fibrous connective tissue stroma
- ★ The outer most cells of islands resemble typical ameloblast and the central cells form a loose network forming stellate reticulum

Plexiform type

- ★ Mature fibrous stroma containing inter digitating cords of columnar cells admixed with poor cellular areas forming loose network of stellate reticulum can be observed

Cystic type

- ★ Cystic spaces are lined by single layer of ameloblasts arranged in different heights to give a serrated outer border
- ★ Cystic spaces may have acidophilic debris or enamel

★ Squamous cell metaplasia may occur to produce squamous cell carcinoma with keratin pearls

★ In most of the ameloblastoma, enamel is not seen and the consistency is soft

Ameloblastic Fibroma

★ This tumour reveals proliferation of both ameloblastic cells as well as supporting stromal connective tissue

★ Epithelial islands or cords are smaller when compared to ameloblastoma

★ The stellate reticular area is very less and cysts formation is not seen

Odontoma

★ Presence of enamel and dentine within the ameloblastoma implies the name Odontoma

★ It is harder than the ameloblastoma

★ Ameloblastic fibroodontoma only differs from ameloblastic fibroma by the presence of enamel and dentine.

32

Kidney Tumours

Adenoma

Rare incidence has been reported in all animals including human.

Gross appearance

- ★ Small (1 – 3 cm) rounded tumours may be observed in the cortical portion of kidney
- ★ Most of the times, they are noticed as embedded masses within the cortex

Histological feature

- ★ Tubules lined by one or more layers of pleomorphic cuboidal epithelium can be observed
- ★ Papillary projections within the lumen of tubules may also be seen in some adenoma
- ★ Widened lumen of tubules may appear as cystic spaces

Adenocarcinoma (Hypernephroma)

This tumour has been reported in animals very rarely, it is so dangerous, because the entire kidney can be completely destroyed by fast proliferation of neoplastic tubular epithelium.

Gross appearance

- ★ This is so large tumour when compared to benign type
- ★ Round to oval in appearance and may fill the entire peritoneal cavity if the size is too large
- ★ Cut sections may reveal lobulations

Histological feature

- ★ Many layered tubules with columnar or cuboidal or polygonal neoplastic epithelial cells can be observed

- ★ Tubular breakage and evasion of epithelial cells may form solid sheet arrangement
- ★ Anaplastic tumour may show highly pleomorphic cells with hyperchromatic nuclei or mitotic figure
- ★ In highly proliferative type, some cells may show clear cytoplasm indicating hydropic or fatty degeneration; these cells are called as **Clear cells**
- ★ These cells are spontaneously formed in this tumour and have no connection with adrenal embryonic cell rest of kidney, so the word Hypernephroma is a misnomer to this tumour

Metastasis

This is highly invasive tumour and metastasis is possible in regional lymphnodes and other organs.

Embryonal Nephroma (Hypernephroma-real, Nephroblastoma, Wilm's Tumour of Children, Adenosarcoma, Round Cell Sarcoma)

- ★ This rare tumour is found in fowl, swine and human (children)
- ★ The origin is pluripotent cells of kidney which have the ability to produce tubules as well as connective tissue
- ★ Since the origin is pluripotent cells, this tumour may contain muscle, cartilage and bone
- ★ This tumour may occur on or within the kidney and usually unilateral. If it is occurring within the kidney, a demarcating capsule around it should be appreciated, otherwise this tumour cannot be differentiated from adenocarcinoma of the kidney
- ★ Multiple tumours have also been reported
- ★ The size varies from 1-20 cm in diameter and weight may go up to 30 kgs
- ★ Smaller tumours may be embedded within the kidney tissue without much elevation
- ★ Thick fibrous capsule divide the tumour into different lobules

Histological feature

- ★ Lobules are consisting of tubular structure lined by flat epithelium, which may project inside the lumen
- ★ Hyaline material may be observed in some of the tubular lumen
- ★ Epithelium and connective tissue dominate in swine and cattle respectively
- ★ Irregularly formed glomeruli like structures may be observed in some places
- ★ Since the fibrous tissue proliferation is also found, this tumour is called as **Adenosarcoma**

- ★ Fibrous tissue area may show round to oval shape young proliferating fibroblasts with round nucleus, which is called as **Round cell sarcoma**
- ★ Isolated areas may show solid masses of proliferating epithelium or cystic spaces lined by neoplastic epithelium

Recurrence and Metastasis

This tumour grow by expansion and destroy the nearby healthy kidney tissue by pressure atrophy, but kidney dysfunction is felt in rare bilateral occurrence. Bulky tumour may cause adhesion and dysfunction of bowel. Metastasis rarely occurs to other organs. Metastasis to peritoneum is possible due to transcoelomic spread.

33

Tumours of Nervous System

Primary neoplasms of the nervous system are relatively rare in most domestic animal species with the exception of dog and cat. Both central nervous system and peripheral nervous system tumours are most prevalent among dogs. Neoplasia of the nervous system in domestic animals is primarily a problem of aged animals. Over 70 % of primary tumours of the CNS of dogs occur over 6 years of age.

Primary Tumours of CNS

Glial Tumour

Astrocytoma

The WHO international classification distinguishes three grades of human astrocytoma based on their degree of differentiation:

1. Diffuse Astrocytoma
2. Anaplastic Astrocytoma
3. Glioblastoma Multiforma

Incidence and site

Glial tumours are the common primary tumours of the CNS in dogs and cats Astrocytoma occurs most frequently in the cerebral hemisphere, predominantly in the temporal piriform region, but they may be located in many areas of CNS including the brain stem, cerebellum and spinal cord.

Gross morphology

Slow growing well differentiated tumours are usually poorly defined and often barely distinguishable from normal brain by their pinkish colour. Rapidly growing tumours are more motile and soft because of frequently associated cyst, necrosis, haemorrhage and edema.

Histological feature

1. Diffuse astrocytoma

- ★ The most common fibrillary astrocytoma is composed of diffusely arranged elongated spindle shaped cells and occasionally polygonal cells
- ★ Neoplastic astrocytes are identified based on their nuclear atypia with enlarged or irregular hyperchromatic nuclei
- ★ Gemistocytic astrocytoma is another subtype which consists of mostly large, irregular globoid cells with eccentric nuclei and abundant eosinophilic cytoplasm with short thick intertwining process
- ★ Protoplasmic type is third type in which small to medium sized cells with poorly defined cytoplasmic borders and round nuclei with a dispersed chromatin pattern and a prominent nucleolus are observed

2. Anaplastic Astrocytoma

- ★ It contains a pleomorphic more dense cell population consisting of fusiform, polygonal or round shaped cells of variable sizes, often with distinct nuclear atypia
- ★ Multinucleate giant cells may be observed
- ★ Nuclei are mostly larger and hyperchromatic than in differentiated astrocytoma
- ★ More anaplastic astrocytomas are highly cellular, fast growing and infiltrative

3. Glioblastoma Multiforma

- ★ It is characterised by marked cellular pleomorphism, nuclear atypia, giant cell formation, high mitotic index and infiltrative growth
- ★ Foci of necrosis surrounded by pseudopalisading radiating glial cells can be observed
- ★ Blood vessel proliferation occurs mostly in the vicinity of necrotic foci or along the tumour margins

Oligodendroglioma

This tumour is the most commonly reported canine primary CNS tumour, especially in brachycephalic breeds. Oligodendroglioma generally occurs in the white or gray matter of the cerebral hemisphere and rarely in the brain stem and spinal cord.

Gross appearance

- ★ Oligodendroglioma are often large tumours with a greyish blue gelatinous or mucoid translucent matrix
- ★ On section, they are usually well demarcated soft and gray to pink coloured mass, and they may protrude through the cortical surface

Histological feature

- ★ It reveals dense sheets of uniform cells or cords or clusters
- ★ A perinuclear halo is commonly seen with delayed fixation and results in the "honeycomb cell pattern" of arrangement
- ★ A prominent microvascular proliferation with the formation of vascular loops or glomeruli like tufts are often arranged in long lines or clusters at the margins or throughout the tumour
- ★ Multifocal microcystic areas containing blue staining mucin like material and foci of recent haemorrhages may be found

Ependymoma

Incidence and site

They are derived from cells lining the ventricular system of the CNS. Ependymomas have been reported in dog, cat, cattle and horse, but are rare tumours.

It occurs mainly within the lateral ventricles, less often in the third and fourth ventricles.

Gross appearance

- ★ Ependymomas are generally large intraventricular masses, mostly well demarcated, gray to red with a smooth texture in the dog, but much more granular in the cat
- ★ Growth is usually intraventricular and it may infilterate the adjacent areas
- ★ Obstructive hydrocephalus may also develop, when the CSF flow is blocked by this tumour

Histological feature

Two subtypes are observed:

1. Cellular
2. Papillary

Cellular Type

- ★ In dogs, they are moderately to densely cellular and well vascularised
- ★ The perivascular zone may show the formation of pseudorosettes
- ★ In feline, this tumour shows densely cellular areas and neoplastic cells reveal minimal cytoplasm with darkly staining basophilic nuclei
- ★ Perivascular pseudorosettes and ependymal rosettes are more in felines than in canines
- ★ In feline, tumour cells contain round to ovoid nuclei and an eosinophilic fibrillar cytoplasm with poorly defined borders. Nuclei are moderately hyperchromatic with a prominent nucleolus and punctuate hyperchromatin

Papillary Type

- ⋆ It has a vascular core forming papillae whose surfaces are covered by single or multiple layers of columnar cells arranged in a pseudorosette pattern
- ⋆ Malignant tumours are characterised by anaplasia, frequent mitosis, necrosis, local neutrophilic infiltration and invasion to surrounding structures

Choroids Plexus Papilloma

Incidence and site

These intraventricular tumours are derived from choroids plexus epithelium and it is a common tumour in dogs. Besides local compression, these tumours may cause hydrocephalus by ventricular obstruction or possibly by excess production of cerebro spinal fluid.

Gross appearance

They are well defined non encapsulated grayish white to red granular or cauliflower like masses that occur either within a ventricle or grow out in the cerebropalatine angle. In dog widespread metastases into spinal cord through CSF is common.

Histological feature

- ⋆ Most of the choroids plexus tumours are papilloma
- ⋆ The typical architecture of the choroids plexus papilloma is the branching tree like pattern with a single layer of cuboidal or columnar cells covering a modest fibrovascular stroma of leptomeningeal derivation

Choroids Plexus Carcinoma

They are rare tumours, but we can distinguish it from papilloma by cellular pleomorphism, nuclear atypia, frequent mitoses and local invasion.

Embryonal tumours

They are mainly grouped under primitive neuroectodermal tumours:

1. Medulloblastoma
2. Neuroblastoma and Ganglioneuroma

Medulloblastoma

Incidence and site

They are common malignant tumours of the cerebellum in children. In animals, they are commonly seen in calves and puppies. In animals they arise from the matrix cells of the external granular layer of the cerebellum and they are exclusively located in cerebellum.

Gross appearance

They are well defined soft grayish or pinkish masses located unilaterally in the cerebellar cortex. Hydrocephalus is commonly linked to an expanding neuroblastoma.

Histological feature

★ It is composed of a fairly uniform and closely packed round to polygonal cell population often arranged in sheets or bands

★ Pallisading of cells and complete or incomplete rosette formation are frequently observed

★ Round to elongated hyperchromatic nuclei and mitoses are frequent and there is mostly a vascular stroma

Neuroblastoma and Ganglioneuroma

Neuroblastoma is a tumour consisting of immature undifferentiated neuroblasts while ganglioneuroma denotes a tumour consisting of well differentiated nerve cells and fibres. The former is rapidly growing and malignant one while the latter is benign.

Incidence and site

These tumours are extremely rare. They have been reported in cattle, horse, dog and fowl. Young animals are more often affected. Though arising from the nervous tissue, these tumours are very, very rare in CNS. They are more commonly found in adrenal medulla (where it is called as 'Sympathoblastoma") and in the sympathetic ganglia of the abdominal and pelvic regions. The cervical and thoracic ganglia may also be affected.

Gross appearance

They are encapsulated and vary in size. They may be white or gray in colour. They are fibrous in consistency.

Histological feature

★ The neuroblastoma is highly cellular and consists of undifferentiated small round cells

★ Large number of mitotic figures are frequently observed

★ Cells often show a tendency toward pallisading and neuroblastic rosette formation

★ The ganglioneuroma consists of more mature nerve cells and their fibres. The cells show nissil substance and no mitoses are noticed

Meningioma

Meningiomas are derived from meningiothelial (arachoidal fibroblasts) cells of the arachanoid and piamater of the nervous system. Predisposing factors in human meningioma are breast tumour, previous trauma, cranial irradiation and a variety of genetic abnormalities.

Incidence and site

These tumours are the most common primary nervous system tumour of both dog and cats. An increasing prevalence with age is noticed. Most of the canine meningioma are intracranial and occur as solitary well demarcated mass that grow either by compression or less commonly by infiltration. It usually occurs over the cerebral hemisphere. In dogs, meningioma is found commonly in the region of the olfactory bulb.

Gross appearance

- ⋆ Meningiomas usually grow as well demarcated, often lobulated firm granular masses that usually have a broad based or pedunculated attachment to the overlying meninges
- ⋆ By local compression behind intact meninges, meningioma generally forms depression in to the brain
- ⋆ Mineralisation may impart a gritty feel on sectioning
- ⋆ In cats, intracranial meningioma are globular well defined masses with a broad meningeal base attachment

Histological feature

- ⋆ Meningiomas are classified based mainly on the WHO classification of human histological subtypes.

Meningiothelial Type

- ⋆ Broad sheets of cells have a elongate to ovoid nuclei
- ⋆ A single prominent nucleolus, abundant cytoplasm and indistinct cytoplasmic borders can be observed

Fibroblastic Type

- ⋆ Cells tend to be more spindle shaped than in meningiothelial subtype and have more elongated nuclei
- ⋆ Cells often forming intersecting bundles or streams between which dense collagen fibres are observed

Transitional Type

- ⋆ This type reveal the picture of mixture of meningiothelial and fibroblastic patterns
- ⋆ There are more syncytial cell clusters or concentric whorls that evolve into well demarcated lobules often interspersed with regions of meningiothelial cells
- ⋆ Occasional psammoma bodies form with a core of central hyalinisation, necrosis and mineralisation within the whorls

Psammomatous Type

★ There is a background transitional pattern with predominant whorl formation with large numbers of psammoma bodies

Papillary Type

★ It is formed by meningiothelial cells radiating around a central vascular core in papillary formation

★ The tapering ends of the meningiothelial cells are terminating on the central vessels creating a prominent perivascular cell free zone resembling the formation of pseudorosettes

★ There are often broad sheets of meningiothelial cells interspersed between the papillary areas

Microcystic Type

★ The cells are spindle shaped with elongated nuclei and processes are loosely arranged and intersecting to form empty intracellular cysts, sometimes containing blue staining mucin like material

Myxoid Type

★ The pattern is of papillary structures with a central fibrovascular stroma and ovoid to fusiform cells radiating away from the vessels

★ The round cells may contain clear vacuoles in an abundant cytoplasm

★ The cells are embedded individually or in clusters in an amorphous myxoid matrix that is positive with mucicarmine alcian blue and PAS stains

Angiomatous Type

★ There are numerous dilated blood vessels on a background of a meningioma

★ This subtype must be differentiated from meningioangiomatosis, which is a vascular malformation within the intracranial leptomeninges with a proliferation of meningiothelial cells around blood vessels

Atypical Type

★ This may be a meningiothelial subtype with aggressive invasion of adjacent neurophils

★ There are solid sheets of meningiothelial cells with multifocal areas of tumour cell necrosis

★ There is a high mitotic index, cellular pleomorphism and individual cell necrosis

Tumours of Peripheral Nervous System

Schwannoma

All peripheral nerve fibres consist of the axon covered with a thin protoplasmic sheath called neurilemma or sheath of Schwann. Sheath of Schwann is a thin tube like membrane or sheath containing a nucleus surrounded by cytoplasm and is also known as Schwann's cell or lemmocytes. The neurilemma forms sheath of the axon in all peripheral nerves and there is no sheath of Schwann in CNS. Benign tumour may arise from these Schwann's cells called Schwannoma.

Incidence and Site

In the dog, Schwannoma tend to occur in older dogs. It commonly occurs in spinal nerves (especially brachial plexus). Multicentric Schwannoma may also occur in older dogs. These tumours have predilection for the autonomic nervous system (nerves which innervates visceral organs). The affected nerve cannot pass impulses, so paralysis may be seen in the respective region.

Gross appearance

In dogs, the gross appearance of Schwannoma is distinctive as nodular masses or fusiform thickening of spinal or cranial nerves. Consistency may be very firm or soft and gelatinous. These tumours show the colour of shiny white to gray and are smooth surfaced.

Histological feature

Two distinct patterns of arrangement of the cells are noticed

1. The Antony type A
2. The Antony type B

The Antony type A

★ In this type, the Schwann cells are elongated and spindle shaped with oval or cylindrical nuclei and fibres form interlacing bundles

★ The cells are arranged parallel to each other

★ A distinct palisade arrangement is obtained by the alternate arrangement of the nuclei of cells and fibres which are nuclei free

★ This palisade arrangements if they take a whorl form, they are called "Verocay bodies". The fibres are derived from the neurilemma cells and are similar to collagen fibres, but are distinct from them

The Antony type B

★ In this variety, cells of varying shades are arranged in a disorderly loose manner

★ Often intercellular vacuoles containing a watery fluid may be seen, which stains blue with haematoxylin

★ In this type fibres are not seen

In the same tumour, the above two varieties may be found together side by side with clear demarcation, but both these tumours never intermingle. Schwannoma can also have single or multiple foci of osseous or cartilaginous or mucoid differentiation.

34

Tumours of Female Reproductive System

Tumours of the Ovary

Tumours of the ovary arise from three embryological origins

1. The epithelium of the ovary which includes the lining epithelium of modified mesothelium
2. The germ cells
3. The ovarian stroma including the sex cords

Epithelial Tumours

Most epithelial tumours arise from the surface epithelium and the subsurface epithelial structures in the bitch.

Gross appearance

- ★ Cystic multinodular tumour can be seen as either unilateral or bilateral growth
- ★ The cut surface typically has multiple cysts that contain thin yellow to brown fluid interspersed between the solid regions
- ★ Carcinomas may appear as proliferative cauliflower like growth that project from the surface of the ovary

Histological feature

- ★ Cystic cavities may show papillary projections into the lumen in both adenomas and carcinomas
- ★ The papillae consists of connective tissue stalks that are lined by single or multiple layers of cuboidal or columnar epithelial cells
- ★ The wall of the cyst is lined by single or multiple layers of epithelium and the lumen may contain proteinaceous material

- ★ Anaplastic carcinomas reveal broad disorganized sheets of neoplastic cells

The common tumours are

- ★ Granulosa cell tumour
- ★ Granulosa theca cell tumour
- ★ Luteoma
- ★ Thecoma
- ★ Sertoli cell tumour of the ovary
- ★ Leydig cell tumour
- ★ Arrhenoblastoma
- ★ Interstitial gland tumour

These tumours are hormonally active and secrete steroid hormones. They produce varying amounts of progesterone, estrogen, testosterone, and inhibin and influence the reproductive behaviour of the affected animal. The animal may exhibit persistent anestrus, intermittent or continuous estrus or masculinisation. Bitches may manifest signs of hyperestronism including endocrine alopecia, bone marrow suppression with consequent anaemia, leucopenia followed by leukocytosis, thrombocytopenia and haemorrhagic diathesis, and cystic endometrial hyperplasia. These changes are reversible by removal of the tumour.

Granulosa cell tumour

It consists of irregular accumulation of granulosa cells separated by a supporting stroma of spindle cells resembling disorganised attempts of follicle formation.

Granulosa theca cell tumour

In some granulosa cell tumours, the stroma resembles thecal tissues and it is designated as granulose theca cell tumour. In some tumours, the follicular pattern is less prominent with the neoplastic granulosa cells being arranged in solid sheets cords or trabeculae or nests. Some granulosa cell tumours closely resembles that of testicular sertoli cell tumours thus called as sertoli cell tumour of the ovary. Lutenisation may occur in some tumours and are characterised by accumulations of polyhedral cells with abundant vacuolated eosinophilic cytoplasm known as **"Call Exner bodies".**

Thecoma

This tumour depicts irregular loosely arranged unencapsulated aggregates of spindle shaped cells. Individual cells have elongated nuclei and the cytoplasm may contain lipid vacuoles indicative of steroid hormone production which can be stained with fat stains such as sudan black.

Germ cell tumours

It includes

- ★ Dysgerminomas
- ★ Teratomas

Dysgerminoma

This tumour is female equivalent of testicular seminoma

Species affected

Most common in the bitch and queen

Age

Older animals are commonly affected

Gross appearance

- ★ Usually large size tumour that cause spherical or ovoid enlargement of the affected ovary
- ★ Cut surface of the tumour reveal white or gray firm and homogenous tissue

Histological feature

- ★ Broad sheets cords and nests of cells are separated by occasional thin connective tissue septa
- ★ Individual tumour cells resemble primitive germ cells
- ★ They are large and polyhedral cells containing vesicular nuclei with prominent nucleoli
- ★ More mitotic figures and multinucleated tumours cells are common feature. Focal aggregation of lymphocytes are also appreciated
- ★ Metastasis may occur

Teratoma

This tumour is composed of abnormal tissue derived from at least two and often all three germinal layers. They arise from pluripotent stem cells that have undergone differentiation.

Gross appearance

- ★ Spherical or ovoid enlargement of the affected ovary with solid and cystic areas on cut surface can be seen
- ★ It may contain sebaceous gland material and hair
- ★ A variety of the tissues may be present including bone, cartilage and teeth
- ★ Teratoma of the bovine ovary are often dermoid cysts

Histological feature

- ★ Most of the teratoma are benign and are composed of well differentiated mature tissues
- ★ Malignant teratoma of the ovary are rarely reported in bitch and mare

Mesenchymal Tumours

Fibromas, haemangiomas, leiomyomas and their malignant counterparts may occur in ovary. These tumours appear grossly as discrete, rubbery, red brown nodules within the affected ovary. Histologically, these tumours consist of numerous endothelium lined channels filled with blood.

Tumours of the Uterine Tube and Uterus

Epithelial tumours

Uterine epithelial tumours are rare in domestic animals and adenoma may occur from glandular elements of uterus.

Uterine carcinoma

In cattle, these tumours are solitary and develop in the uterine horn. It is observed as discrete firm enlargement of the uterus composed of very firm dense white to yellow tissue.

Histology

Nests and cords of anaplastic epithelium among abundant fibrous connective tissue stroma can be seen. From the endometrium it extends into the myometrium early in the disease and metastasize to other parenchymal organs such as lungs, liver and abdomen later.

Mesenchymal tumours

It includes leiomyoma, leiomyosarcoma, fibroma, fibrosarcoma, fibroleiomyoma and fibroleiomyosarcoma. They occur as firm nodular multiple proliferations within the myometrium that may project into the uterine lumen.

Lymphosarcoma

Lymphosarcoma may also seldom occur that appear as homogenous gray or yellow mass. Histologically accumulation of neoplastic lymphocytes within the endometrium and disruption of normal tissue can be seen.

Tumours of the cervix vagina and vulva

Epithelial tumours

Virus induced papilloma (wart) appear as papillary projections of epithelium with a scant fibrovascular stroma. Squamous cell carcinoma are common in ruminants especially in vulva of sheep, goats and cattle in areas where they are exposed to high levels of solar radiation. Squamous cell carcinoma is occasionally invasive, but rarely metastasize to other organs.

Mesenchymal tumours

Leiomyoma, fibroma, lipoma, canine transmissible venereal tumour and melanomas in gray horses may occur in external genitalia.

35

Tumours of Male Reproductive System

Tumours of the Testis

Sertoli Cell Tumour (Sustentacular tumour)

Incidence

This tumour is commonly seen in dogs, especially in retained testes, rare in cat, bull and horse. Average age of occurrence in dog is 8-11 years, but in cryptorchid condition, younger ones are also affected.

Clinical characteristics

Unilateral or bilateral, common in testes those are extrascrotal in the inguinal canal or abdominal cavity. The uninvolved testis will be atrophied, small, flabby and brown. Bilateral symmetrical alopecia, atrophy of hair follicles and sebaceous glands can be seen. The skin of affected dog depicts dark purple melanin pigmentation in the hairless areas. Enlargement of prostate gland, gynaecomastia and feminization in male dogs are other features.

Gross appearance

- ★ Sertoli cell tumours may grow about 5 cm in diameter and are discrete tumours
- ★ External surface is smooth or nodular and is enclosed by thick capsule
- ★ Cut surface is irregularly lobulated and the lobules are separated by thick fibrous tissue
- ★ Consistency is harder than seminoma

Histological feature

Two main patterns are observed

- ★ Intratubular type
- ★ Diffuse type

Intratubular type

* ⋆ This type reveals well formed tubules separated by connective tissue septa and the tumour cells are multilayered in the tubules and are arranged with their long axes perpendicular to the basement membrane
* ⋆ The tumour cells are long and fusiform with thin cytoplasmic prolongations and show indistinct cell borders
* ⋆ Elongated round or oval small nuclei are seen within the pallisading cells
* ⋆ The cytoplasm may be vacuolated in some cells
* ⋆ In some areas, intratubular neoplastic cells spill out of the tubules into the stroma forming solid infiltrating nests of cells outside the tubules

Diffuse form

* ⋆ Malignant type often show the diffuse arrangement
* ⋆ The tumour cells may invade the tunical albuginea, rete testis, epididymis and even scrotal skin
* ⋆ Anisocytosis and poikilocytosis are common features and the neoplastic cells possess larger more hyperchromatic nuclei
* ⋆ Cytoplasmic vacuolation are frequently observed

Metastasis

Metastasize to regional lymph nodes, liver, lungs, kidneys, spleen, adrenals and pancreas.

Interstitial Cell Tumour (Leydig cell tumour)

Incidence

This tumour is very common in dog, rare in bull, cat, stallion, boar and ram. Older dogs are commonly affected and incidence increases with the age. No breed prevalence is known.

Clinical characteristics

Alopecia and perineal hernia may be noticed.

Gross appearance

* ⋆ Round, discrete and encapsulated tumour, which is soft and bulge on cut section
* ⋆ Solitary or multiple growths in the same or opposite testis can be seen
* ⋆ The size vary from 1 to several cm in diameter

Histological feature

The tumour cells are arranged in three main patterns.

Solid diffuse type

The cells are arranged either diffusely in large sheets of uniform cells or as cords separated by thin delicate septa.

Pseudoadenomatous type

The cells are arranged as groups surrounding empty spaces that are not lined by endothelial cells, but may contain acidophilic staining material.

Cystic vascular type (Angiomatoid type)

- ★ Interconnecting strands of few cell wide tumour cells surround spaces filled with pink fluid and erythrocytes
- ★ The neoplastic cells shape may be polyhedral, cuboidal or columnar and the cytoplasm reveal dull acidophilic ground glass appearance with small or large vacuolar spaces containing lipid
- ★ Some of the cells contain cytoplasmic lipochrome pigment
- ★ The nuclei are small and hyperchromatic
- ★ Mitotic figures are rarely seen
- ★ Metastasis to regional lymph nodes and lungs is noticed

Germ Cell Tumours

It includes:

1. Seminoma
2. Embryonal carcinoma
3. Gonadoblastoma
4. Teratoma

Seminoma

Incidence

This tumour is commonly observed in dogs and rare in other species. Aged dogs are affected and no breed predisposition is noticed. Unilateral or bilateral with solitary or multiple occurrence can be observed. More incidences are noticed in right testis than the left. This tumour is mostly associated with cryptorchid testicles. This tumour may concurrently occur with sertoli cell tumour.

Gross appearance

- ★ The size may vary, bulging masses depict softness while palpation
- ★ The colour may vary from creamy white or pinkish gray and cut surface may show lobulations

Histological feature

Intratubular type

- ★ It originates from spermatogenic epithelium in seminiferous tubules
- ★ Proliferating tumour cells replace the spermatogenic epithelium within the tubule
- ★ The fast proliferating neoplastic cells may invade the interstitial stroma in between the tubules and the tumour becomes the diffuse type

Diffuse type

- ★ The proliferating cells are arranged as diffuse sheets or islands of cells
- ★ The neoplastic cells are larger and uniform in size and shape and are round or ovoid or polyhedral with discrete cellular outlines
- ★ The nuclei are prominent, large, ovoid and hyperchromatic
- ★ Multinucleated cells can be seen commonly
- ★ Since the nucleus is larger, cytoplasm appears scanty
- ★ Most of the cells reveal mitotic figures
- ★ Scattered vacuolated histiocytes may show starry sky appearance to the diffuse type
- ★ Metastasis occur less commonly to regional lymph nodes and lungs

Diffuse type of seminoma in a three year old Pomeranian dog was reported by **Sivaseelan** *et al.* (IJVP, 2015, 39-4: 360-362), which showed tendency to infiltrate blood vessels. Secondary growth was noticed in regional lymph-node. Immunohistochemically, it depicted more than 80 per cent positivity to Ki-67 proliferation antigen pointing to a high proliferation potential proving an unfavourable course of the tumour.

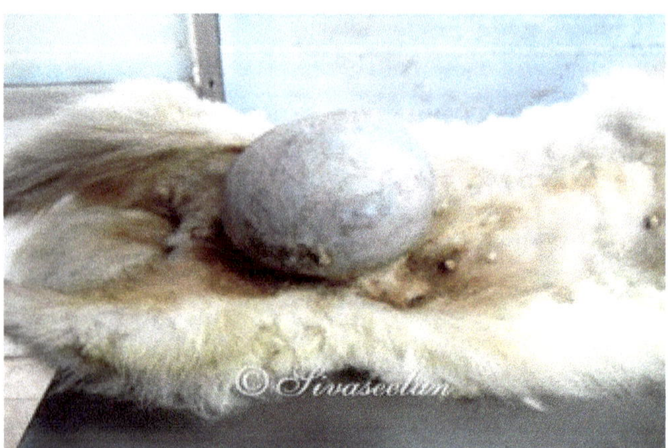

Fig. 153: A dog showing a large Seminoma involving right testis causing atrophy of left testis.

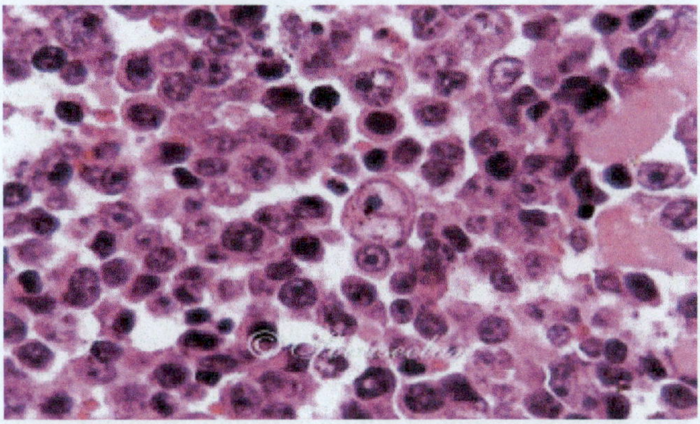

Fig. 154: Diffuse sheet arrangement of neoplastic round to polyhedral germ cells with large nuclei leaving scanty cytoplasm. Twin nuclei and large nucleoli are also seen.

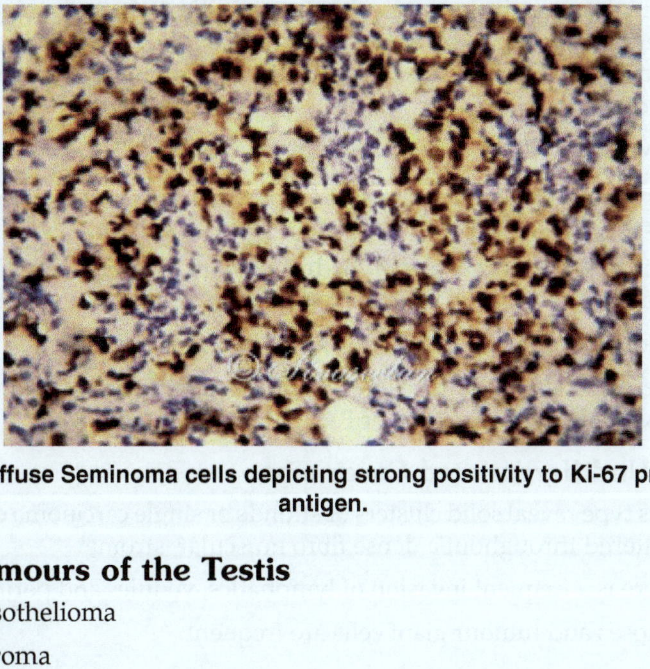

Fig. 155: Diffuse Seminoma cells depicting strong positivity to Ki-67 proliferation antigen.

Other Tumours of the Testis

1. Mesothelioma
2. Fibroma
3. Haemangioma

Tumours of the prostate

Adenoma and adenocarcinoma

Incidence

This tumour is reported only in dog and cat. Aged dogs are commonly affected, no breed predisposition is known.

Clinical characteristics

The affected dog become emaciated, show rear limb weakness or lameness, has lumbar pain and strain to defecate or urinate. Extension of growth leads to adhesion with surroundings sites.

Gross appearance

- ★ The involved prostate is usually enlarged and the surface is nodular
- ★ Size may vary from few millimetre to centimetre
- ★ Consistency varies from hard or rubbery
- ★ The tumours are focal or diffuse and located in any part of the gland
- ★ Cut surface appears greyish white or yellow in colour

Histological feature

- ★ The picture will be intra-alveolar papillary type consisting of large irregularly shaped alveoli filled with papillary projections of prostatic glandular epithelium and occasionally containing cell clusters, debris and mucin
- ★ Alveoli and lobes are separated by fibrous septa
- ★ In adenocarcinoma, the tumour cells infiltrate basement membrane of alveoli and proliferate in between alveoli also
- ★ The cells are round or polyhedral or oval or elongated, the nuclei are located in the base of the cells and are hyperchromatic with large nucleoli
- ★ Moderate numbers of mitotic figures are seen
- ★ The cells are vacuolated and produce mucinous secretions that stains positive with alcian blue or PAS

Prostatic Undifferentiated Carcinoma

- ★ This type reveal solid clusters or strands or single carcinoma cells diffusely scattered throughout a dense fibro muscular stroma
- ★ There is a frequent invasion of lymphatics, venules and perineural spaces
- ★ Mitoses and tumour giant cells are frequent

Growth and metastases

- ★ Metastasize to pelvic and sublumbar lymph nodes and lungs. It can also metastasize to bone, kidneys, brain, adrenal glands, spleen and liver.

Tumours of the External Male Genetalia

Fibropapilloma of cattle

It is a transmissible benign tumour of fibrous connective tissue with varying amounts of pseudo epitheliomatous hyperplasia of the overlying mucosa.

Incidence

This tumour is common in cattle in the USA. Incidence is more in bulls of 1-2 years of age. Older animals seldom show this tumour. Both dairy and beef animals are equally affected. No breed predisposition is known.

Clinical characteristics

Haemorrhage during copulation or erection is noticed. The affected animal may refuse to copulate because of severe pain. Large tumours may cause retention of urine. This tumour is mostly found on the glans-penis and prepuce at the point of its reflection from the glans. Occur mostly as solitary and few as multiple tumours.

Gross appearance

- ★ This tumour appear as lobulated or fungi form or cauliflower like mass and they are soft in younger animals and firm in older cases
- ★ They are pedunculated and the size vary from 2 to 5 cm in diameter
- ★ Due to ulceration haemorrhagic inflammation can be seen on the surface
- ★ Cut surface shows pinkish or grayish white colour with the central area of necrosis

Histological feature

- ★ The multilayered epithelium make finger like projections of epidermal pegs, extending deep into the fibromatous tissue
- ★ Ulceration leads to granulation tissue formation
- ★ Extensive proliferation of connective tissue can be seen
- ★ Interwoven bundles and whorls of fibroblasts and collagen fibres are typically observed

Etiology and Transmission

Bovine papilloma virus is proved as an etiological agent. This tumour is transmitted naturally during copulation. Recurrence is commonly noticed.

Transmissible Genital Papilloma (Condyloma)

These tumours are found on the genetalia of pigs. They are circular, round and project about 1 cm from the mucosal surface. Some are pedunculated and others are filiform with secondary papillary formation.

Histological feature

- ★ Affected skin shows excessive thickening of the stratum spinosum and marked prolongation of the rete pegs
- ★ Mitotic figures are frequent

Squamous Papilloma and Carcinoma of the penis-horse

These tumours are found in adults and aged ones. No breed predilection is reported. They occur on the glans penis and inner lining of the prepuce. Their shape may vary from cauliflower to mulberry shape.

Histological feature

Typical papilloma metastasizes rarely.

Index

D

E

F

G

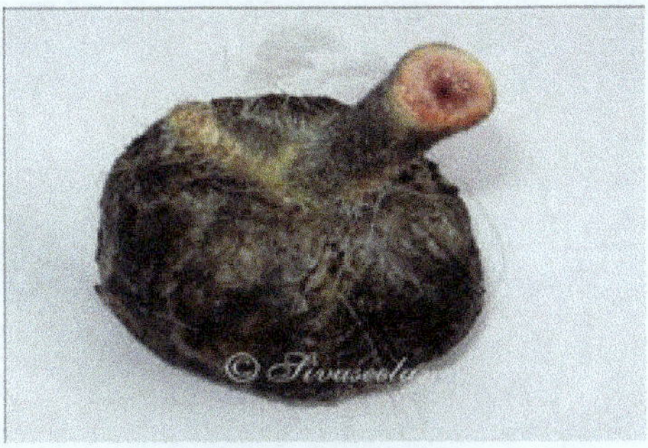

Fig. 1. A round solitary fibroma amputated from tip of the tail of a dog. (p. 80)

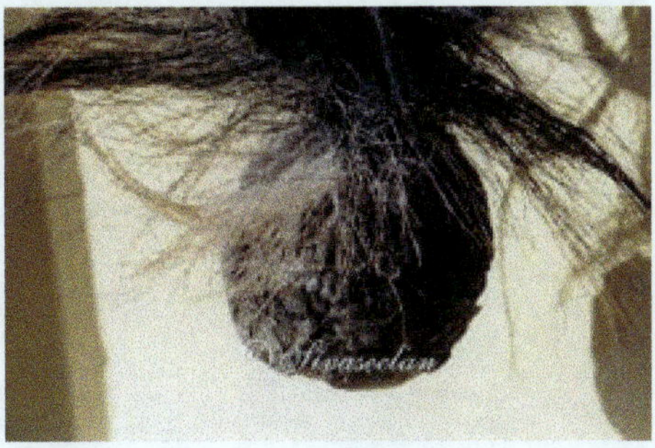

Fig. 2. A fibroma arising from the tail of a cow (p. 80)

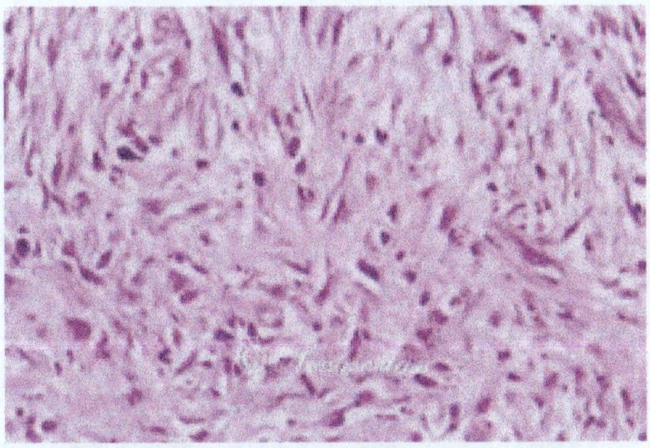

Fig. 3. Histological appearance of the fibroma shown in fig. 1 & 2 revealing loosely arranged fibroblasts and fibres. (p. 80)

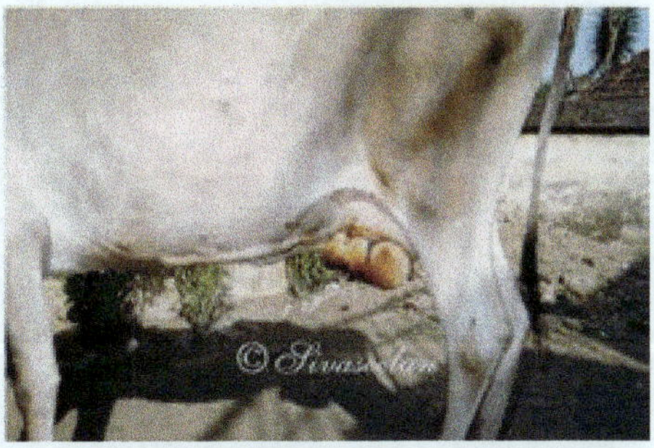

Fig. 4. An ulcerated fibrosarcoma of the udder of a cow (p. 82)

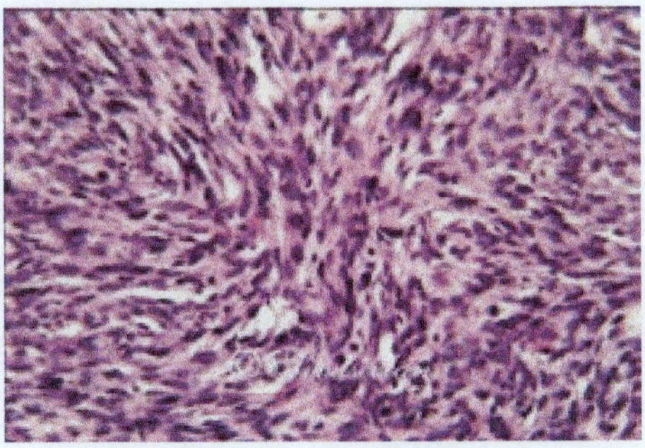

Fig. 5. Fibrosarcoma shown in fig. 4 histologically revealing criss-cross pattern of fibroblasts with hyperchromatic nuclei and fibres. (p. 82)

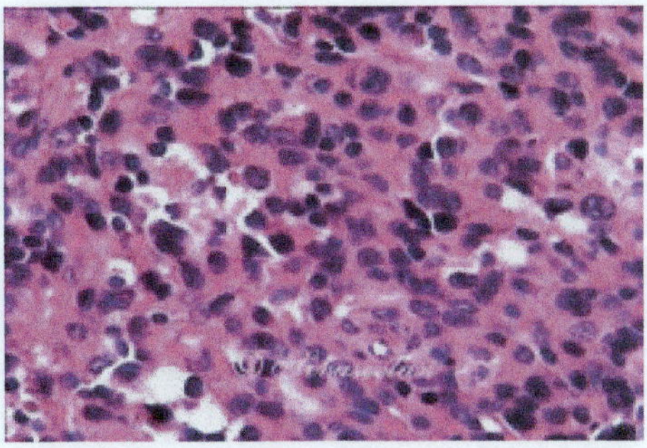

Fig. 6. A malignant fibrous histiocytoma of a cat depicting bizarre cells resembling fibroblast as well as histiocytes with atypical mitotic figures (p. 83)

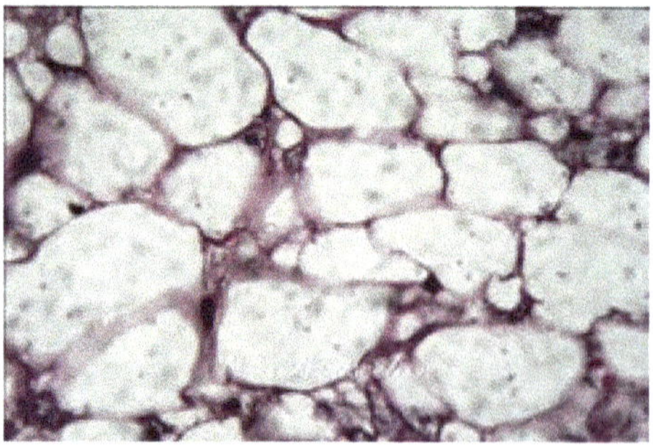

Fig. 7. A lipoma of subcutis of dog revealing lipocytes with large lipid vacuoles (p. 87)

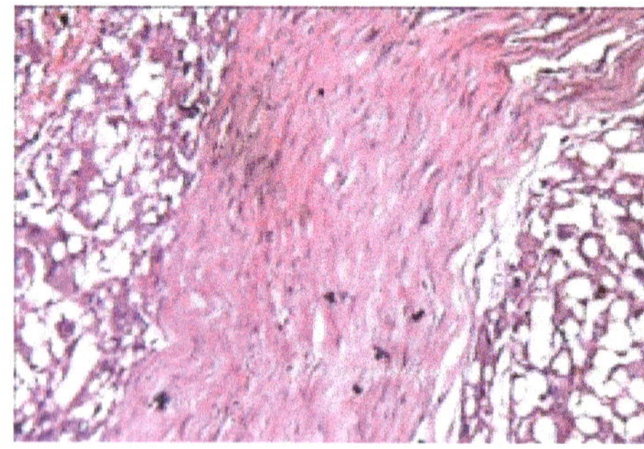

Fig. 8. A fibro-lipoma of skin of a dog showing neoplastic lipocytes divided by thick fibrous septa (p. 88)

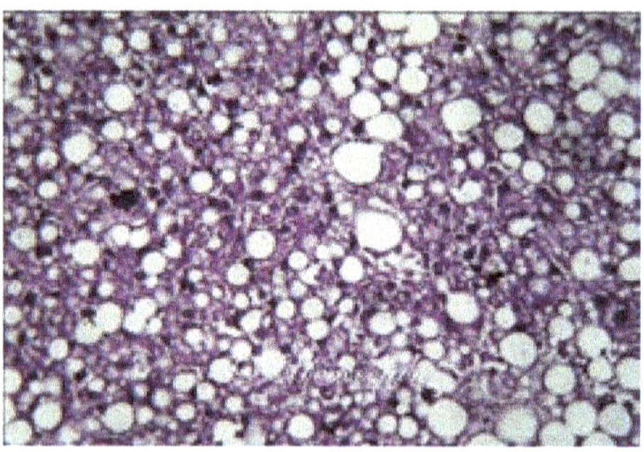

Fig. 9. Liposarcoma of skin of a dog depicting pleomorphic lipocytes with hyperchromatic nuclei and variably sized cytoplasmic vacuoles (p. 88)

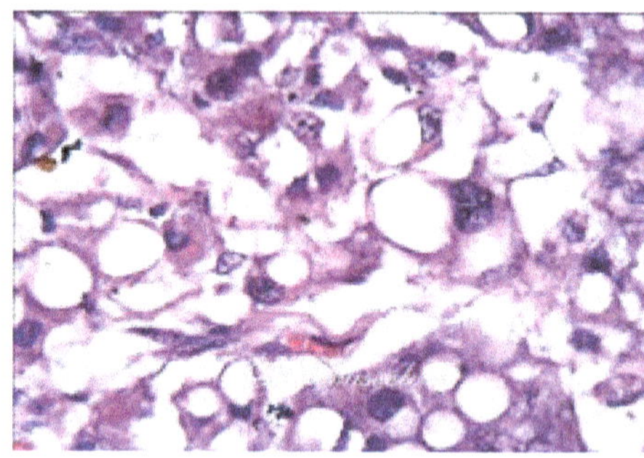

Fig. 10. Liposarcoma of skin of a dog showing lipocytes with multiple nucleoli within the anisokaryotic and poikilokaryotic nuclei (p. 89)

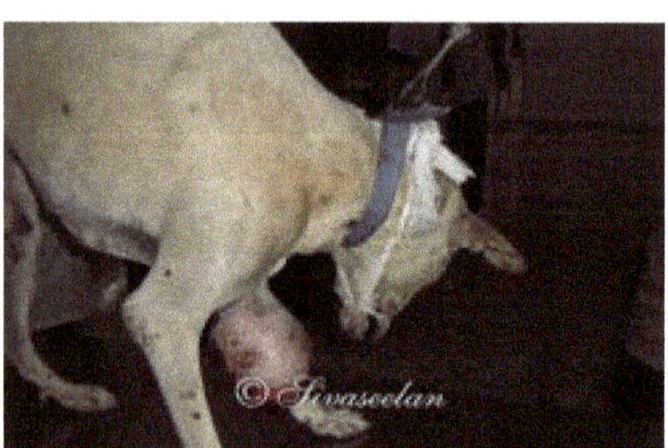

Fig. 11. A large infiltrative lipoma of the skin of a dog showing ulceration (p. 89)

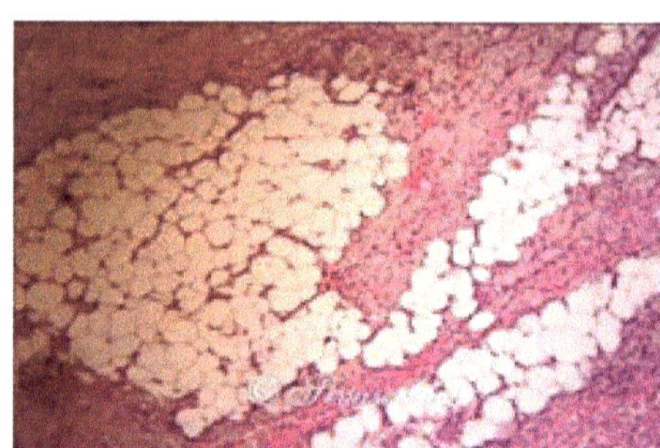

Fig. 12. Infiltrative lipoma of the skin of a dog showing lipocytes infiltrating between and atrophying the muscle fibres. (p. 90)

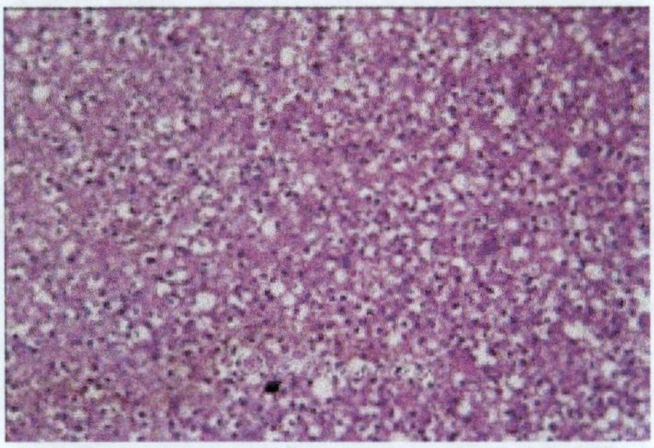

Fig. 13. Chondrosarcoma of mammary tissue of a dog showing pleomorphic individual chondrocytes arranged as sheet (p. 94)

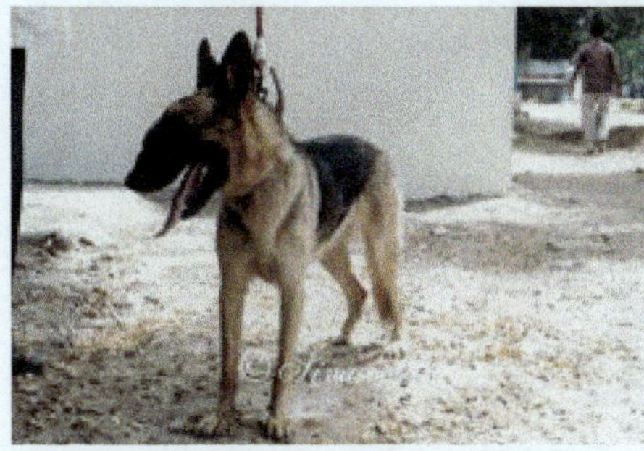

Fig. 14. Osteosarcoma of facial bone of a dog causing disfigurement of face (p. 96)

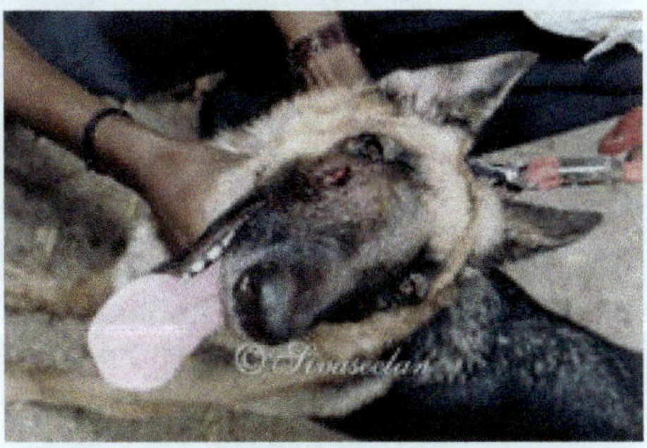

Fig. 15. Osteosarcoma shown in fig. 14 revealing ulcer on the tumour (p. 96)

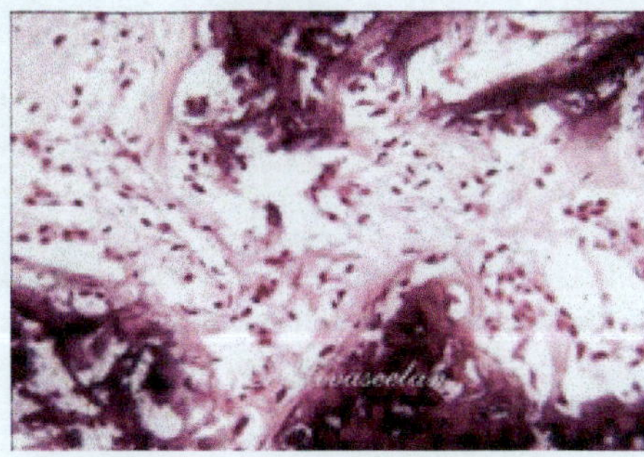

Fig. 16. Osteosarcoma revealing neoplastic osteocytes arranged as sheet without lacunae (p. 97)

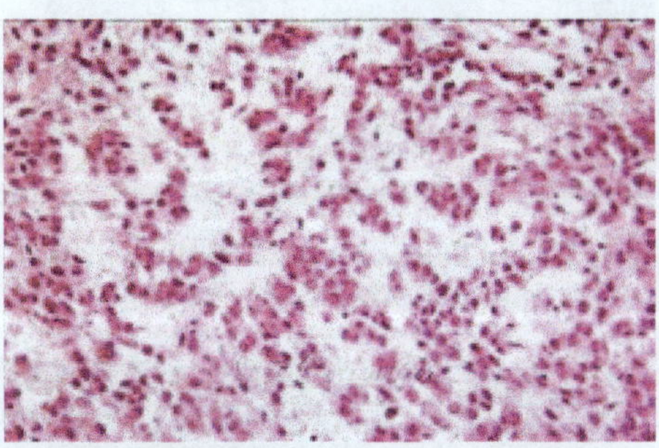

Fig. 17. Osteoblastic osteosarcoma showing osteoblasts with angular borders (p. 97)

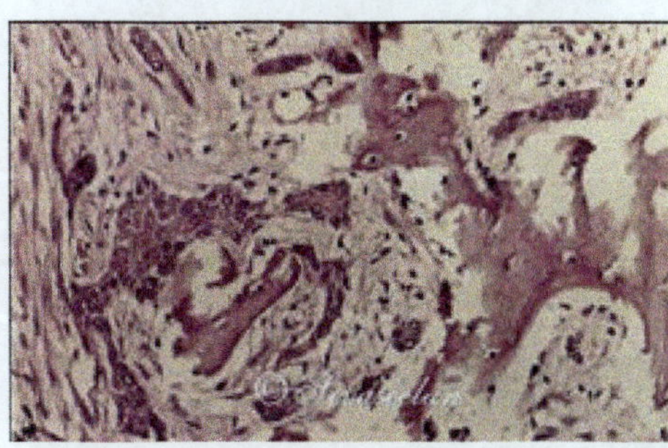

Fig. 18. Osteoclastoma depicting variably sized giant cells (p. 98)

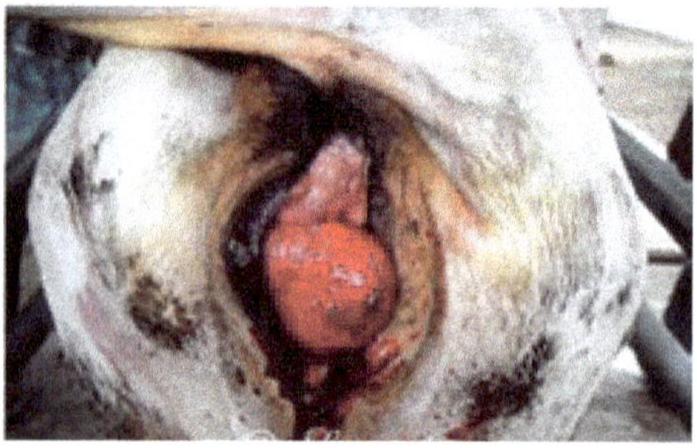

Fig. 19. A solitary pedunculated Leiomyoma protruding from the vagina of a cow. (p. 99)

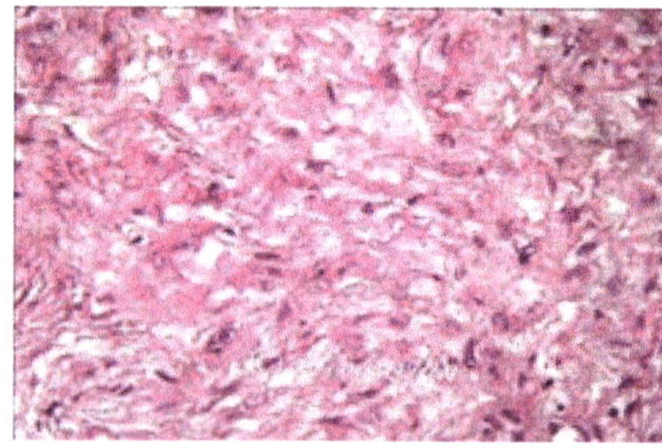

Fig. 20. Leiomyoma of the vagina of cow revealing elongated muscle fibres and scattered neoplastic leiomyocytes (p. 100)

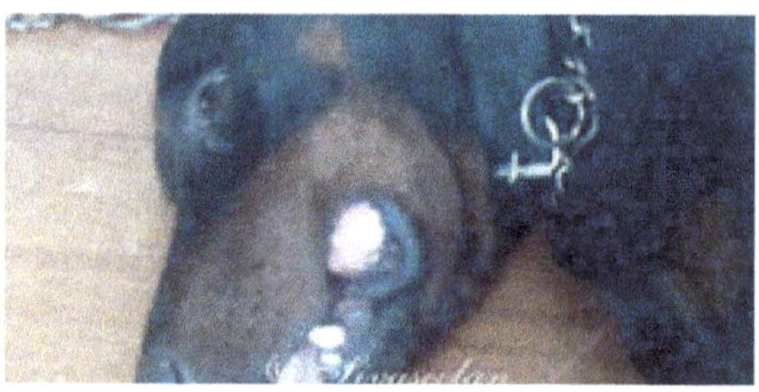

Fig. 21. Ossifying solitary mandibular Epulis of a dog. (p. 105)

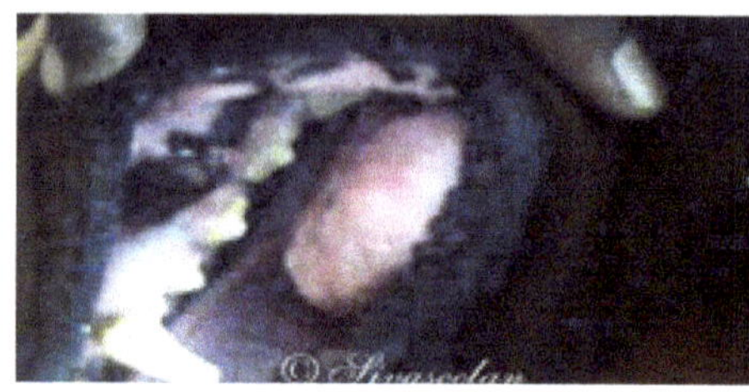

Fig. 22. Closure view of the Epulis shown in fig. 21 revealing a solitary mass occupying about 5 cm in length on the mandibular gum. (p. 105)

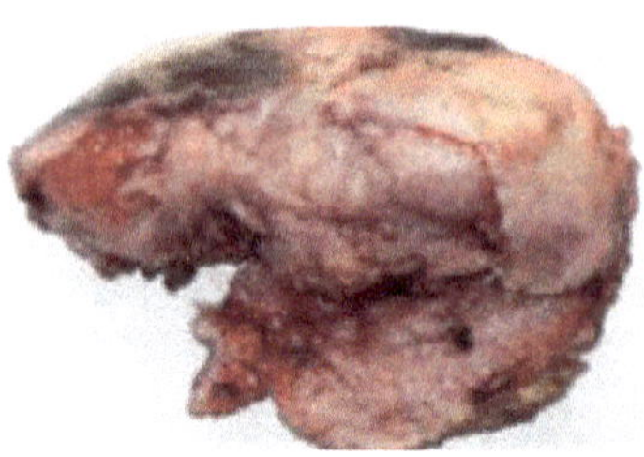

Fig. 23. Removed Epulis mass shown in fig.22 revealing lobulations. (p. 105)

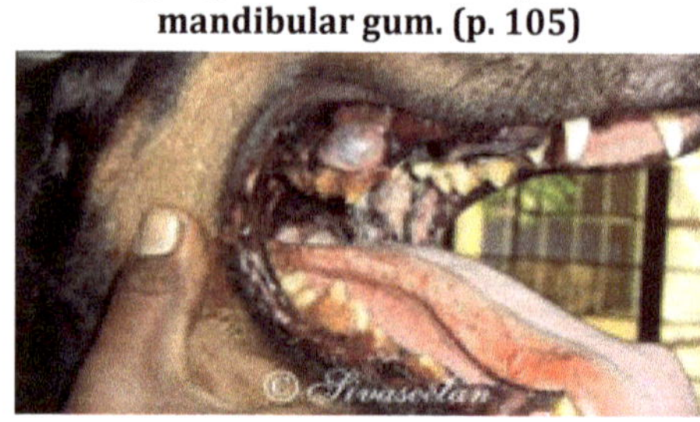

Fig. 24. An Epulis on the maxillary molar gum region of a dog. (p. 105)

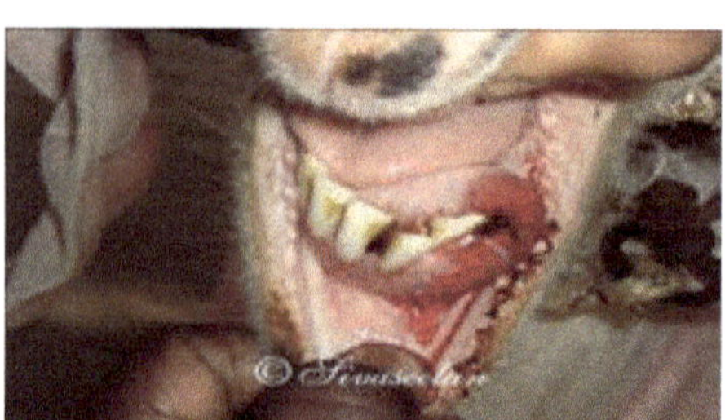

Fig. 25. An Epulis on the mandibular premolar gum region of a goat revealing disruption of orientation of teeth. (p. 106)

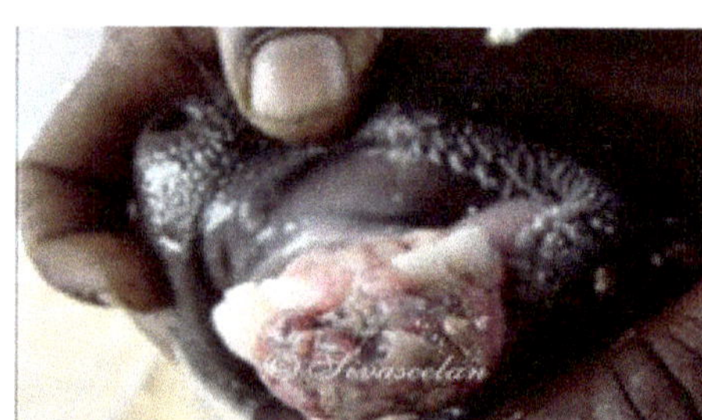

Fig. 26. An ulcerated large acanthomatous Epulis growing inside as well as outside of the incisor region of a cow. (p. 107)

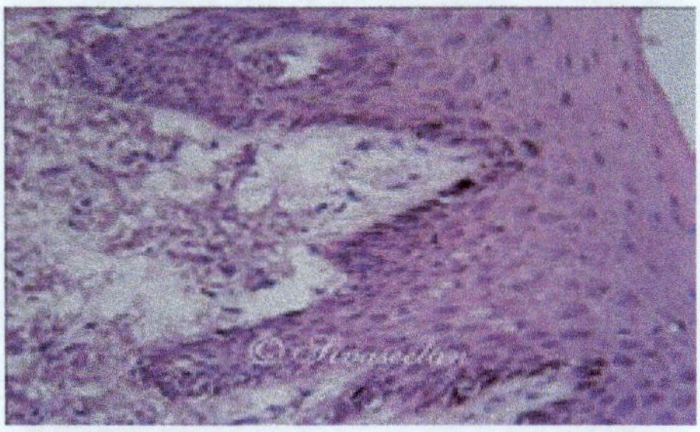

Fig. 27. Ossifying Epulis shown in fig. 22 revealing rete pegs of proliferating surface epithelium bordered by palisading arrangement of the cells. (p. 107)

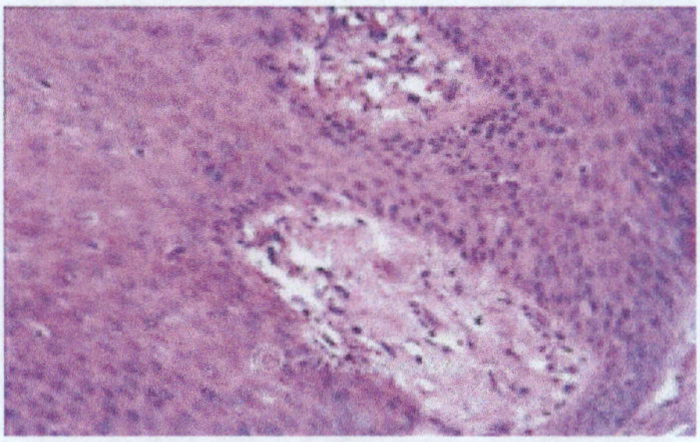

Fig. 28. Ossifying Epulis shown in fig. 22 depicting pseudo cyst formation Among proliferating epithelial cells. (p. 107)

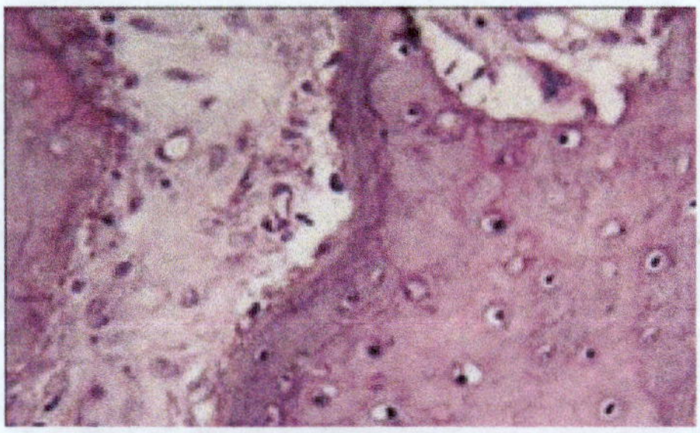

Fig. 29. Ossifying Epulis shown in fig. 22 revealing ossifying regions in the deeper areas. (p. 108)

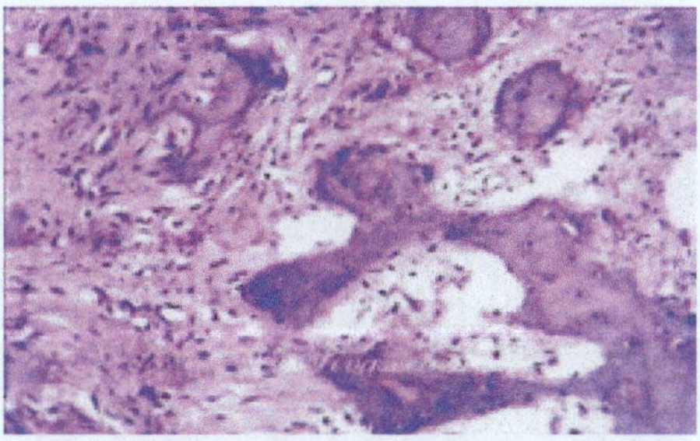

Fig. 30. Ossifying Epulis shown in fig. 22 revealing proliferation of fibroblasts and ossification in the deeper areas of the mass. (p. 108)

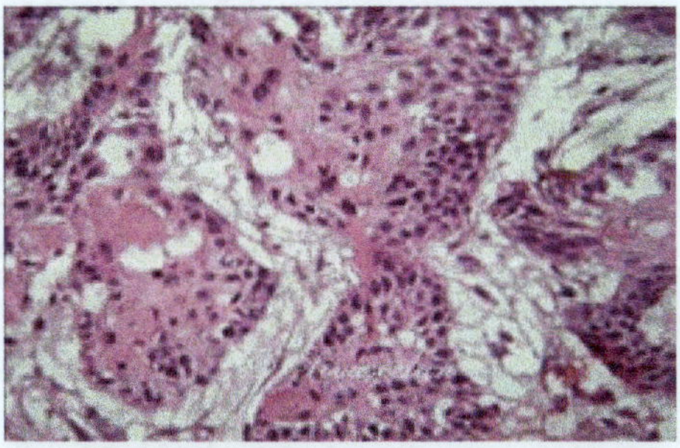

Fig. 31. Acanthomatous type of Epulis shown in fig. 26 revealing island arrangement of keratinocytes that depict anisocytosis, anisokaryosis, hyperchromatic nuclei with variable number of nucleoli and rare mitotic figures. (p. 108)

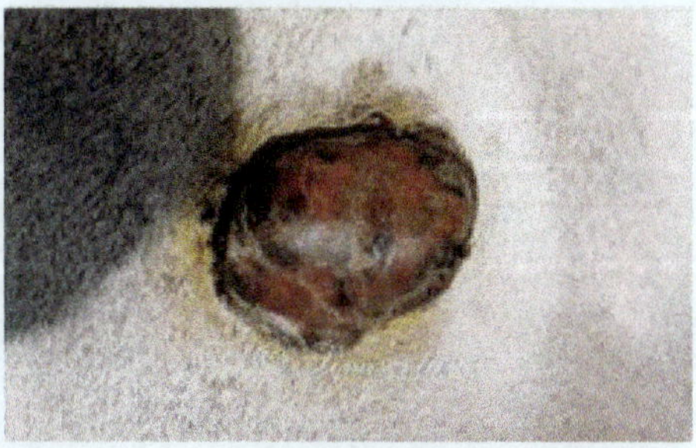

Fig. 32. A subcutaneous haemangioma of cattle revealing dark red colour (p. 110)

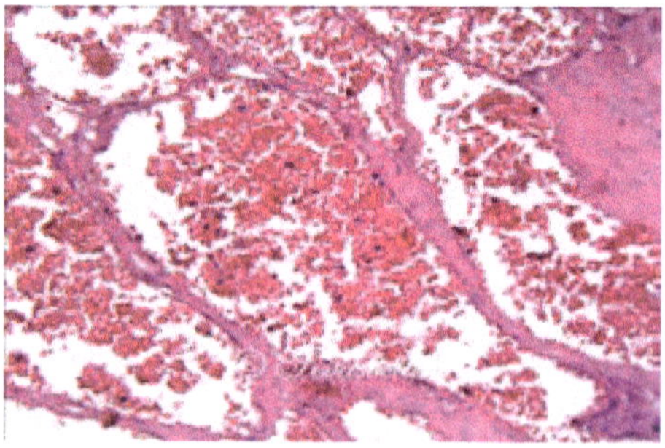

Fig. 33. Cavernous haemangioma of the subcutis of cattle shown in fig. 32 revealing irregular spaces filled with blood cells and separated by fibrous bands. (p. 111)

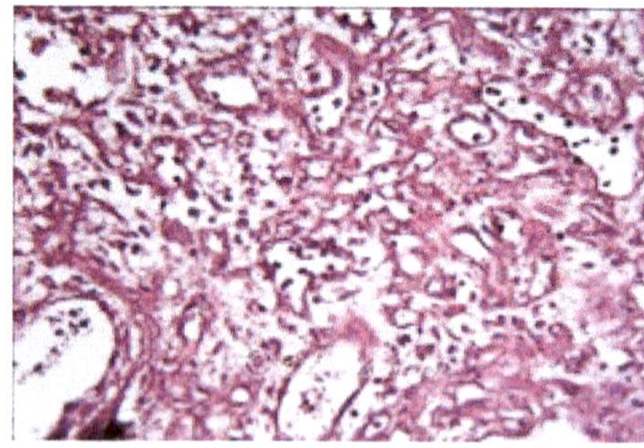

Fig. 34. Capillary haemangioma of subcutis of a dog depicting numerous capillaries lined by endothelial cells and few capillaries reveal blood cells. (p. 112)

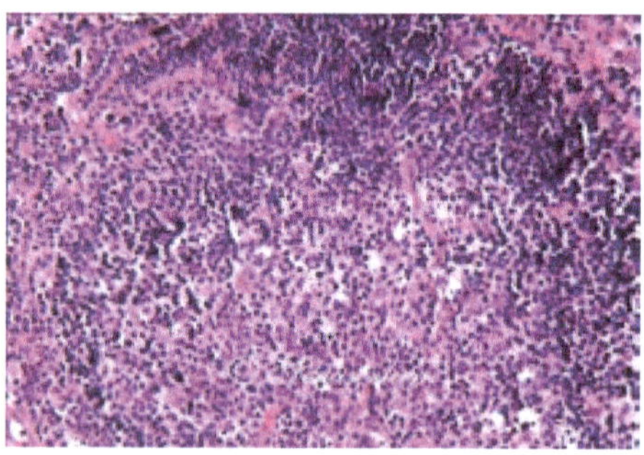

Fig. 35. Histiocytoma of the skin of a dog revealing densely populated cells in the dermis and loosely arranged cells in the epidermis. (p. 115)

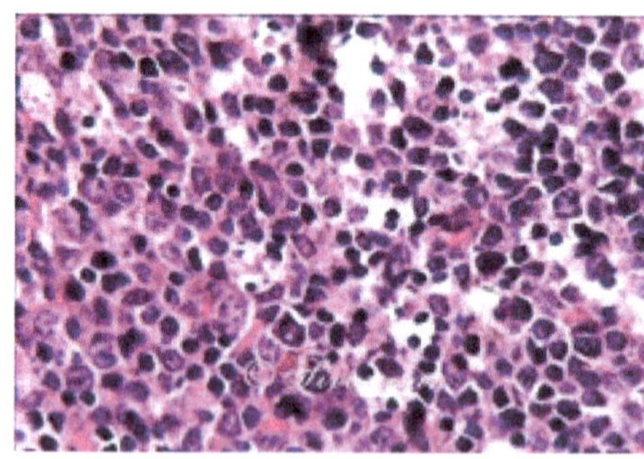

Fig. 36. Higher magnification of the fig. 35 depicting cellular as well as nuclear pleomorphism with prominent multiple nucleoli in the loosely packed cells. (p. 115)

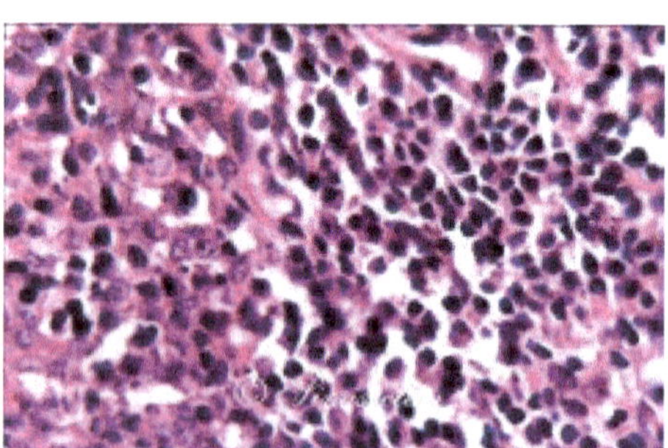

Fig. 37. Histiocytoma of the skin of a cow revealing mixture of round, ovoid and polygonal cells with pleomorphic nuclei. (p. 116)

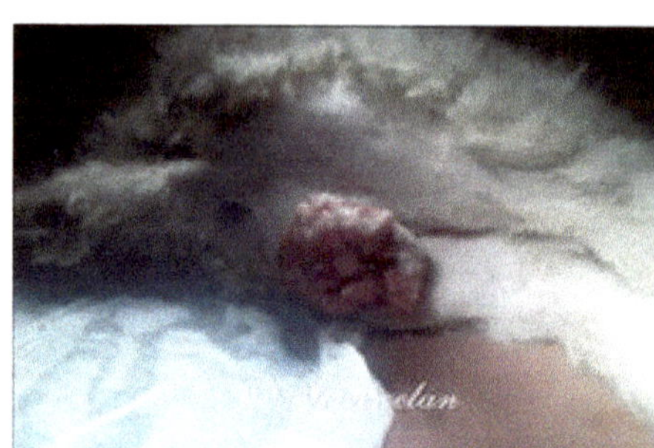

Fig. 38. Multilobulated TVT protruding from the vagina of a dog. (p. 117)

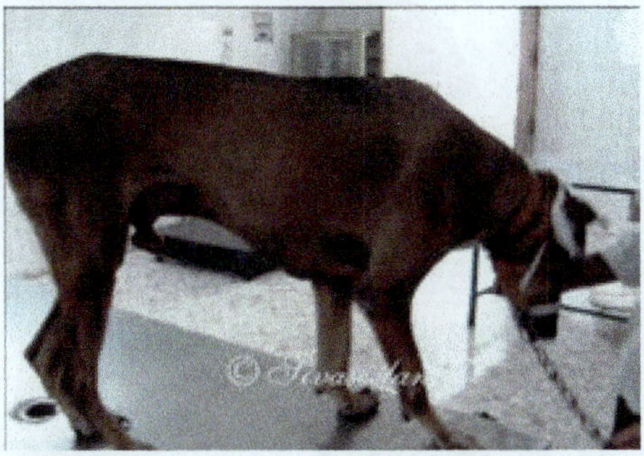

Fig. 39. TVT arising from the glans-penis of a dog. (p. 117)

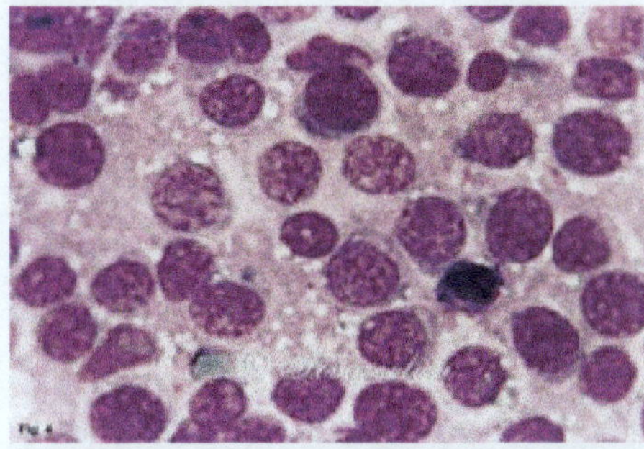

Fig. 40. Cytology of the vaginal TVT of a dog revealing sheet arrangement of round cells with cytoplasmic punctate vacuoles. p. (118)

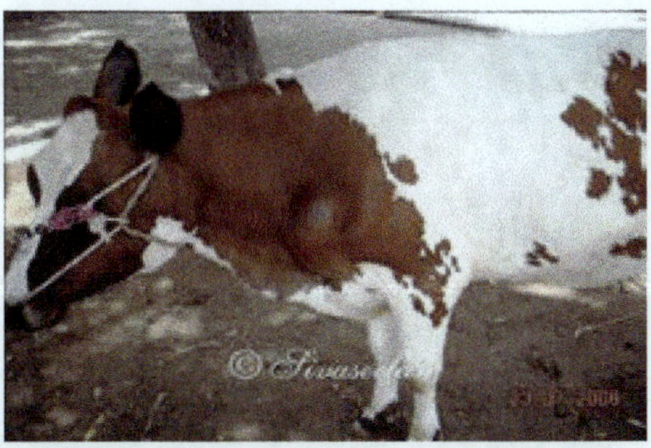

Fig. 41. Prescapular lymph node lymphoma of a cow. (p. 120)

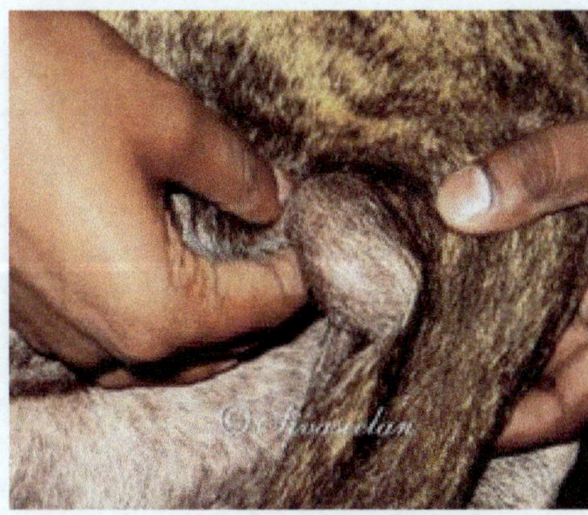

Fig. 42. Pre-crural lymph node. (p. 120)

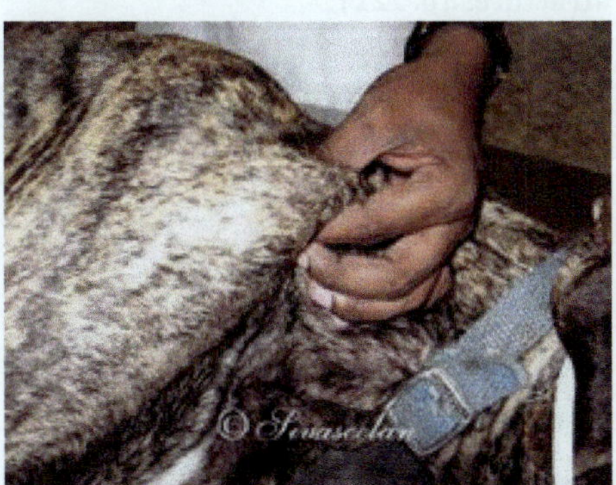

Fig. 43. Pre-scapular lymph node. (p. 120)

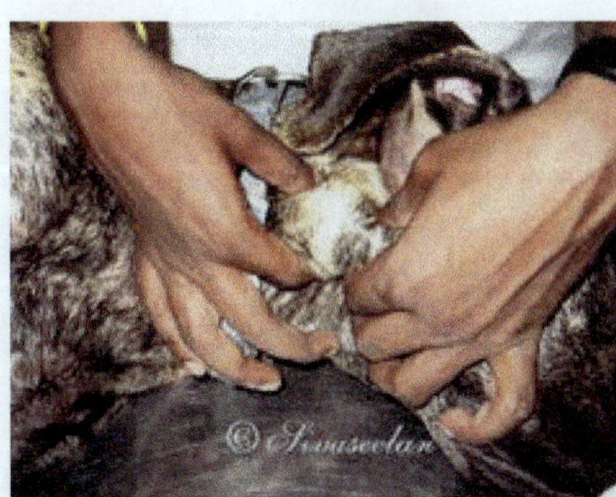

Fig, 44. Sub-mandibular lymph node. (p. 121)

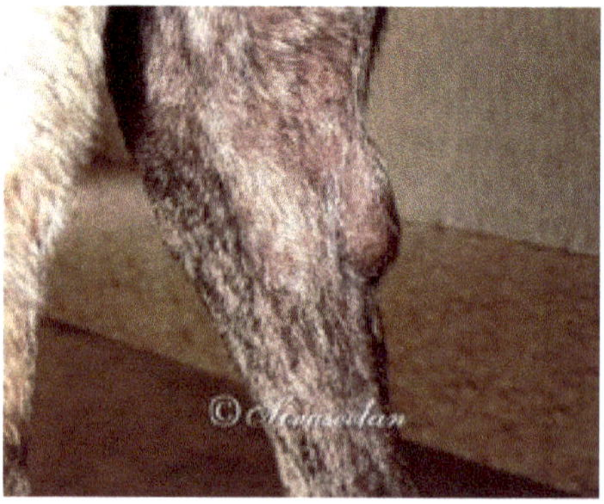

45. Popliteal lymph node. (p. 121)

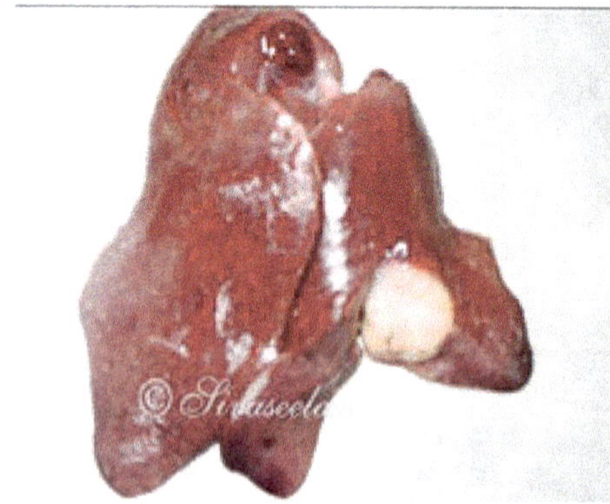

Fig. 46. Solitary lymphoma of the liver of a fowl. (p. 121)

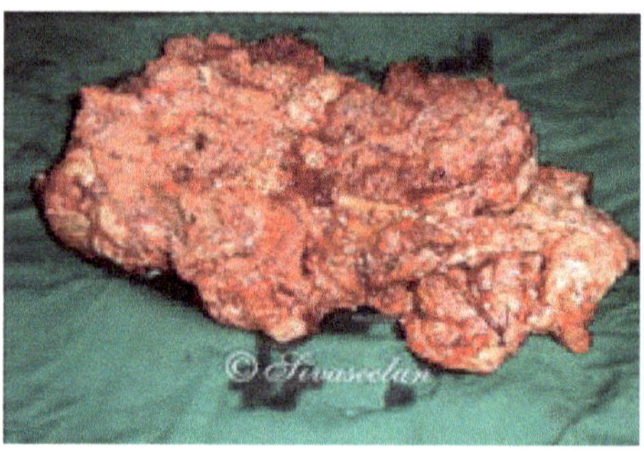

Fig. 47. Multicentric lymphoma of the mesentery of a dog revealing fusion of lymphnodes causing concretion of intestine. (p. 121)

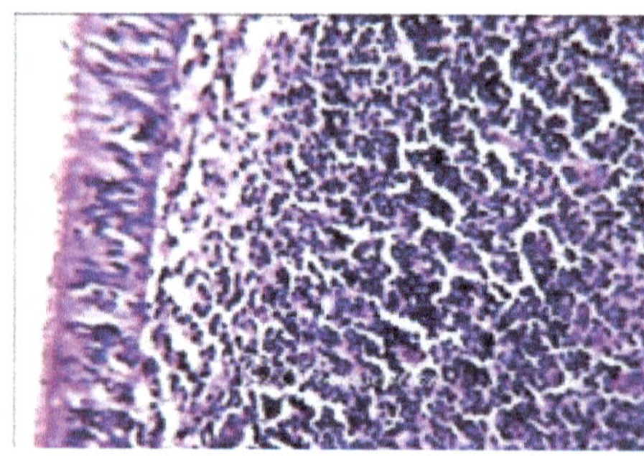

Fig. 48. Well differentiated lymphoma of the intestine of a dog revealing uniform sheet arrangement of infiltrating small lymphocytes replacing sub-mucosal structures.(p. 122)

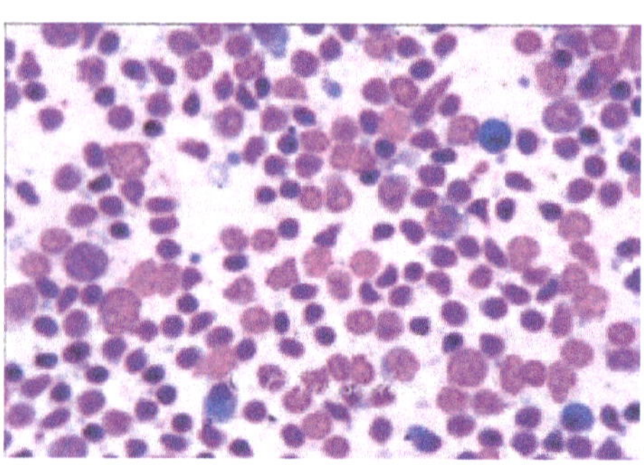

Fig. 49. Poorly differentiated lymphoma of prescapular lymph node of a cow revealing more number of lymphoblasts and few irregular anaplastic cells with multiple angular nucleoli. (p. 123)

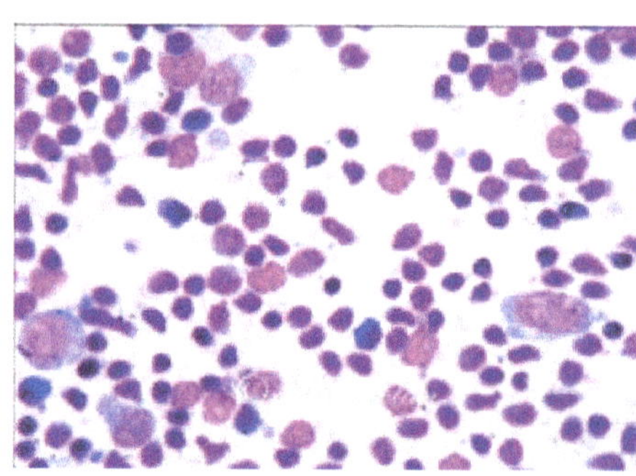

Fig. 50. Intermediate lymphoma of prescapular lymph node of a cow revealing more number of small lymphocytes, few lymphoblasts and rare irregular anaplastic cells with multiple angular nucleoli. (p. 123)

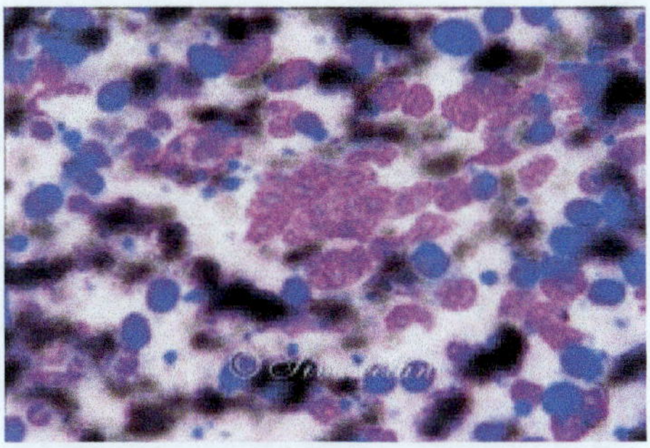

Fig. 51. Anaplastic lymphoma of multicentric origin of a dog revealing more number of anaplastic cells with multiple angular nucleoli adhering with each other. (A special stain was developed and used to differentiate neoplastic cells from normal cells). (p. 124)

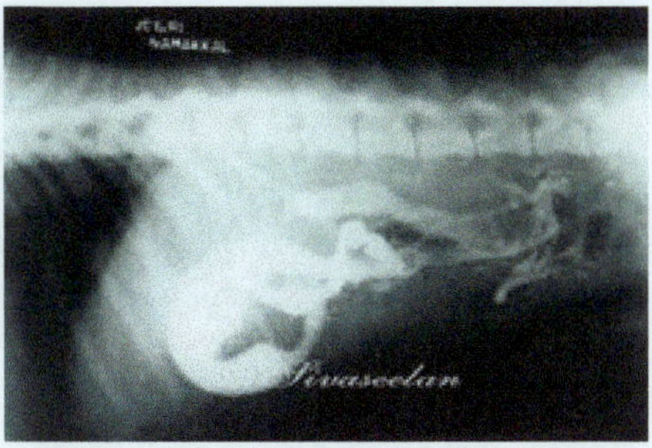

Fig. 52. An abdominal radiograph of a dog showing abnormal thickness of the intestine wall, which was confirmed as plasma cell tumour histopathologically. (p. 126_

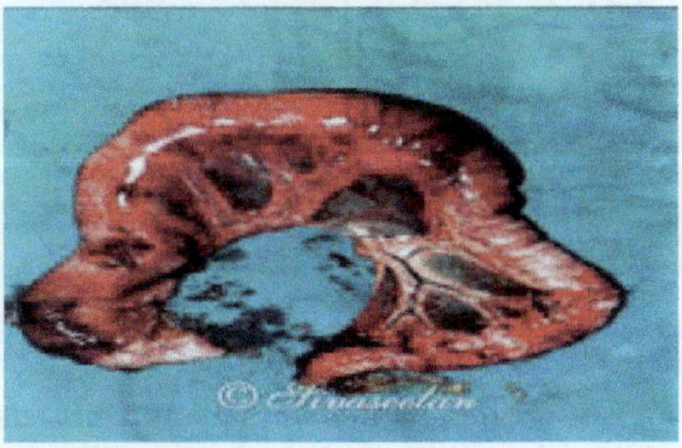

Fig. 53. An excised portion of the affected intestine shown in fig. 52. (p. 126)

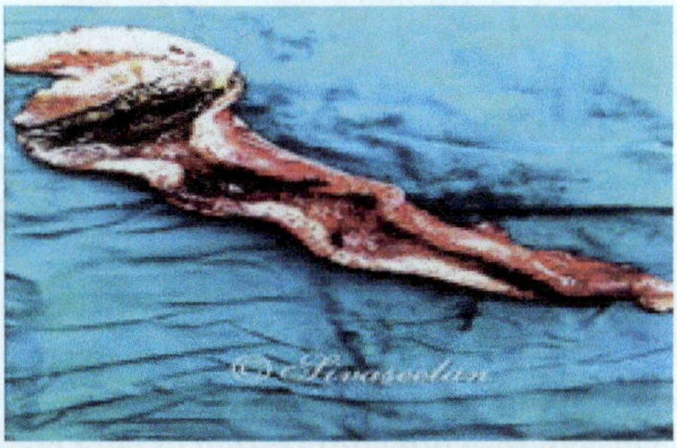

Fig. 54. Cut opened intestine shown in fig. 52 revealing markedly thickened wall. (p. 126)

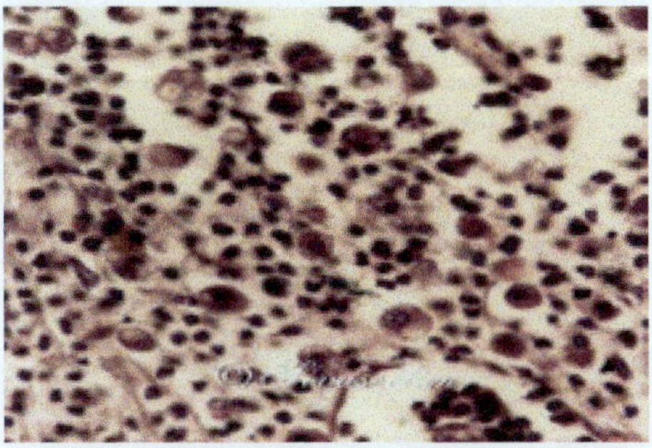

Fig. 55. Plasma cell tumour shown in fig. 53 revealing loosely arranged pleomorphic plasma cells. (p. 127)

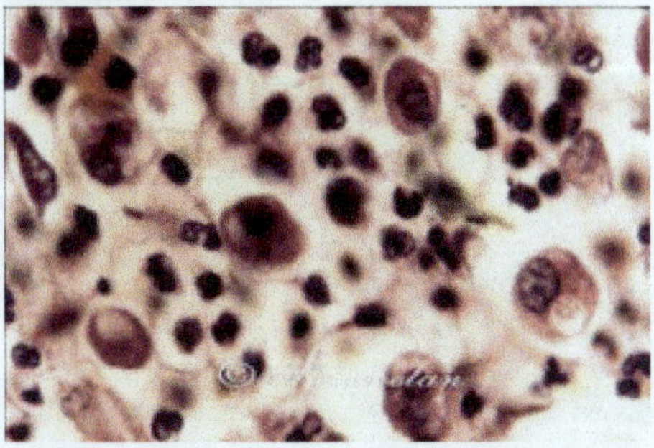

Fig. 56. Plasma cell tumour shown in fig. 54 revealing pleomorphic plasma cells with eccentrically placed nucleus and cytoplasmic immunoglobulin vacuole. (p. 127)

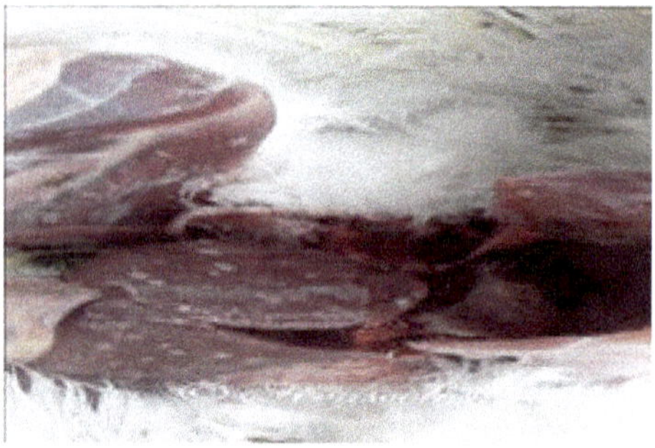

Fig. 57. Avian Leucosis affected liver of a chicken revealing multiple foci of studded tumours without elevating from the surface of the organ. (p. 130)

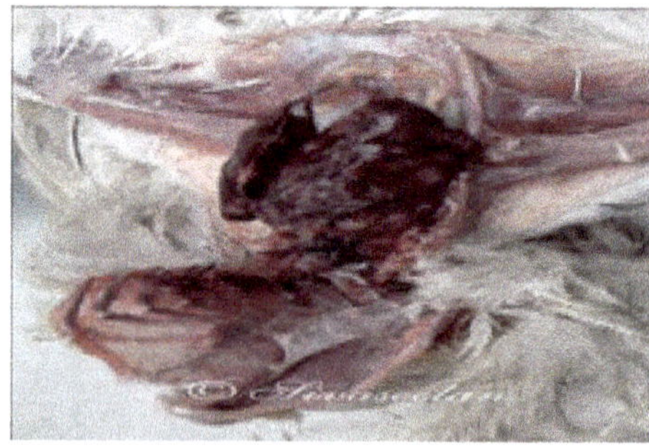

Fig. 58. Avian Leucosis affected liver of a turkey revealing multiple foci of tumours elevating from the surface of the organ. (p. 130)

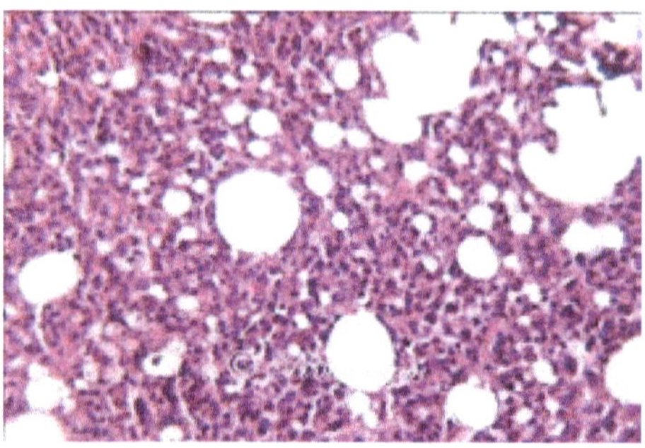

Fig. 59. Avian Leucosis affected lung of a chicken revealing infiltration of neoplastic lymphocytes in the interstitial areas. (p. 131)

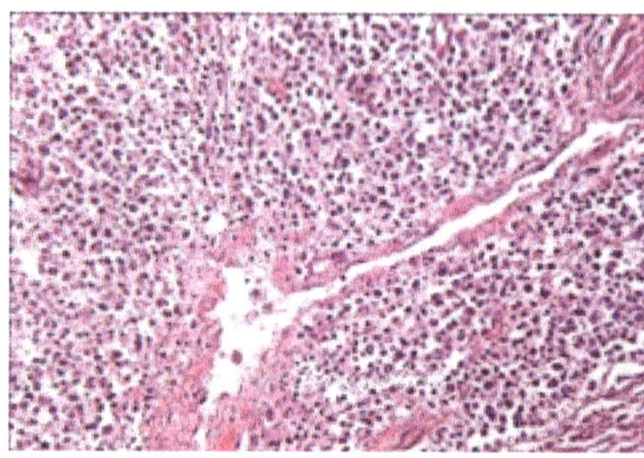

Fig. 60. Avian Leucosis affected uterus of a chicken revealing infiltration of neoplastic lymphocytes in the myometrium replacing the normal sturctures. (p. 131)

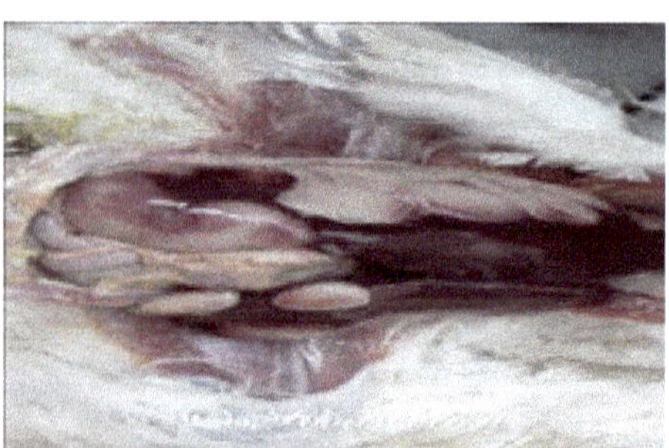

Fig. 61. Marek's Disease affected liver of a chicken revealing multiple elevated nodular growths resembling fat deposits. (p. 131)

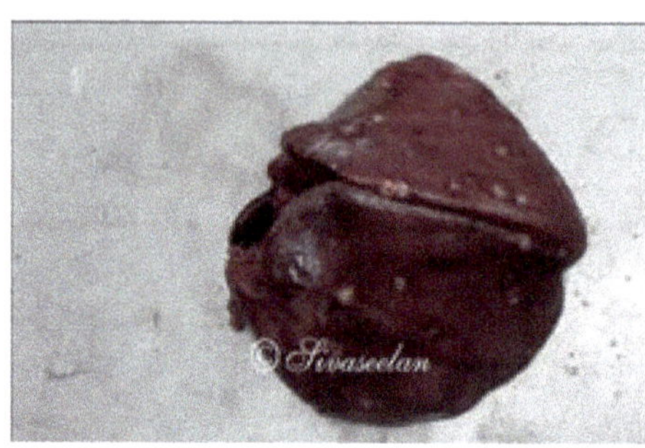

Fig. 62. Marek's Disease affected liver of a chicken revealing multiple studded growths without elevating from the surface. (p. 132)

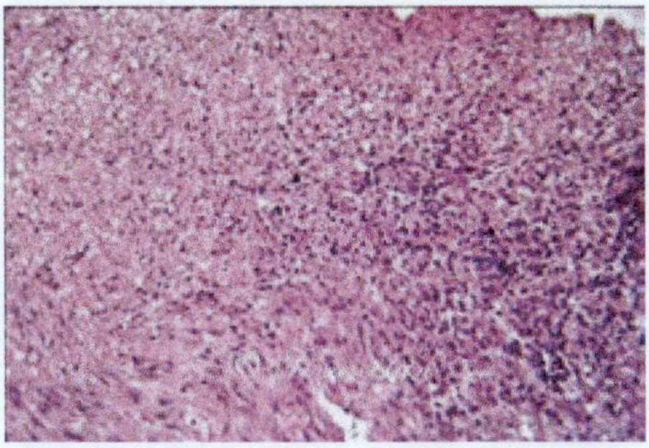

Fig. 63. Marek's Disease affected peripheral nerve of a chicken revealing Infiltration of lymphocytes. (p. 132)

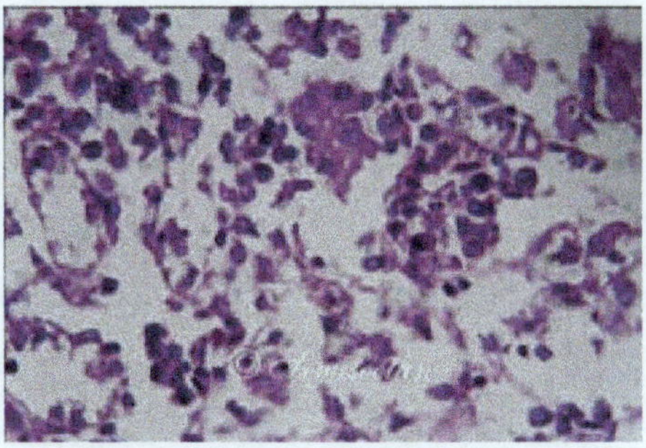

Fig. 64. Marek's Disease affected liver of a chicken revealing infiltration of lymphocytes and MD cell. (p. 132)

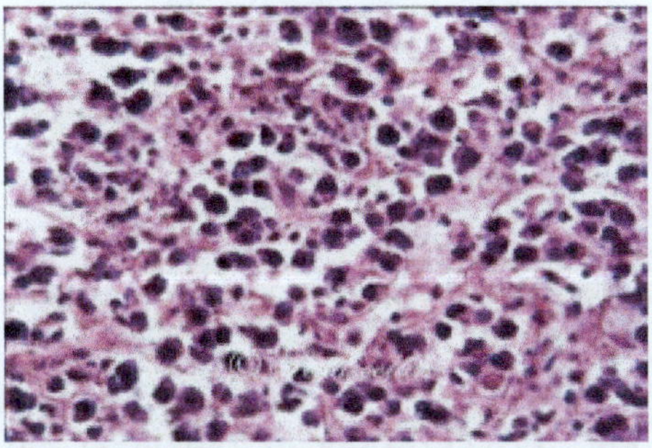

Fig. 65. Marek's Disease affected Bursa of a chicken revealing infiltration of pleomorphic lymphocytes. (p. 133)

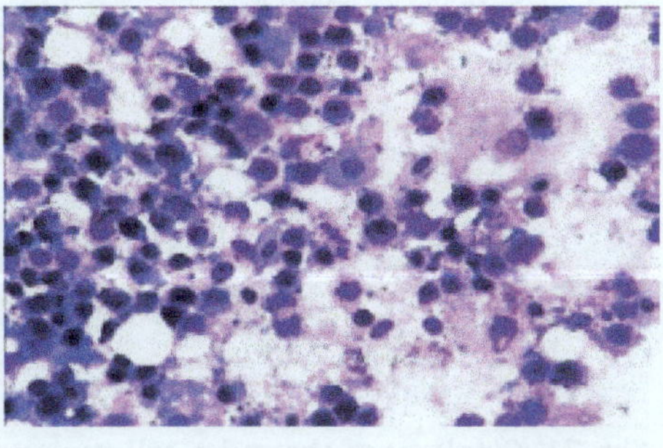

Fig. 66. Cytology of Marek's Disease affected liver of a chicken revealing pleomorphic lymphocytes. (p. 133)

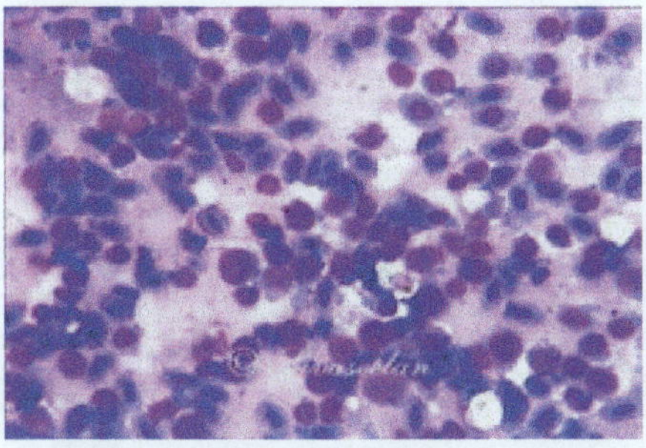

Fig. 67. Cytology of Marek's Disease affected kidney of a chicken revealing pleomorphic lymphocytes. (p. 133)

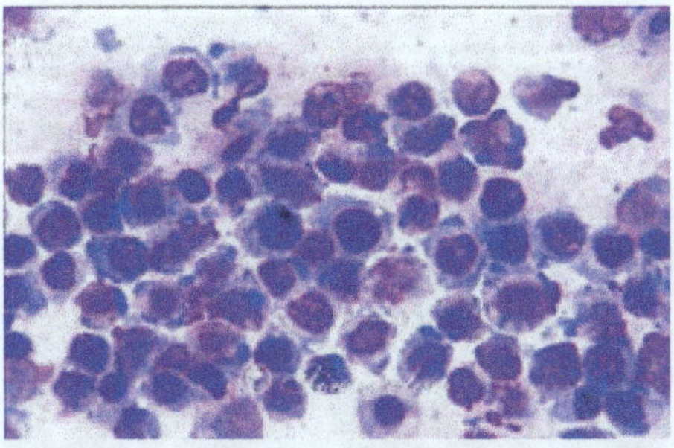

Fig. 68. Cytology of Marek's Disease affected hair follicle of a fowl revealing almost same size lymphocytes. (p. 134)

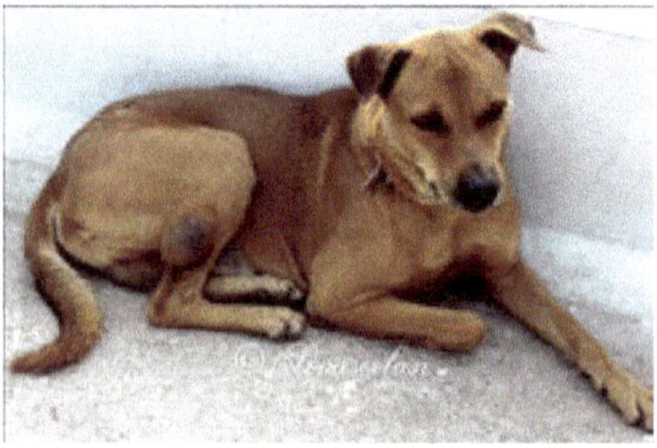

Fig. 69. A Mast cell tumour on the thigh region of leg of a dog. (p. 135)

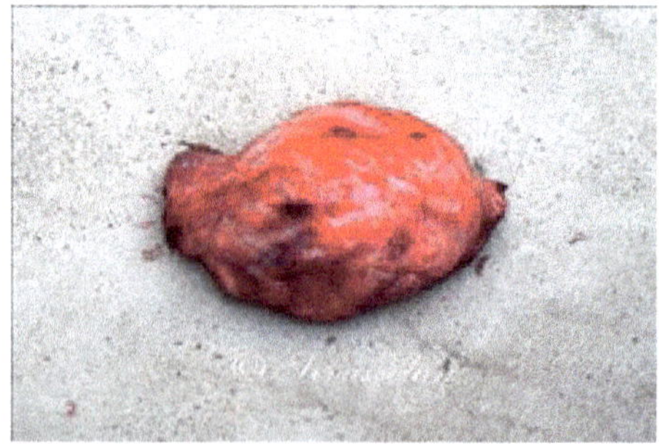

Fig. 70. Removed mast cell tumour shown in fig. 69 revealing non-encapsulation and invasion into the muscle. (p. 135)

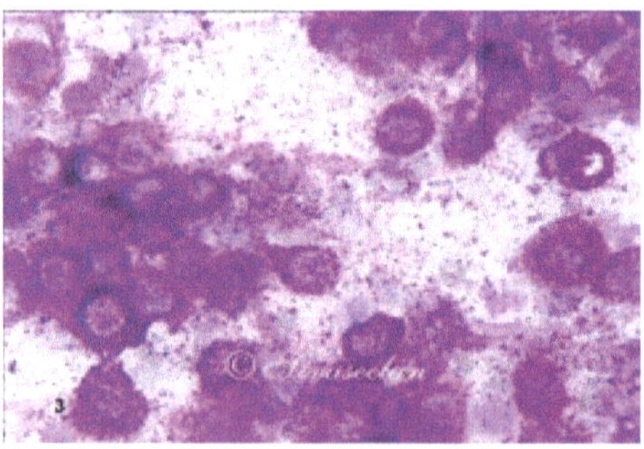

Fig. 71. Cytology of the mast cell tumour shown in fig. 69 revealing enormous number of granules in the cytoplasm of the cells under Giemsa staining. (p. 136)

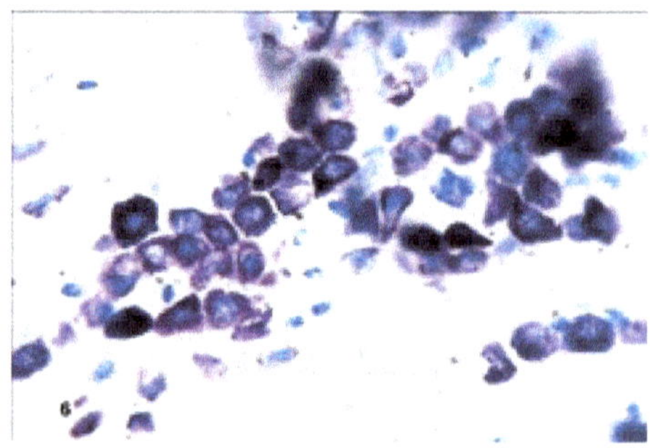

Fig. 72. Cytology of the mast cell tumour shown in fig. 69 revealing enormousnumber of metachromatically stained granules in the cytoplasm of the cells under Toluidine blue staining. (p. 136)

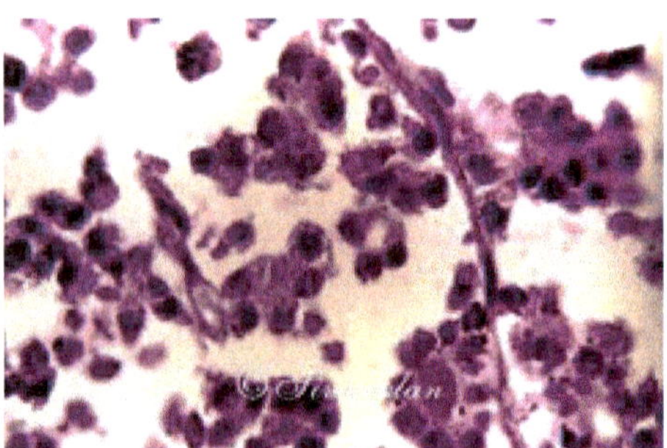

Fig. 73. Poorly differentiated type (grade III) mast cell tumour of the skin of a dog revealing pleomorphic cells with indistinct cytoplasmic borders and the cytoplasm contains only a few large granules . (p. 137)

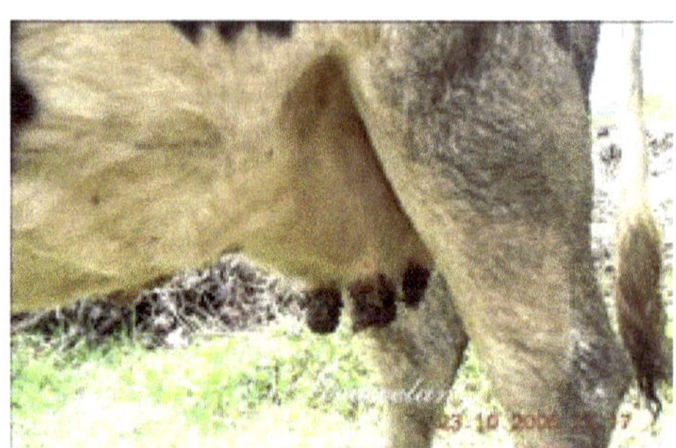

Fig. 74: Bovine Cutaneous Papilloma -Teat. Multiple papillomatous warts on the teat of a milch cow. (p. 140)

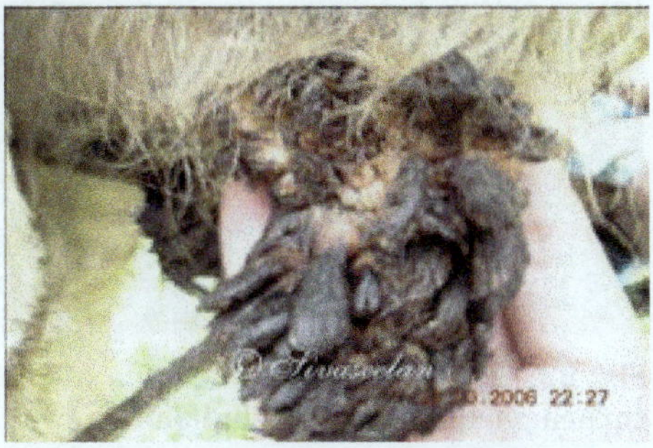

Fig. 75: Bovine Cutaneous Papilloma – Teat. Mutilated teat due to multiple warts. (p. 140)

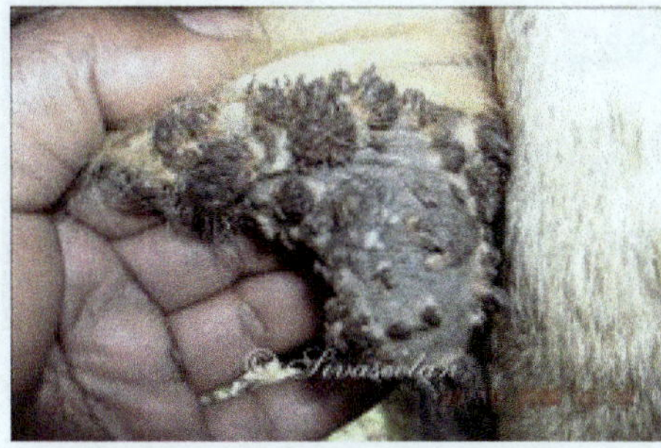

Fig. 76: Bovine Cutaneous Papilloma – Teat. Spontaneous regression of tumour shown in fig. 75. (p. 141)

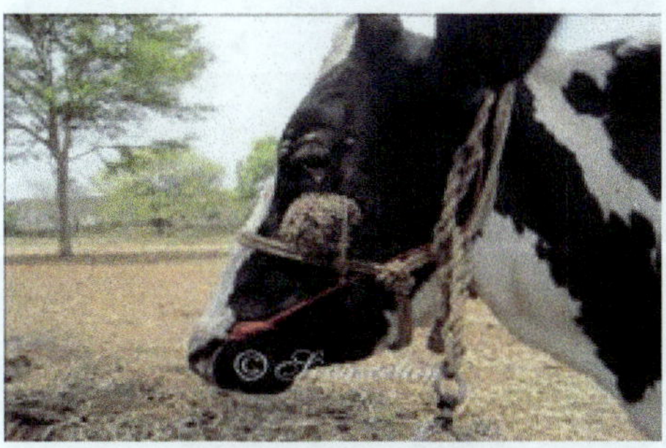

Fig. 77: Bovine Cutaneous Papilloma. Multiple tumours collectively forming a cauliflower like appearance. (p. 141)

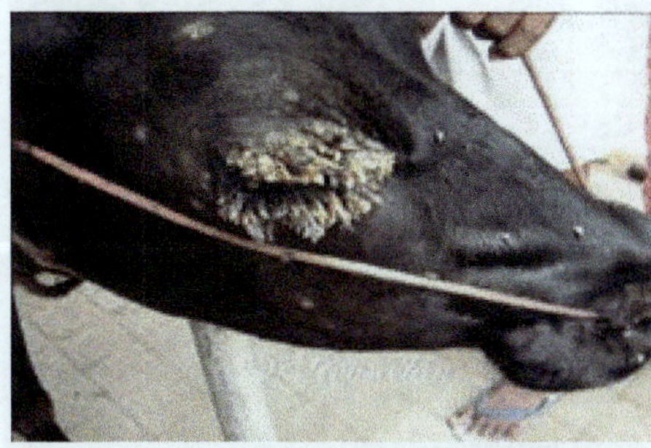

Fig. 78: Bovine Cutaneous Papilloma. Multiple warts arising from both eyelids of a cow masking the vision. (p. 141)

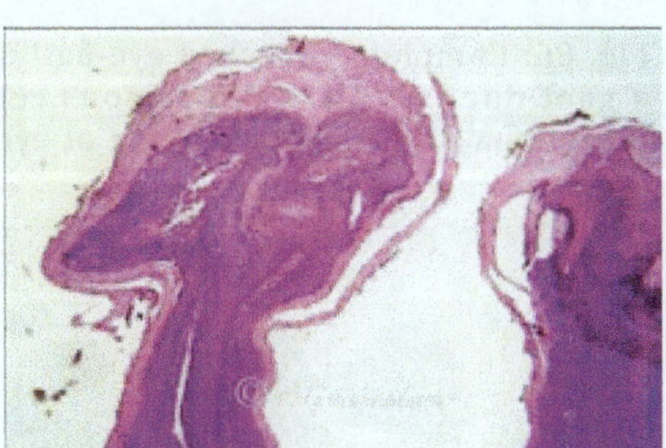

Fig. 79: Papilloma showing proliferating cutaneous epithelial cells forming finger like growth covered by hyperkeratotic layer. (p. 142)

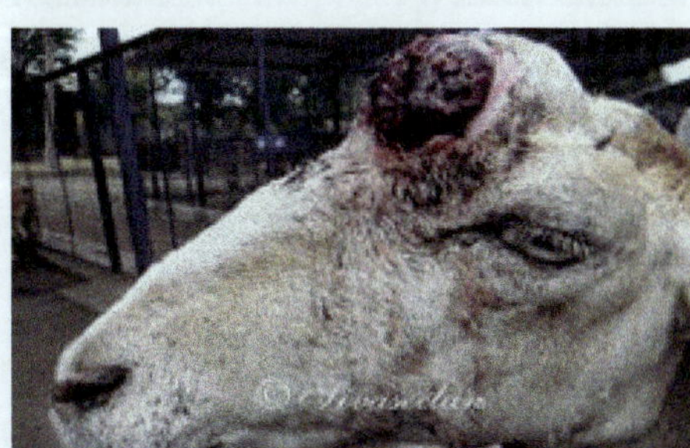

Fig. 80: Squamous cell carcinoma on the head of a sheep revealing ulceration and bleeding. (p. 143)

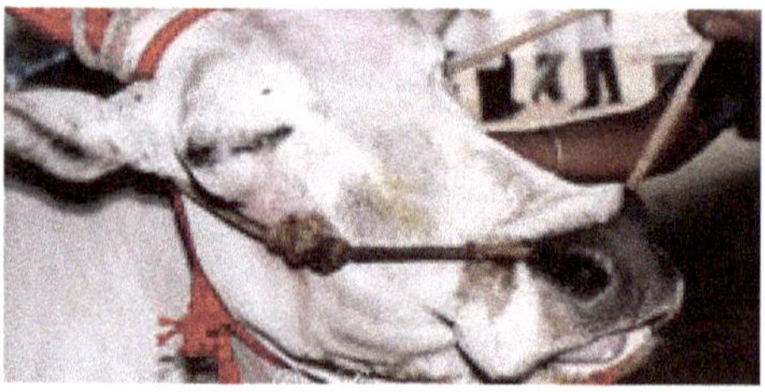

Fig. 81: Squamous cell carcinoma of the eye of a bullock causing fusion of eyelids. (p. 145)

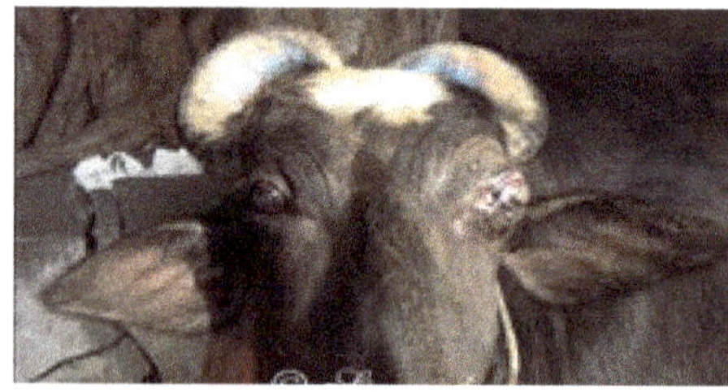

Fig. 82: Squamous cell carcinoma of the cornea portion of eye of a buffalo. (p. 145)

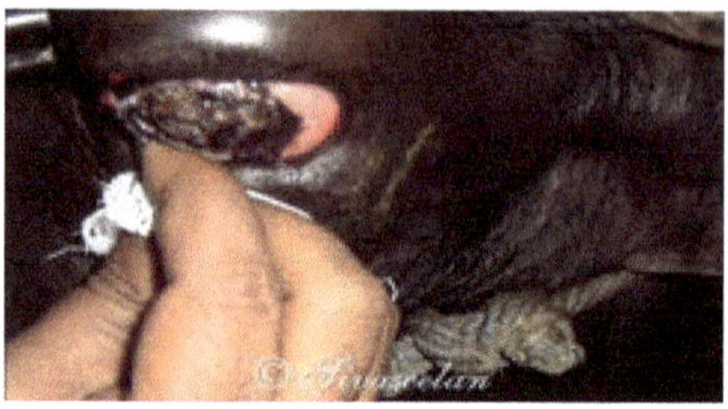

Fig. 83: Closure view of the tumour shown in fig. 81depicting total destruction of cornea. (p. 145)

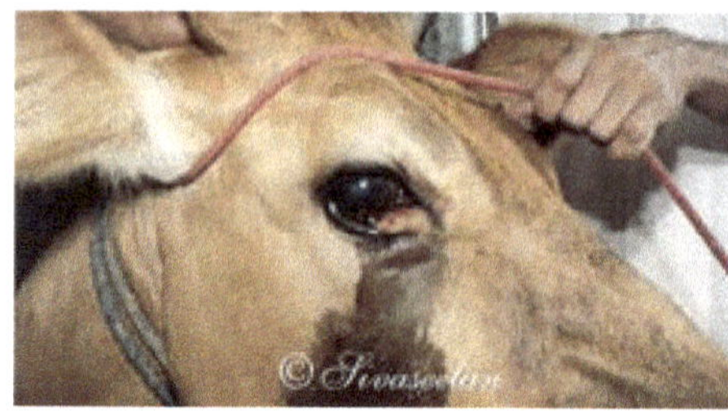

Fig. 84: Squamous cell carcinoma of the inner-canthus of eye of a Jersey cow. (p. 146)

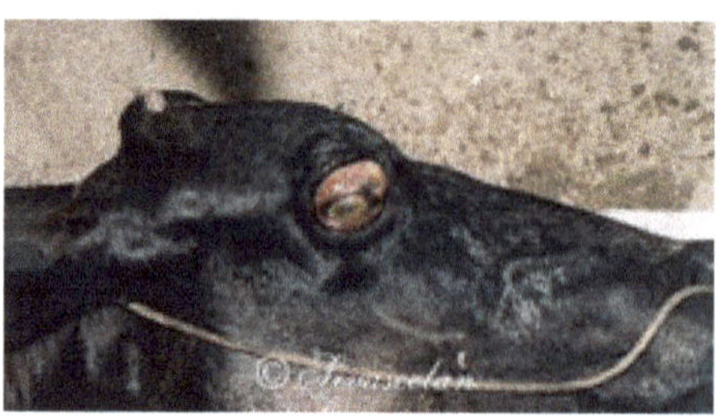

Fig. 85: Squamous cell carcinoma of the sclera portion of eye of a cow. (p. 146)

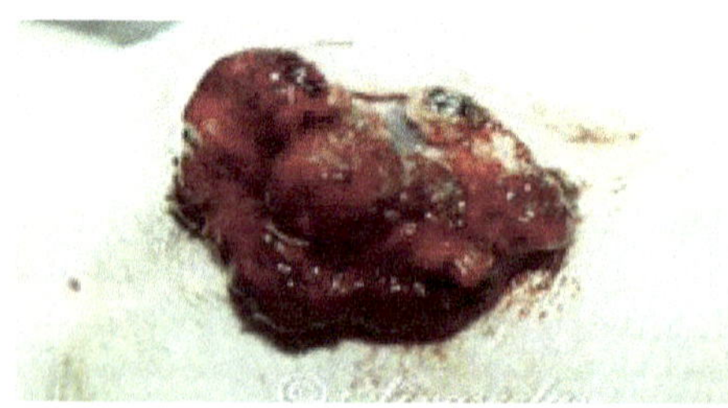

Fig. 86: Completely masked eye-ball of a goat due to multiple Squamous cell carcinoma of the sclera portion of eye. (p. 146)

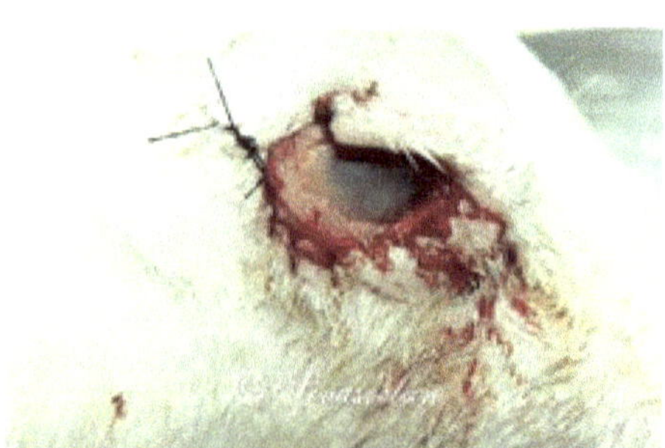

Fig. 87: Squamous cell carcinoma affected eye shown in fig. 86 after surgical removal of tumours. (p. 147)

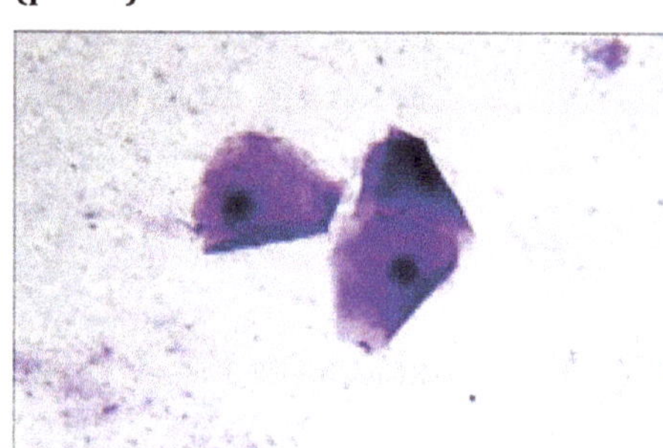

Fig. 88: FNAC smear of non-tumour mass showing normal squamous epithelial cells with uniformly tiny nucleus. (p. 148)

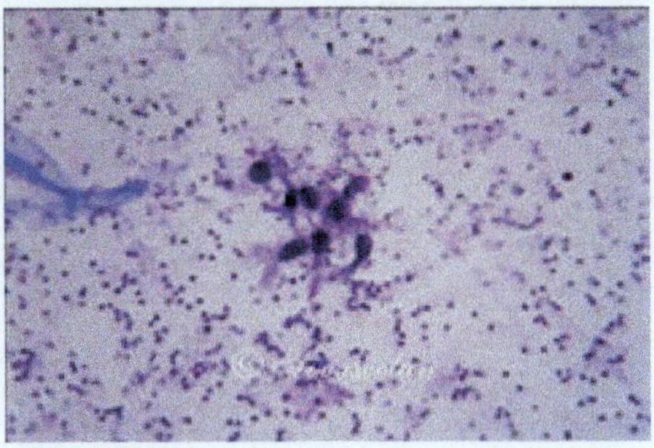

Fig. 89: FNAC smear from squamous cell carcinoma depicting neoplastic squamous cells with anisokaryotic and poikilokaryotic nuclei. (p. 148)

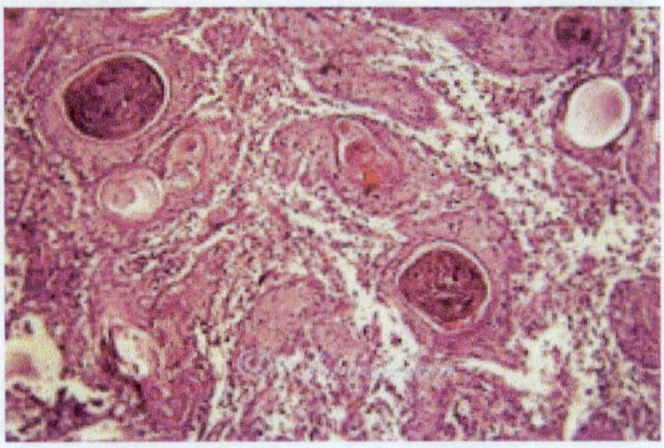

Fig. 90: Squamous cell carcinoma of the eye revealing cell nests with keratin pearls. Almost equal proportion of cell nest and pearl indicates moderately proliferating tumour. (p. 148)

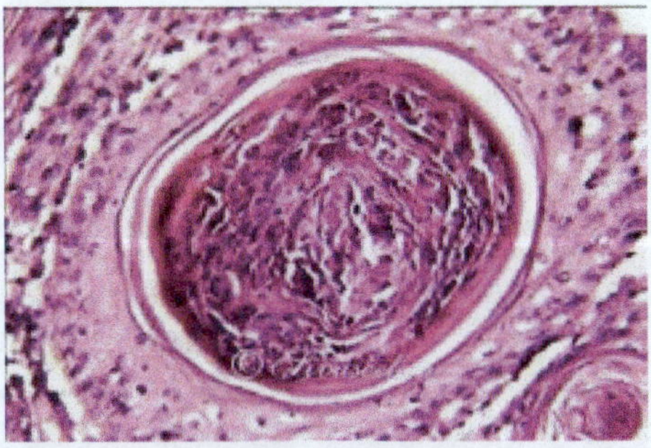

Fig. 91: Magnified view of single cell nest with keratin pearl. (p. 149)

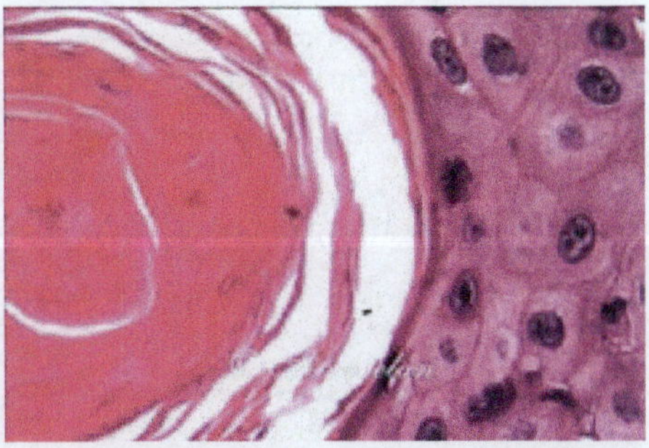

Fig. 92: Highly magnified cell nest and pearl revealing the neoplastic squamous cells with enlarged nucleus. Multiple angular nucleoli are also seen within nucleus. (p. 149)

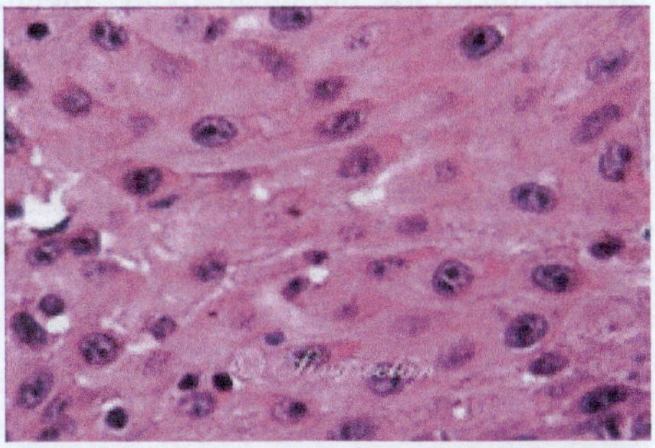

Fig. 93: Neoplastic squamous cells (prickle cells) of a cell nest revealing typical intercellular bridges and anisokaryosis with multiple angular nucleoli. (p. 149)

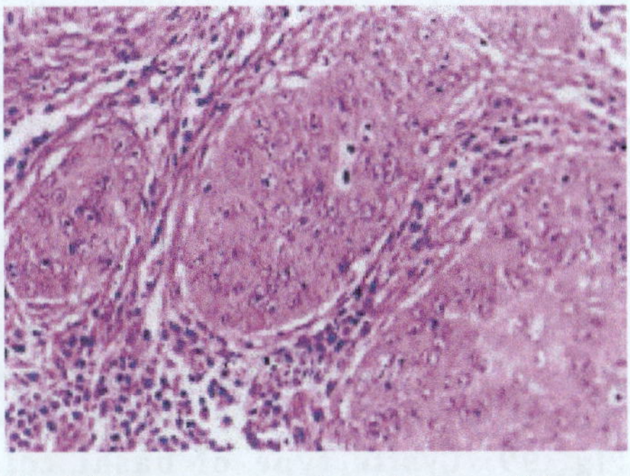

Fig. 94: Squamous cell carcinoma of the eye of cow revealing cell nests without keratin pearl indicating fastly proliferating tumour. (p. 150)

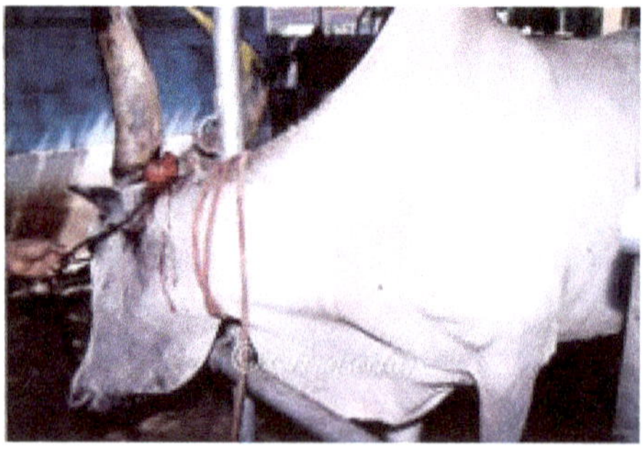

Fig. 95: Squamous cell carcinoma arising from the horn of a bullock (horn cancer) showing tendency to bleed easily. (p. 151)

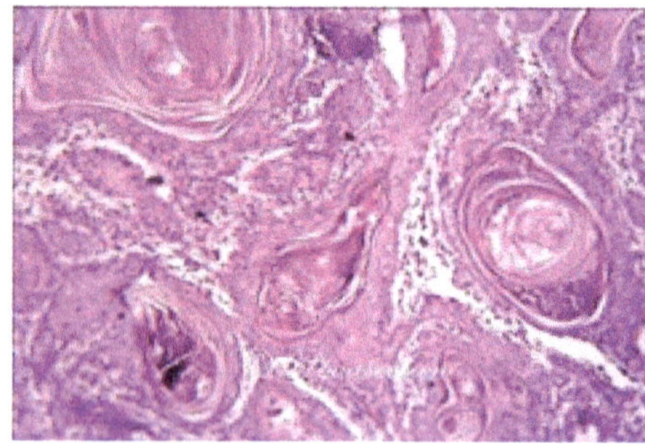

Fig. 96: Squamous cell carcinoma of the horn shown in fig. 95 depicting lesser cellular component than pearl indication slowly proliferating tumour. (p. 151)

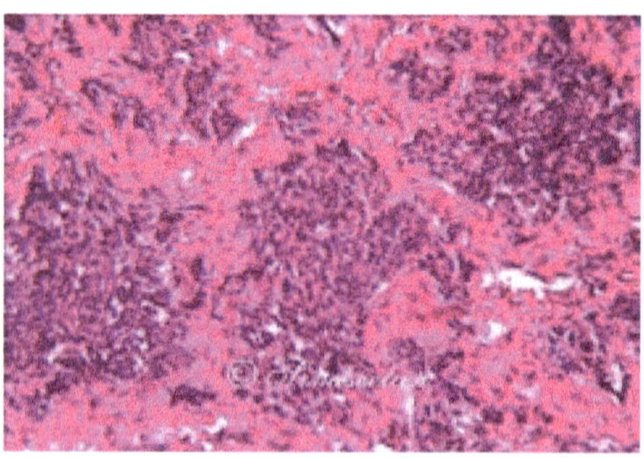

Fig. 97: Solid type of basal cell tumour revealing islands of cellular masses of variable sizes. The cells are indistinguishable from each other due to prominent nuclei and scanty cytoplasm. (p. 153)

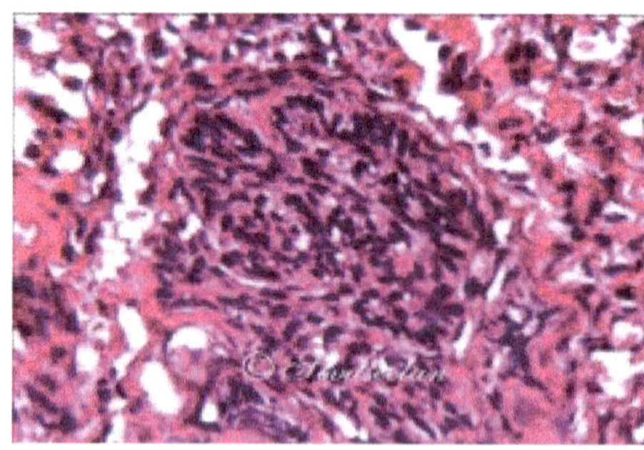

Fig. 98: In the outer layers of an island, the basal cell nuclei are pallisading, but in the inner layers, nuclei are haphazardly arranged. (p. 153)

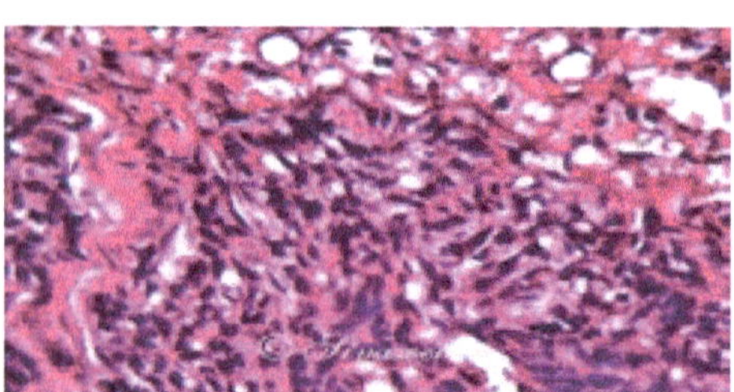

Fig. 99: Cystic type of basal cell tumour showing the neoplastic basal cells encompassing the cystic spaces. (p. 154)

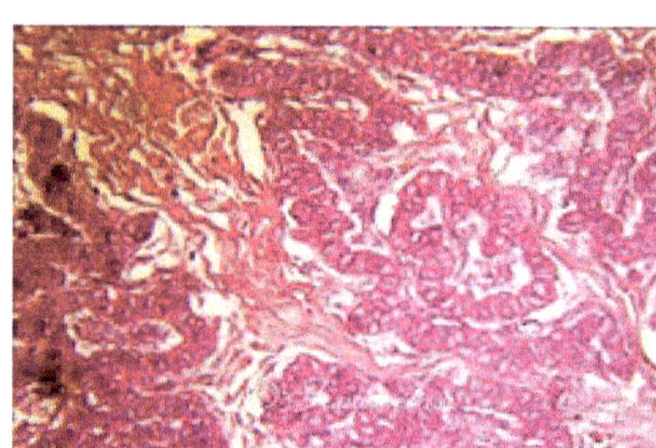

Fig. 100: Ribbon type of basal cell tumour showing strands consisting of one or two rows of basal cells resembling ribbon intervening to exert snake like appearance. (p. 154)

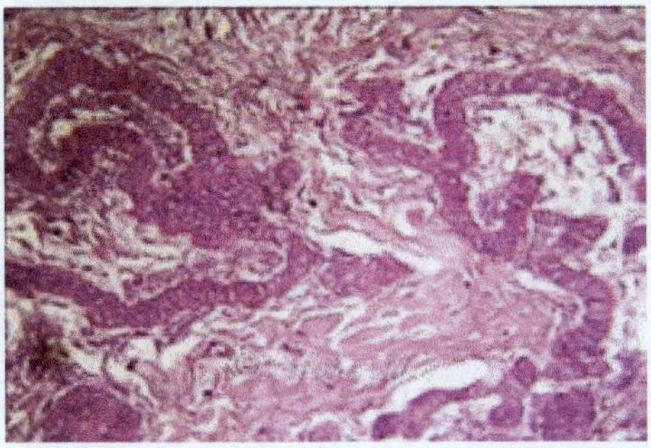

Fig. 101: A mixed type of basal cell tumour showing both Medusoid appearance of radiating strands of basal cells from a central mass of parallel arrangement of group of basal cells (left) and ribbon like arrangement (right). (p. 155)

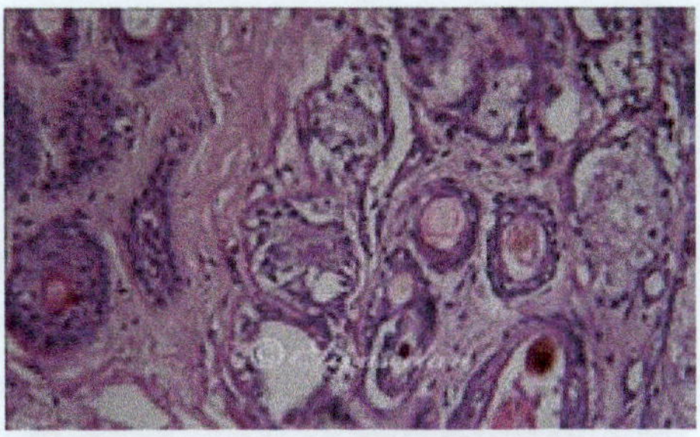

Fig. 102: Trichoepithelioma of a dog showing many layered hair follicle basal cells encompassing the keratin material. (p. 157)

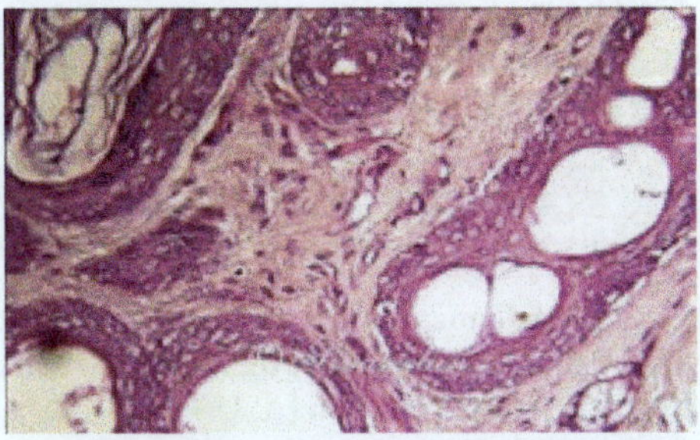

Fig. 103: Magnified view of Trichoepithelioma of a dog showing proliferation of hair follicle basal cells. (p. 157)

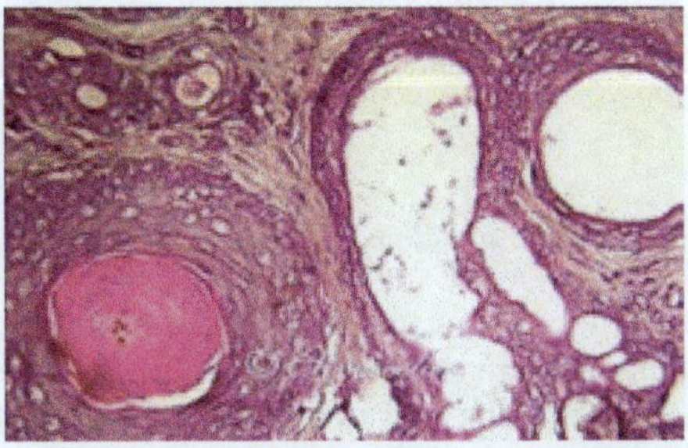

Fig. 104: Trichoepithelioma of a dog showing many layered neoplastic hair follicle basal cells encompassing the keratin centre making a horn cyst. (p. 158)

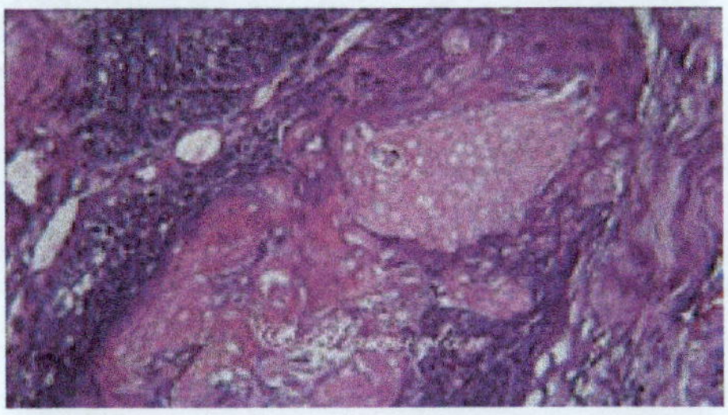

Fig. 105: Pilomatricoma of a dog revealing proliferating darkly stained basal cells and faintly stained shadow cells. (p. 158)

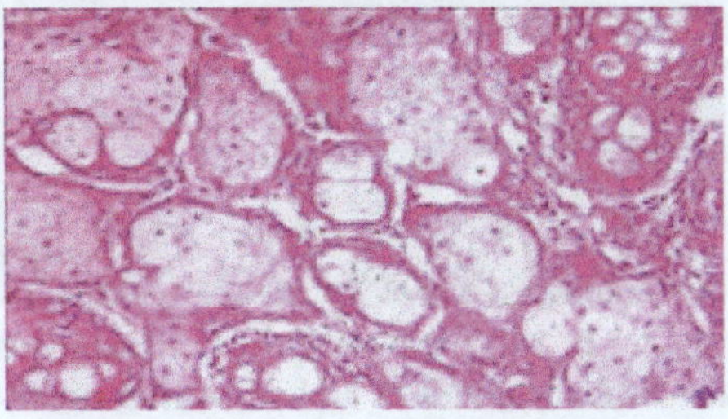

Fig. 106: Sebaceous Gland Adenoma of a dog showing irregularly shaped and sized lobules containing matured sebaceous cells. (p. 160)

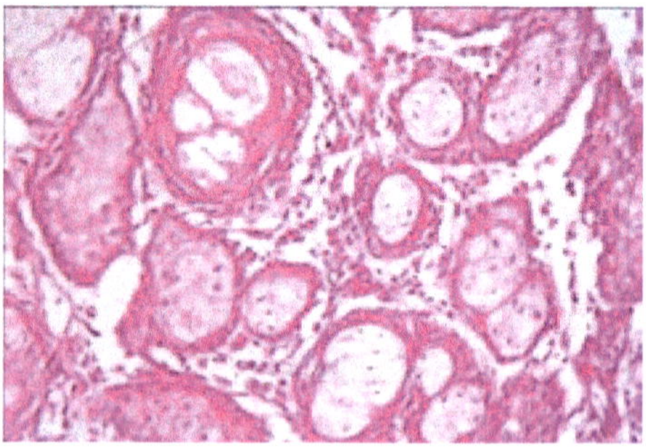

Fig. 107: Sebaceous Gland Adenoma of a dog showing degenerating sebaceous cells indicating regressive type. Undifferentiated generative cells are seen in-between the lobules. (p. 160)

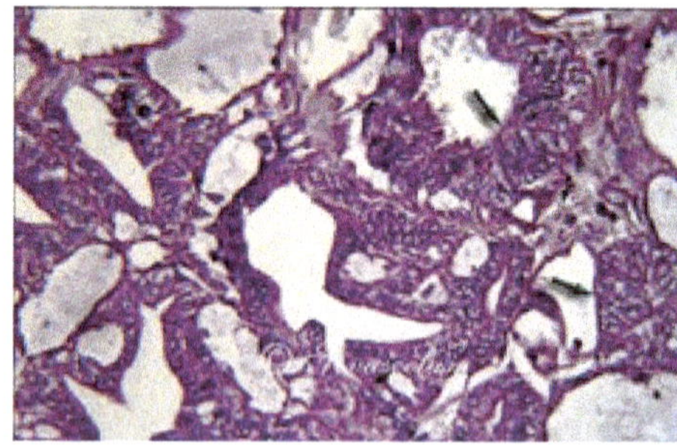

Fig. 108: Adenoma of the mammary gland of a cow showing proliferating epithelial cells confined within the basement membrane of acini. (p. 162)

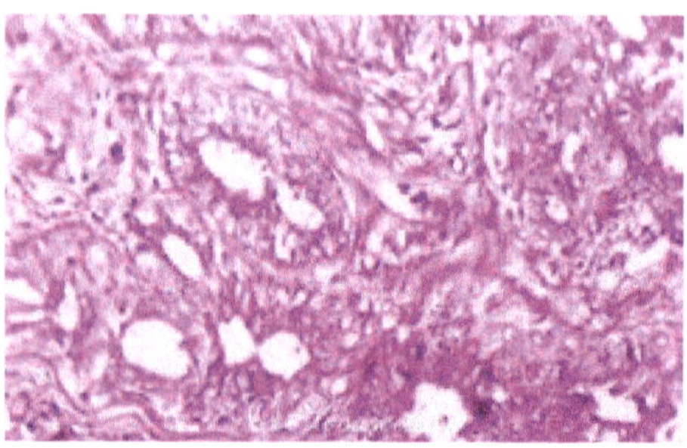

Fig. 109: Adenocarcinoma of the mammary gland of a cow showing proliferating acinar cells breaking and evading the basement membrane. (p. 163)

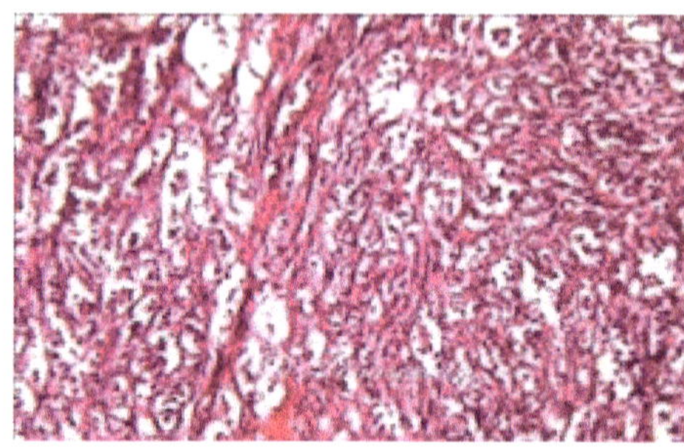

Fig. 110: Adenocarcinoma of the intestine of a fowl showing proliferating epithelial cells forming irregular acini. (p. 164)

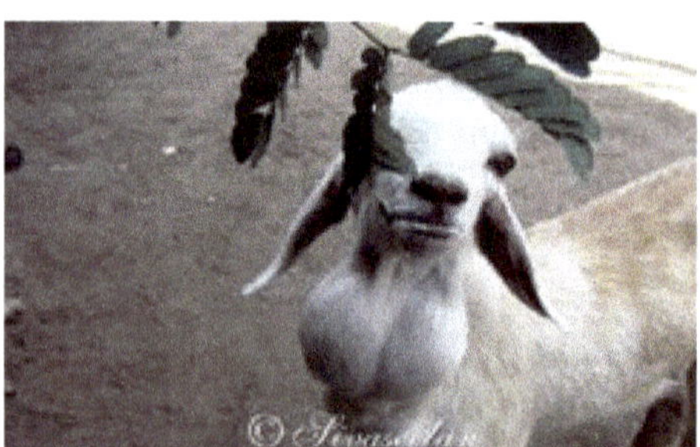

Fig. 111: Bilateral Adenocarcinoma of the salivary gland of a kid showing highly prominent enlargement of the gland. (p. 166)

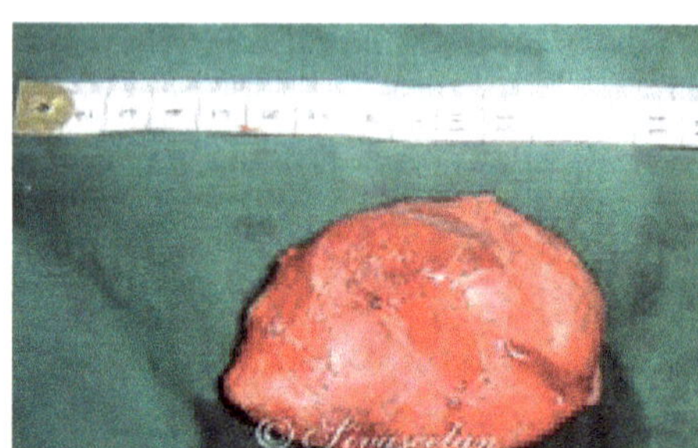

Fig. 112: Removed tumour shown in fig. 111. (p. 166)

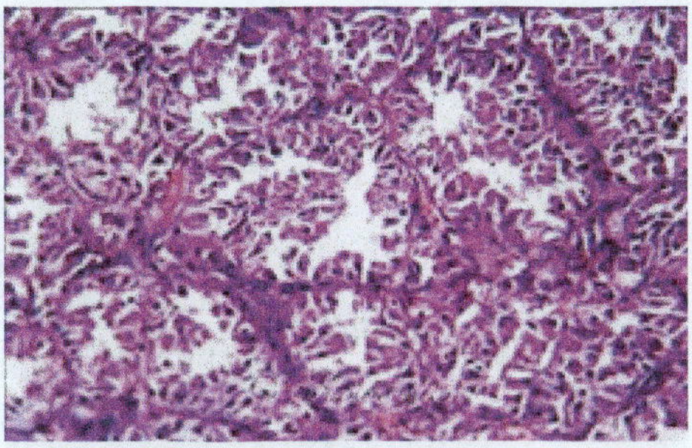

Fig. 113: Histological photomicrograph of the tumour shown in fig. 112 revealing irregular acini formed due to proliferating secretory epithelial cells. (p. 166)

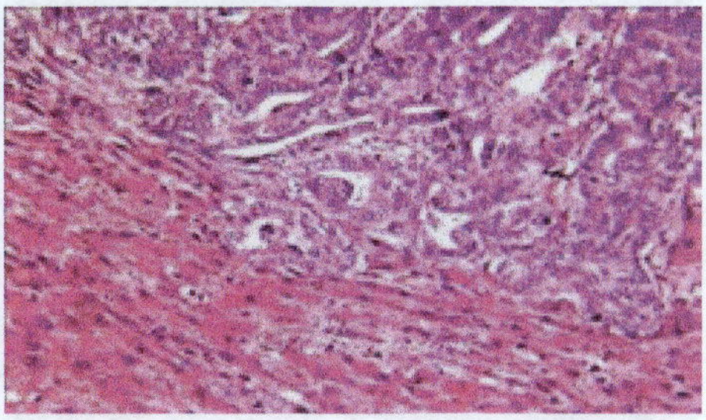

Fig. 114: Metastasis of the salivary gland shown in fig 111 to liver (Irregular acini formed due to proliferating neoplastic salivary gland cells growing into the hepatic cells by infiltration (p. 167)

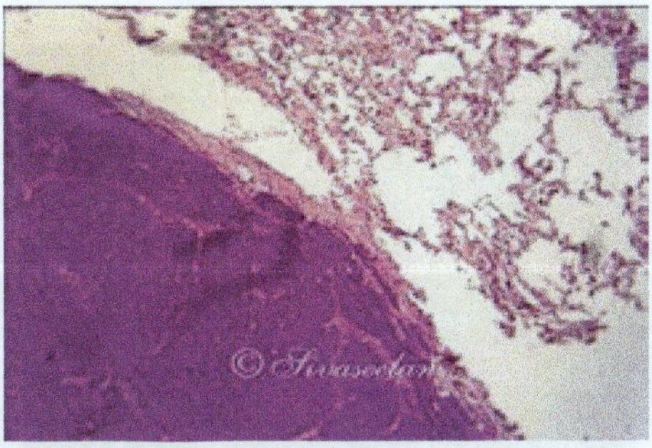

Fig. 115: Metastasis of the salivary gland shown in fig 111 to lung (Irregular acini formed due to proliferating neoplastic salivary gland cells growing into the lung parenchyma). (p. 167)

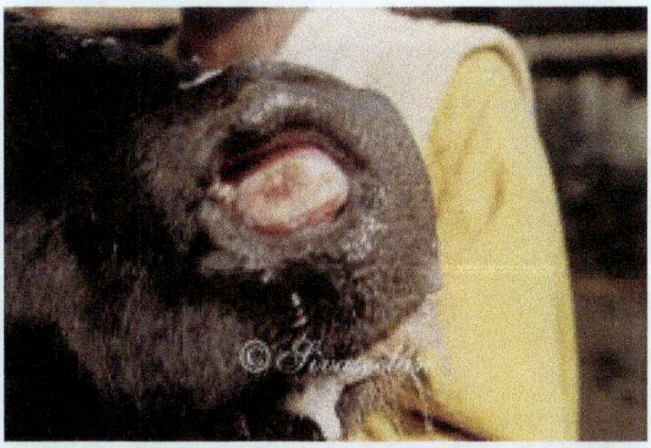

Fig. 116: Nasal septum of a cow revealing a carcinoma protruding from nasal cavity. (p. 168)

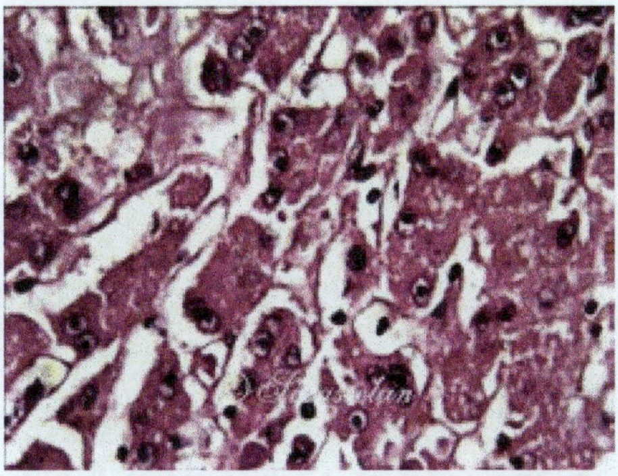

Fig. 117: Nasal septal tumour shown in fig. 116 depicting sheet arrangement of pleomorphic neoplastic epithelial cells with prominent nucleoli within vesicular nuclei. (p. 169)

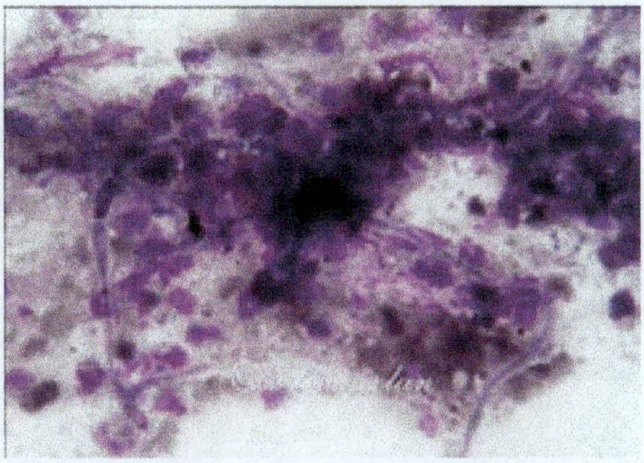

Fig. 118: Urine smear of a dog revealing pleomorphic carcinoma cells admixed with fungal filaments. (p. 171)

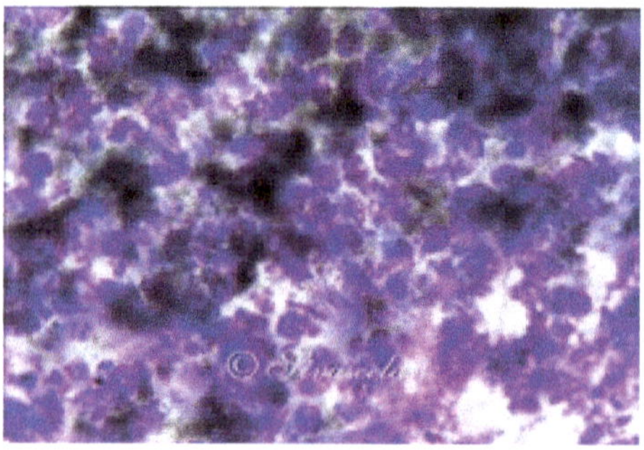

Fig. 119: Urine smear of a bitch showing pleomorphic carcinoma cells with multiple angular nucleoli. (p. 171)

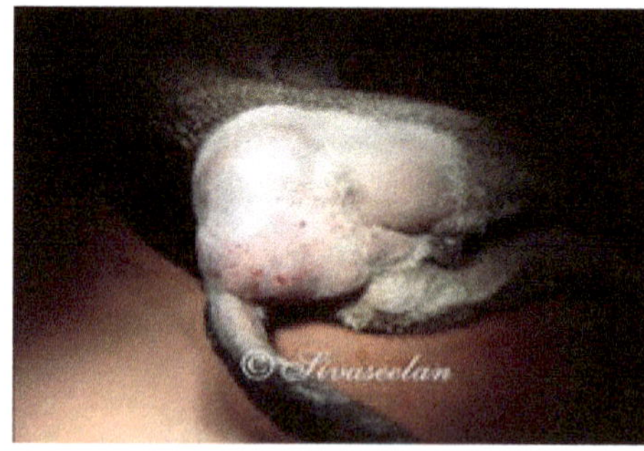

Fig. 120: Multiple Perianal gland tumours around the anus of a native breed dog. (p. 172)

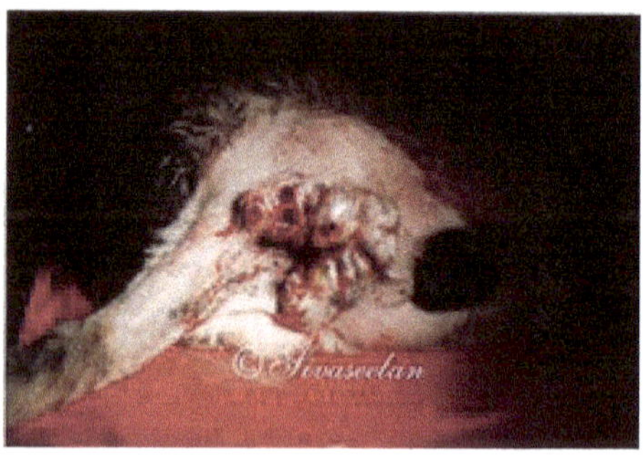

Fig. 121: Multiple Perianal gland tumours around the anus of a dog revealing haemorrhage. (p. 173)

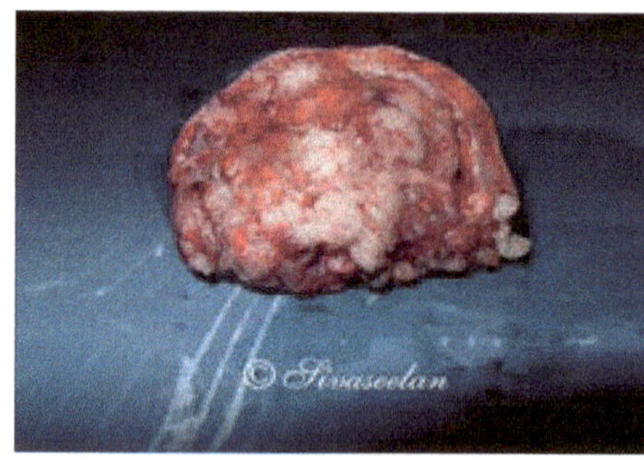

Fig. 122: An excised single tumour shown in fig. 121 depicting easily bleeding nature of Perianal gland tumour. (p. 173)

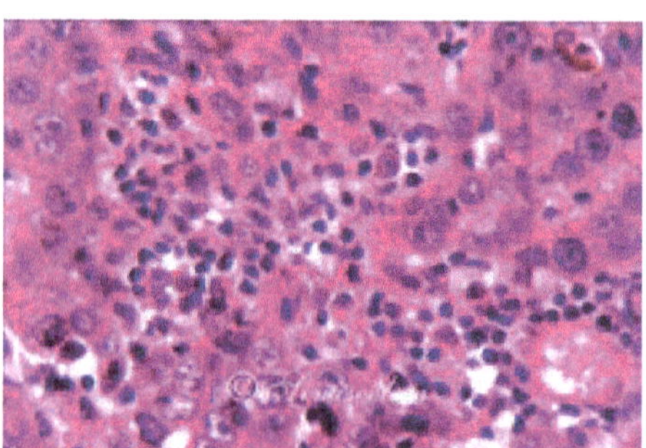

Fig. 123: An adenocarcinoma of Perianal gland of a dog showing Hepatoid cells and Reserve cells arranged as a mixed cell sheet. (p. 174)

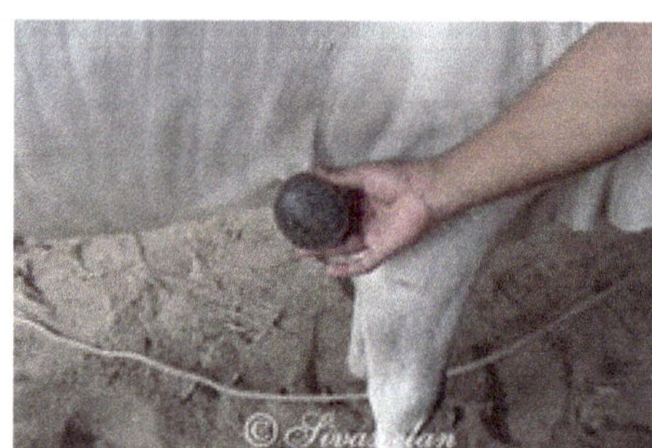

Fig. 124: A bullock showing a tennis ball size circumscribed and pedunculated melanoma on the skin. (p. 176)

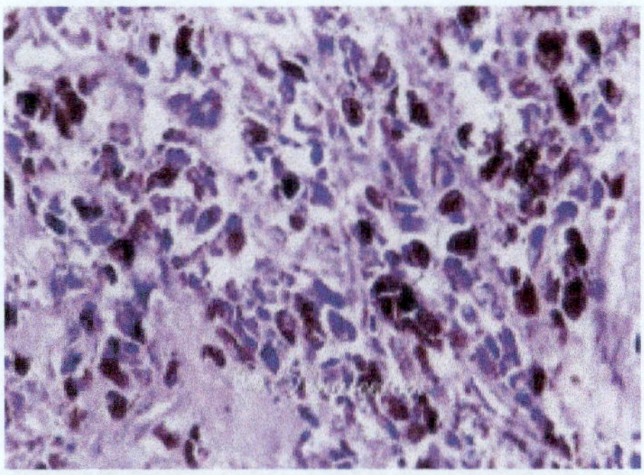

Fig. 125: Tissue section of the tumour shown in fig. 124 revealing pleomorphic darkbrown melanin pigment containing neoplastic melanoblasts. (p. 176)

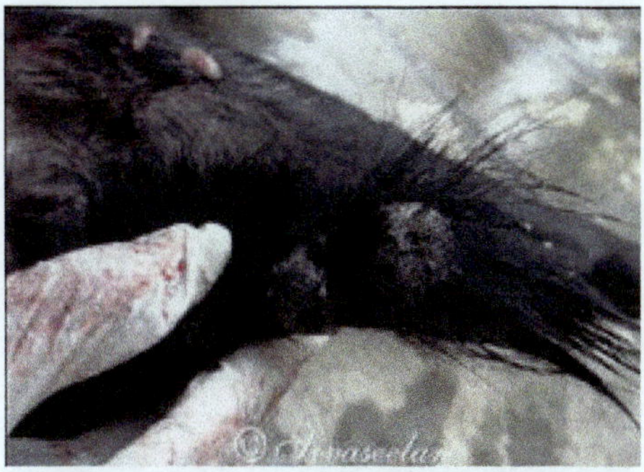

FIg. 126 (p. 177)

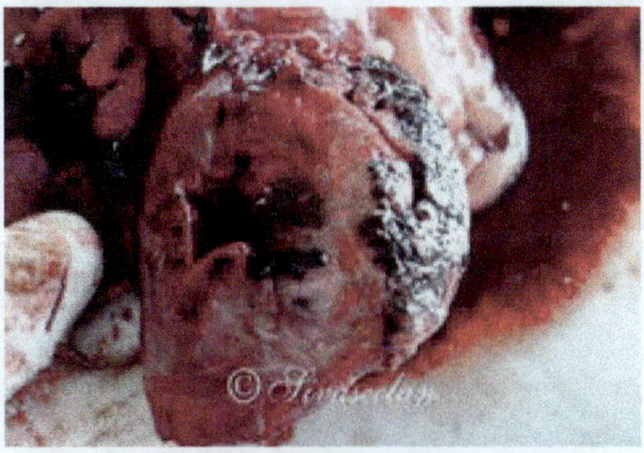

FIg. 127 (p. 177)

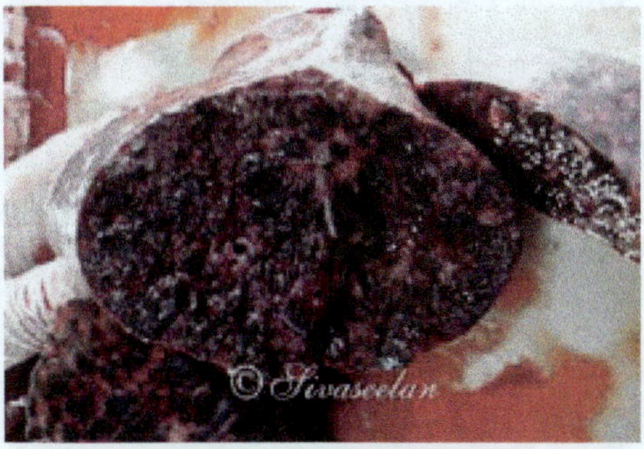

FIg. 128 (p. 177)

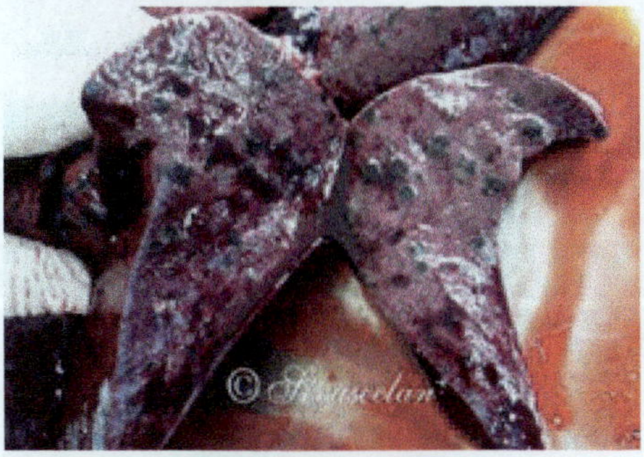

FIg. 129 (p. 177)

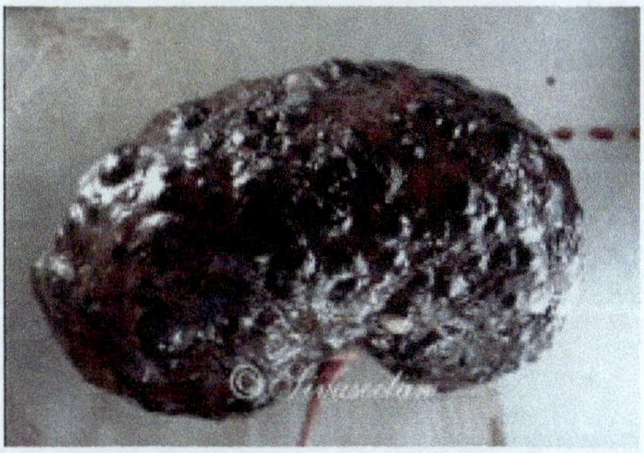

FIg. 130 (p. 177)

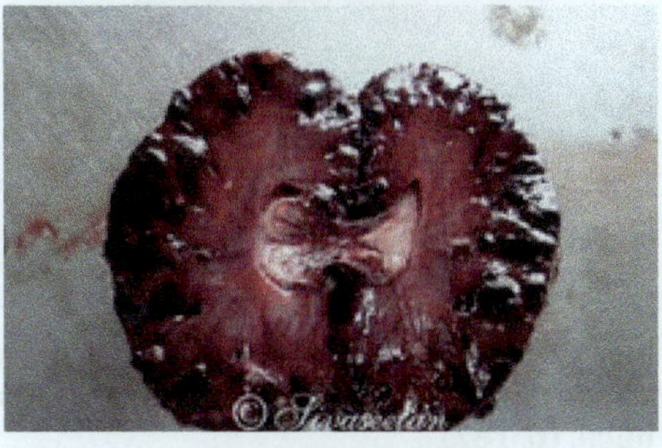

FIg. 131 (p. 177)

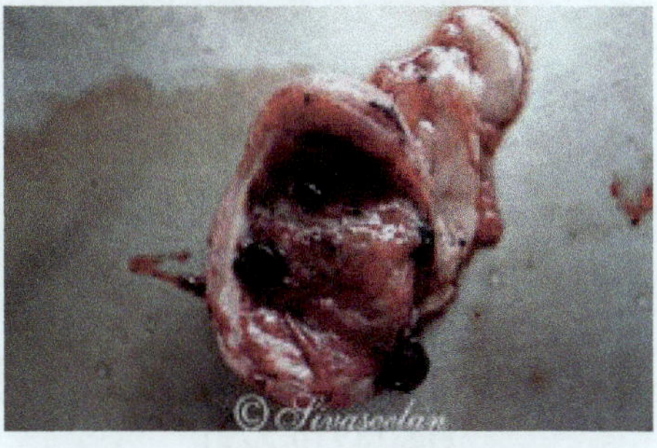

FIg. 132 (p. 178)

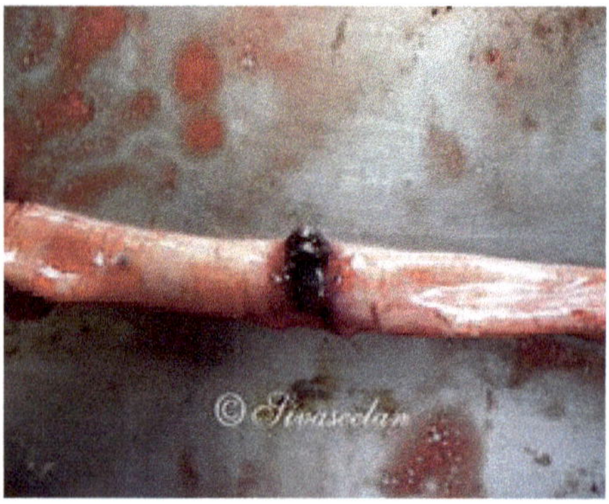

FIg. 133 (p. 178)

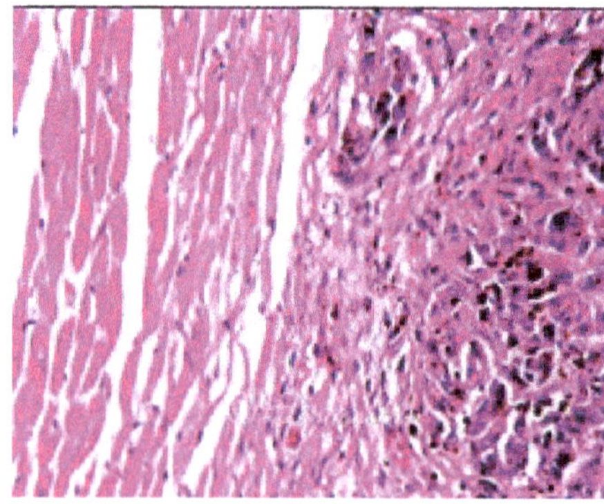

FIg. 134 (p. 178)

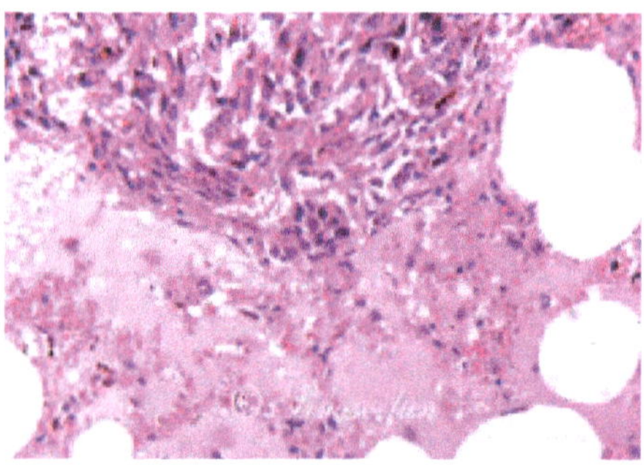

FIg. 135 (p. 178)

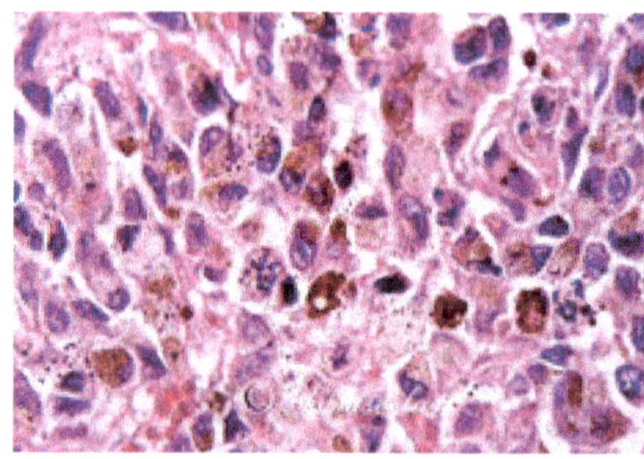

FIg. 136 (p. 178)

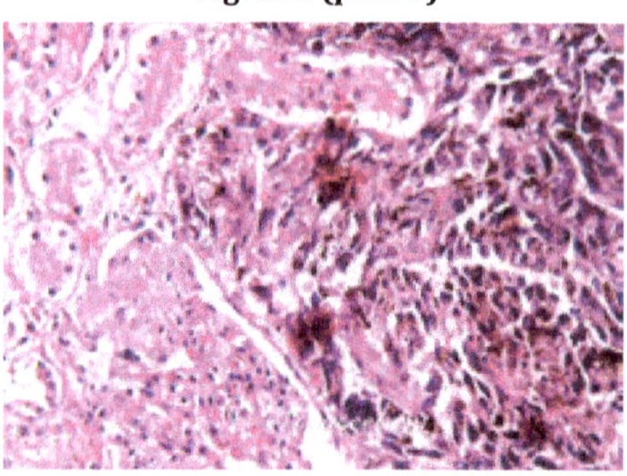

FIg. 137 (p. 178)

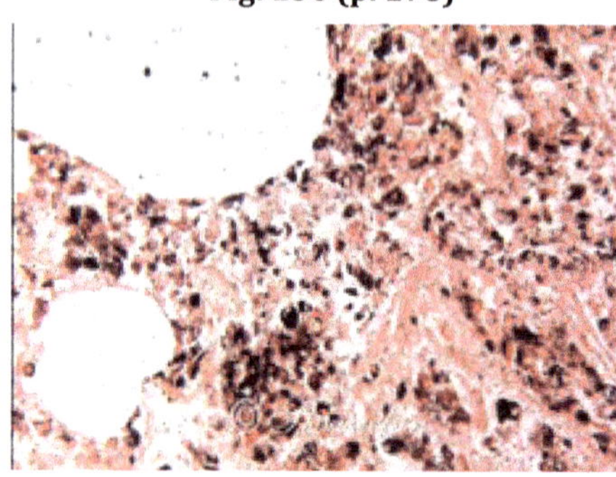

FIg. 138 (p. 179)

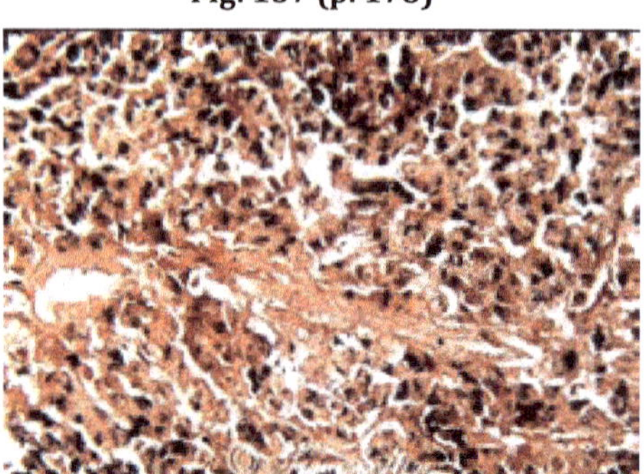

FIg. 139 (p. 179)

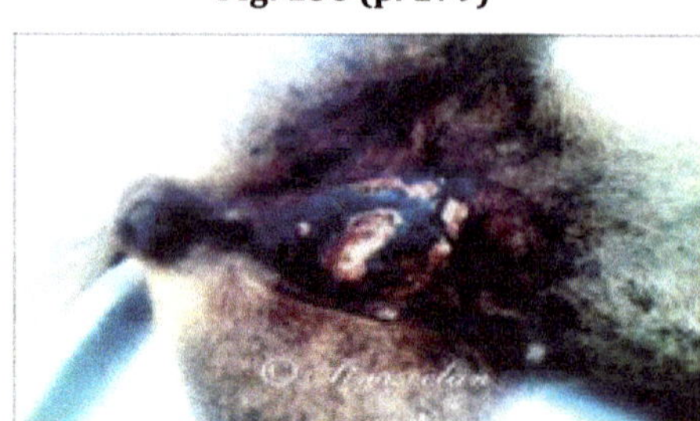

Fig. 140: Mammary tumour arising from the posterior pair of mammary gland of a bitch. (p. 182)

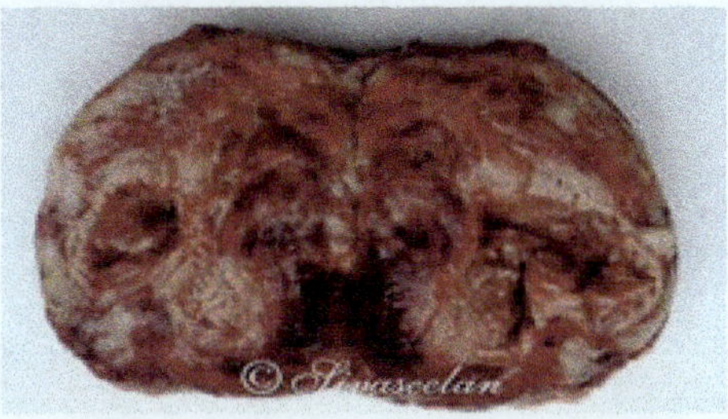

Fig. 141: Mammary tumour shown in fig. 140 revealing intermixed congested and necrotic areas. (p. 182)

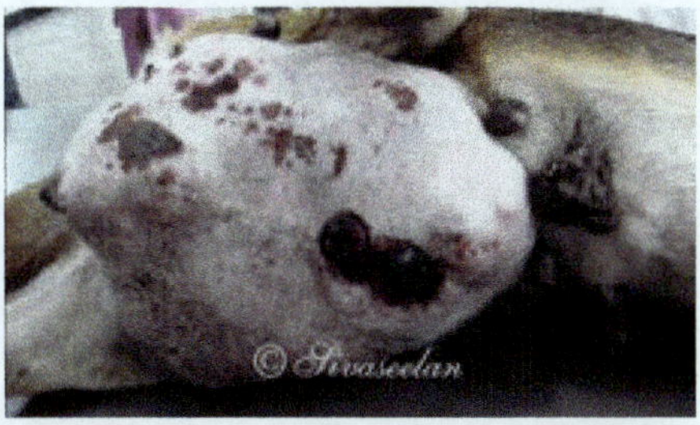

Fig. 142: A massive mammary tumour of a bitch involving posterior quarters. (p. 183)

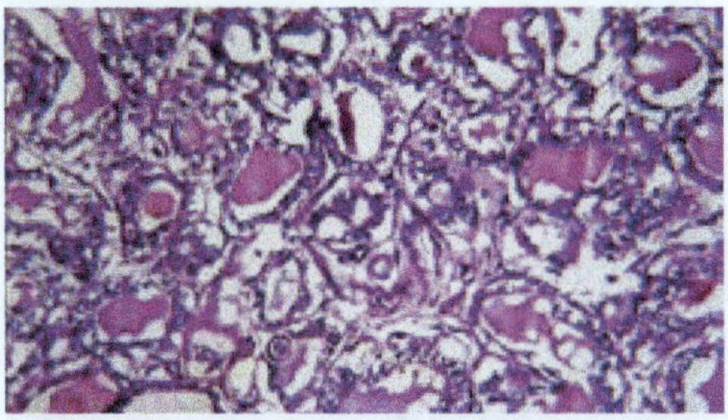

Fig. 143: Mammary tumour shown in fig. 142 depicting cystadenoma (note: variable size and shape of acini with retained secretion due to lack of outlets to release the secretion) (p. 183)

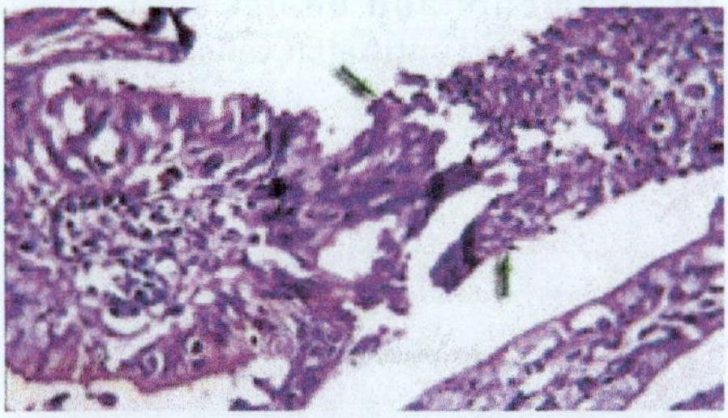

Fig. 144: Tissue from yet another location of Mammary tumour shown in fig. 142 depicting metaplastic transformation of myo-epithelium into chondrocytes (arrows) to form chondroma. (p. 183)

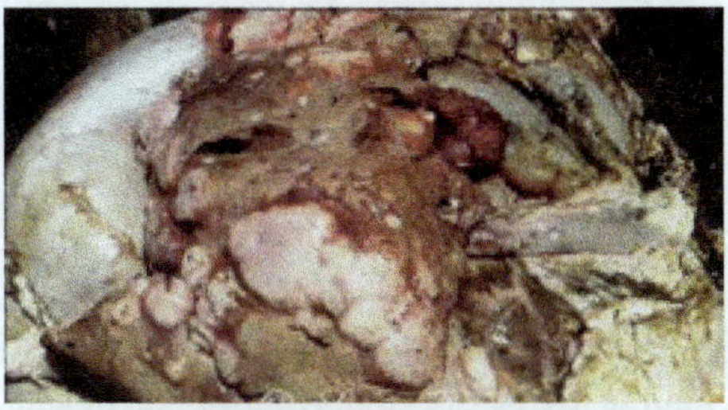

Fig. 145: Hepatocellular carcinoma of a rabbit revealing multiple tumours involving the whole liver. (p. 185)

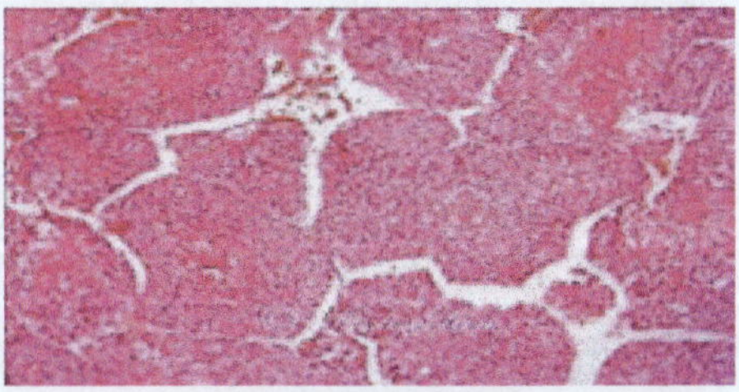

Fig. 146: Hepatocellular carcinoma revealing pseudo-glandular arrangement of neoplastic hepatocytes. (p. 185)

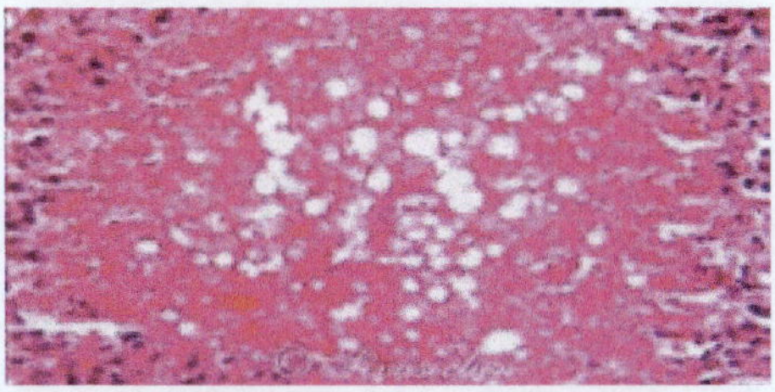

Fig. 147: A pseudo-gland depicting central necrosis with cystic changes (p. 185)

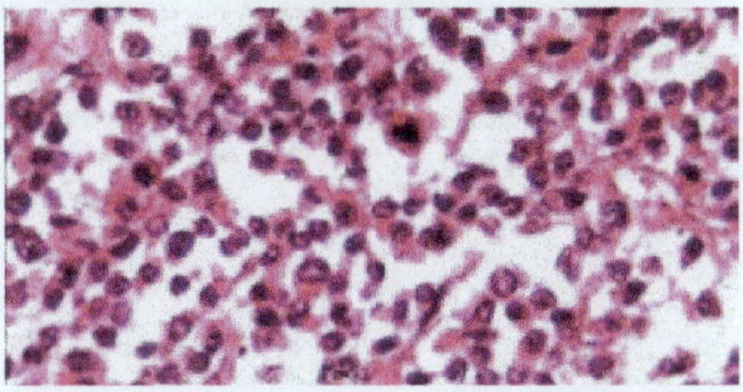

Fig. 148: Hepatocellular carcinoma revealing aniso and poikilo karyosis. Nucleoli are multiple in some cells depicting angularity. (p. 186)

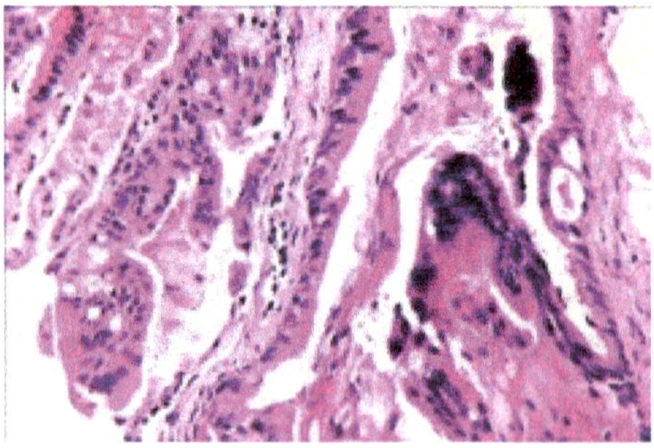

Fig. 149: Lung revealing loss of alveolar arrangements and depict solid sheet arrangement of epithelial cells. (p. 189)

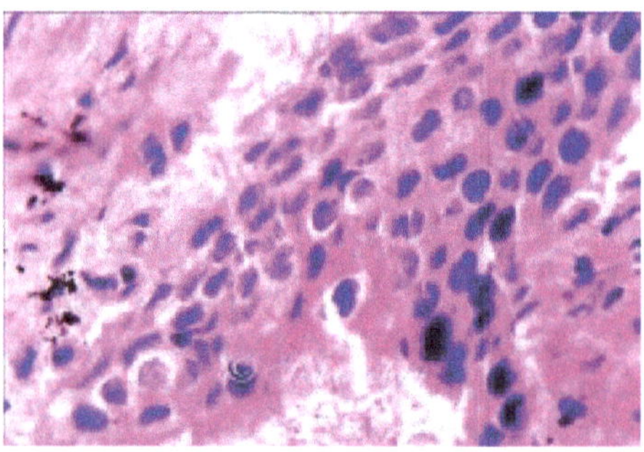

Fig. 151: Lung revealing solid sheet arrangement of epithelial cells with granular cytoplasm indicating accumulation of secretion. (p. 190)

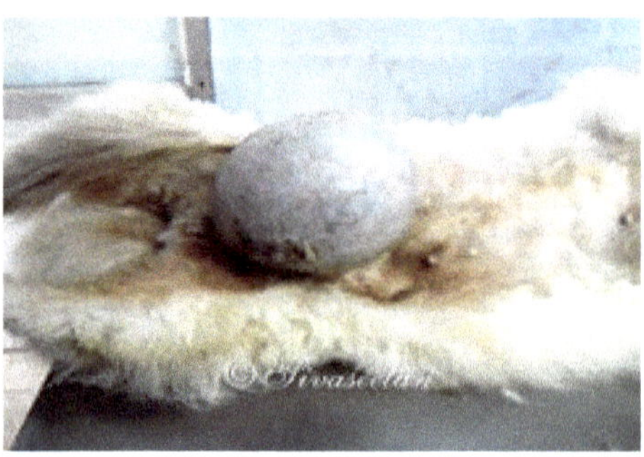

Fig. 153: A dog showing a large Seminoma involving right testis causing atrophy of left testis. (p. 214)

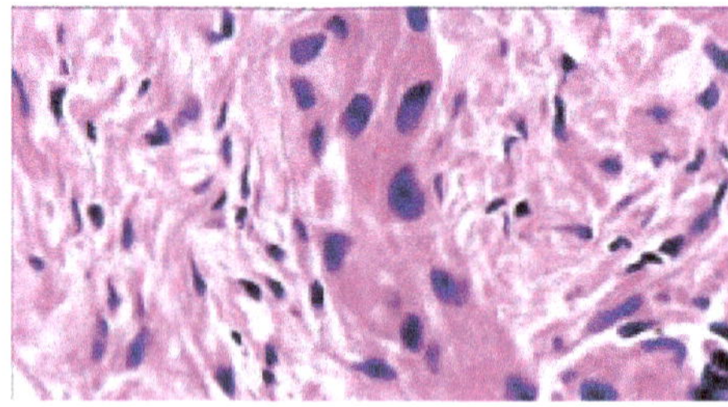

Fig. 150: Lung revealing solid sheet arrangement of epithelial cells (oat cells) (p. 189)

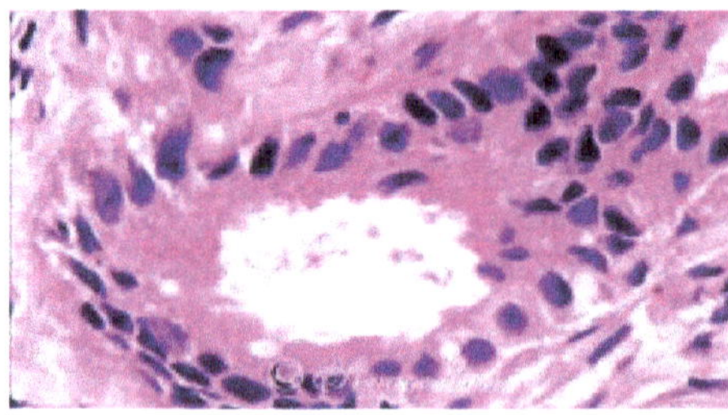

Fig. 152: Adenocarcinoma of lung showing formation of typical acini with multiple layers of epithelial cells. (p. 190)

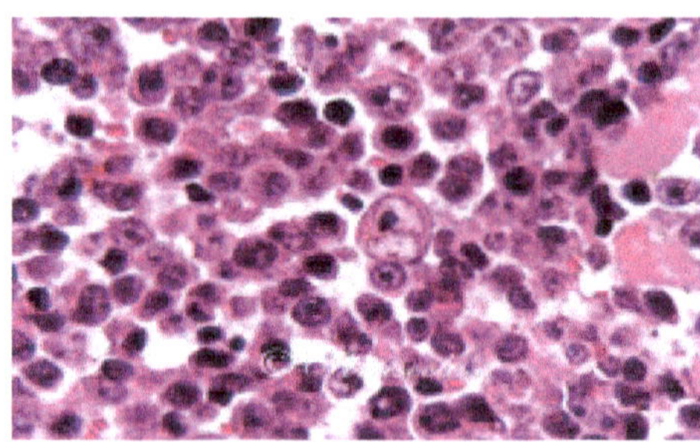

Fig. 154: Diffuse sheet arrangement of neoplastic round to polyhedral germ cells with large nuclei leaving scanty cytoplasm. Twin nuclei and large nucleoli are also seen. (p. 215)

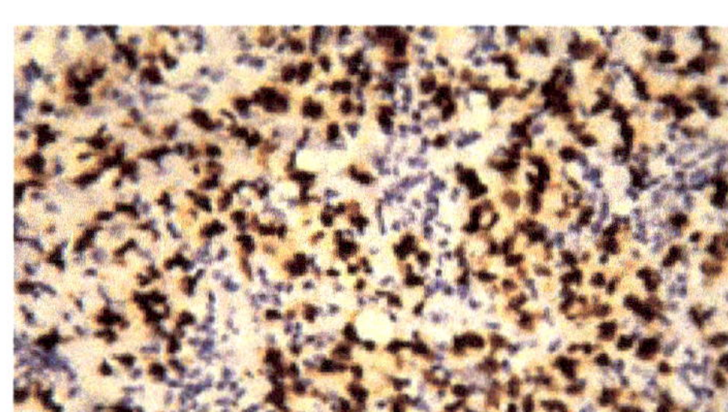

Fig. 155: Diffuse Seminoma cells depicting strong positivity to Ki-67 proliferation antigen. (p. 215)

www.ingramcontent.com/pod-product-compliance
Ingram Content Group UK Ltd.
Pitfield, Milton Keynes, MK11 3LW, UK
UKHW021322190726
13845UKWH00003B/24

9 789390 371365